# Earlier works of Janine Roberts

## Massacres to Mining: the colonization of Aboriginal Australia

'She handles her history with a restraint that makes it deserving to be a classic in our history. Every revelation, whether openly bloody-handed or covertly mean-souled, is authenticated from official records. The effect on myself was profound. It should be required reading for everyone not of the Aboriginal race.'
– Xavier Herbert, a great Australian literary figure, in *The National Times*

'Jan Roberts does not look like the sort of woman you would find sitting in the bush having a feed of lizard or file snake. The only indication that the British born sociologist roughs it was a mass of mosquito bites on her legs – for the rest, she was pretty much haute couture. Her book *Massacres to Mining* has already inspired the Grenada production *Strangers in their own land.* Now it is to be the basis for a joint BBC-ABC television production for the *prestigious* BBC program, *Everyman* ... Her book is essential reading for anyone who wants a balanced view of Australian history.'
– *The Alice Springs Star* - Republished in 2008.

## Jack of Cape Grim

'Jan Roberts has found an unused "treasure trove" of material. A well researched tapestry of the early colonial years' about a 'natural leader' of the Aborigines. – *The Age*
The inspiring story of a final stand by a band of Tasmanian Aborigines, three men and two women, against British settlers and the three military expedition launched against them.
– Republished in 2008.

## Munda Nyuringu: He's taken the land.

'What happened to the Aborigines at Menzies [as told in this film] was a microcosm of what happened all over Australia.' – *The Age*
A powerful film telling of the last major Australian gold rush from the viewpoint of the Aborigines invaded. Janine Roberts co-produced this in the West Australian goldfields with Aboriginal Elder Robert Bropho, jointly winning an Australian Film Institute Nomination for Best Documentary. The *Sydney Morning Herald* gave it a full-page spread, calling it the television film of the week. In 2008 the Australian government said 'Sorry' for some of the atrocities documents in this film.

## The Diamond Empire

A two-part investigative television movie, shot in six continents, which uncovered the worldwide greed and corruption behind the romantic diamond industry. The author created and produced this for WGBH Boston, the BBC and ABC (Australia). It has been credited with starting the campaign against blood diamonds. After a highly controversial release that the De Beers cartel tried to prevent, she was invited to show the film and to testify on diamonds and human rights at a US Congressional Hearing. The Professor of Communications at the University of Massachusetts, Sut Jhally, said of this: 'In all my years of teaching, this is the single most important video I have ever shown to my students… This movie changes the way we see the world."

## Glitter and Greed`: The secret world of the Diamond Cartel

'Formidably well researched and widely sourced account of the global diamond trade by the investigative journalist Janine Roberts. It strikes this lay reader as one of most dogged and damning exposes of a near-monopolistic industry to appear in years. The great wonder is that it appeared at all. Her gripping book for once deserves the epithet "brilliant."'
 – *The Independent.*


'Like the miners shuffling down deep shafts to search for the earth's bounty, Roberts plumbs the depths to come up with the damning truth.'
– *The Minnesota Daily*


'Roberts delivers her information without any apprehension. It is a life's work, a piece to admire.'
– *New City Chicago*


'Janine Roberts' book is a must read for every African.'
– *New African.*


'Brides-to-be hoping for a diamond ring are advised to keep *Glitter and Greed* out of their fiancés' hands.'
– *The Boston Globe*


'If you are in the market for a tale of murder, intrigue, gem smuggling and international smuggling, diamonds has it all. I can recommend *Glitter and Greed.*
– *The Observer*


'Janine Roberts is the rare individual who unflinchingly speaks truth to power. She battles her way past all the obstacles and provides us with a glimpse of those who are in the innermost circles of global power. But instead of being seduced by their power and wealth, she exposes what they do and how they do it and how it comes to hurt us all. … I count myself among the privileged in this world to know Janine and her works.
 – *Former Congresswoman Cynthia McKinney*


## The Seven Days of My Creation

'Robust scholarship runs throughout this passionate and honest autobiography. She has delved deep into spiritual philosophy, science and history to put her unique experience of life into context. Hers is a strong voice that both challenges and touches the heart.'
 – Kay Bridger.
'Janine's story is one of personal courage, conviction, sacrifice and triumph.'
'Fascinating and inspirational. Definitely a must read.'
 – Suzanna Read

**For information about these works – contact** jan@janineroberts.com
**For information about this book see** www.fearoftheinvisible.com

# Fear of the Invisible

## An Investigation of
## Viruses and Vaccines
## HIV and AIDS

## Janine Roberts

**Published by Impact Investigative Media Productions**

**Acknowledgements.**

We are very grateful for Professor Emeritus
Etienne de Harven for his scientific checking of this work.
If any errors remain, they entirely ours.

We also wish to thank the many medical scientists and
Biologists whose work we have cited in this work
And our proof readers
Carla O'Haris. Gina Roberts and Cathy van Miert


**Cover Design
By
Katie Roberts**

**ISBN 978-0-9559177-2-1**

**Website:**   www.fearoftheinvisible.com

**2nd Edition 2009 Minor revisions and addition of chapter on Vaccine Plagues.**


**Published by Impact Investigative Media Productions**
**Leonid, Bristol Marina,**
**Hanover Place, Bristol, BS1 6UH.**
**U.K.**
**Tel.   (44) (0)117 925 6818**
**Cell   (44) (0)7970 253931**
**Email**     impactmedia@fearoftheinvisible.com

Impact was founded in 1985 in Australia and moved to the UK in 1990. It has produced
investigative films seen on the BBC, WGBH, ABC (Australia) and Channel 4 in the UK,
as well as numerous features and investigative works on spiritual, historical, health,
environmental and human rights issues. It has also produced films and  books on the
colonization of Aboriginal Australia.

Cataloguing Information

History: Virology
Ethics:  Medical
Health: Vaccination
Indexed.

# Preface

## DEMOLISHING FEAR

People do not die of AIDS, they die of fear! This volume by Janine Roberts constitutes an invaluable instrument that individuals might employ once they sincerely decide to overcome the fear of the phantom virus, HIV.

The World Health Organization and UNAIDS, agencies of the United Nations, take their cue from agencies of the United States federal government, the Centers for Disease Control and Prevention and the National Institutes of Health, in their parroting the unexamined equation, HIV = AIDS = DEATH.

Similarly, taking their lead from the above federal agencies, the global media spread the unfounded belief that there is still no cure for AIDS. Thus AIDS is included in the list of so-called "incurable diseases" such as cancer, multiple sclerosis, Alzheimer's, psoriasis, lupus, etc. The tragic result is that, from the very moment that an individual reacts positively in one of the erroneously named "tests for HIV," that person's mind is immediately programmed to anticipate an inevitable death from AIDS. This belief is the true tragedy!

Since at least the time of Galen in the 2nd century, it has been common knowledge that the mind influences the body (1) and plays a vital role in diseases related to immune responses (2-4). Only in recent decades have we clarified the innermost biochemical mechanisms through which mental stress can weaken the immune system and cause immune deficiency. The inverse has also been identified; the biochemical reactions that occur when we successfully cope with mental stress, thereby stimulating our immune responses; mechanisms that today are employed in the treatment and prevention of a variety of immunological conditions. (5-13)

We now know we are made of cells that are extraordinarily capable and adaptable. Lymphocytes, 'white' blood cells, produce hormones and neurotransmitters, contrary to the previously long-held belief that only neurons can produce neurotransmitters and only endocrine glands produce hormones. (14,15) Similarly, lymphocytes have receptors for all kinds of hormones and neurotransmitters, even for the endorphins and enkephalins that block pain from disabling us (15,16). Furthermore, neurons and cells of the endocrine glands have receptors for cytokines (lymphokines), messenger molecules that tell immune cells where they are needed. (16) Therefore, our brain cells, our endocrine glands and the cells of our immune system are all woven into a biochemical network that is a vitally important part of our defence mechanism against internal or external intruders. (17-20)

Psychoneuroimmunology is a new branch of knowledge that studies the effects and consequences of positive and negative emotions on our immune system (9,10,12). The immune system senses all our emotions (14); it feels fear, guilt, doubt, insecurity, lack of confidence, anxiety, depression, lack of self esteem, panic, intolerance, pride, arrogance, envy, anger, hate, rancour, laziness, gluttony, lust, remorse, fury, revenge, love for material things, and disloyalty. But it also feels happiness, joy, security, confidence, self-esteem, tranquillity, gratitude, tolerance, admiration, love, compassion, pardon and so forth (14). Our emotions depend on our principles, beliefs and values, which are dynamic processes that can be modified if we sincerely wish.

Undoubtedly, immunological stressor agents of external origin (chemical, physical, biological, nutritional) affect our health. However, mental stressors - those that we feel as a threat and depend on the state of our consciousness - have much more importance in the genesis of all illnesses. (21)

Furthermore, since the beginning of the AIDS epidemic, numerous scientific publications have explained how the different manifestations of fear constitute powerful stressor agents, factors that play a crucial role in the generation of the clinical manifestations of AIDS, including the complications that kill AIDS patients. Additionally, the consciousness status of 'seropositive' people (those who react positively on the so-called 'tests for HIV') and of patients with AIDS (those with opportunistic infections, tumours and metabolic diseases) can determine both the course of the illness and its prognosis (22-28). Therefore healing from, or dying of, AIDS depends greatly on our fear of HIV and AIDS, a factor emanating from the patients themselves, not from doctors or miraculous therapies!

Our positive and negative emotions stimulate biochemical processes that can either heal or harm many of the body's tissues, organs and systems, especially the immune system. (9,10,12) Therefore, the power of the mind and of our consciousness has a great capacity for good as well as for ill.

The myths concerning AIDS, that it is sexually transmitted and incurable, stigmatize both 'seropositive' individuals and those with AIDS, subjecting them to a new and terrible shame. For example, 'seropositive' persons are frightened of infecting their partners with 'the virus' that they are condemned to carry to their graves. Seropositive mothers panic at the thought of transmitting the same virus to their infants through pregnancy, delivery and breastfeeding. Thus these myths have converted mother's milk into something terribly dangerous, to the great detriment of many tens of thousands of children. (30)

This means that "seropositive" individuals and patients with AIDS, together with persons who belong to the groups at risk for AIDS, are being made to live the worst of torments, a Calvary of fear.

Fear is the preferred tool of those in positions of power, of those who would control and manipulate humans. In the case of AIDS, fear is employed by the pharmaceutical companies, the World Health Organization, UNAIDS, the CDC, and the NIH, and used to promote toxic and unnecessary antiretroviral medications. The media echo this message. They all uncritically proclaim: "If you are HIV-positive and do not ingest the antiretroviral cocktails, you will get AIDS and die of it." Fear serves only the enemies of our species. We must vanquish fear!

We must bear in mind that no physician or natural therapy can heal us unless we perceive and are aware of the problems in our consciousness, in our psychopathology (22,23). We are born with a gift from God; our inner physician and our inner pharmacy. Hippocrates (460-337 B.C.) said that "the power of the patient's self healing is essential and we must stimulate it." The father of homeopathy, Samuel Hahnemann (1755-1843) said "the homeopathic remedies work by stimulating the patient's defence mechanisms." Dr. Albert Schweitzer (1875-1965) explained: "In the interior of each patient there is a physician and we accomplish our mission when we help our patients stay in contact with their inner physician." Similarly, Dr. Keppe (1927-) says that "man spends a whole life waiting to receive the wellness to come from outside, when that wellness already exists in our interior" (22). In this volume, Janine Roberts rightly explains the fact that "why most children are not falling ill from this dangerous vaccine contamination is, it seems, because most are thankfully gifted by nature with very effective immune systems – and because these viruses are generally not as dangerous as these scientists believe."

It is very comforting to read in *Fear of the Invisible*: "We all have been taught to greatly fear viruses – and yet scientists are now discovering that they are fundamental parts of life, made by the millions by all healthy cells. I hope this book will help by combating this fear, this damning of the invisible because we do not understand it.

Without this fear, hopefully the focus in medical research will shift to looking more at the environmental toxins that really put us, and our world, gravely at risk."

Certainly, "what we do know is that there is not much difference between maintaining the health of our planet and the health of our inner world. Give your cells the natural foods they need. Keep your internal and external environments healthy. Try not to be stressed out. Keep positive. Respect your body – all parts of it, even the nano world within. Enjoy having both a marvellous inner world and planet to explore – and keep them both unpolluted."

In *Fear of the Invisible* Janine Roberts describes with elegant detail and in a most accessible manner how to combat fear, or, should I say, how to overcome "seropositivity" and AIDS itself. Thank you very much Ms. Roberts for having the courage to write a great book of infinite helpfulness to those who live the martyrdom of AIDS.

Roberto Giraldo, M.D.   New York, April 2008

### *REFERENCES*

1.   Holden C. Cancer and mind: how are they connected? Science 1978; 200: 1363-1369.

2.   Solomon GF, Moos RH. Emotions, immunity and disease. Speculative theoretical integration. Arch General Psychiatr 1964; 11: 657-674.

3.   Rasmussen AF. Emotions and immunity. Ann NY Acad Sci 1969; 164: 458.

4.   Justice BJ. Who gets sick. How beliefs, moods, and thoughts affect your health. Los Angeles: Jeremy P. Tarcher, Inc.; 1988: 407.

5.   Locke SE et al. The influence of stress on the immune response. Annual Meeting of the American Psychosomatic Society. Washington, D.C. 1978.

6.   Goetzl EJ. Neuroimmunomodulation of immunity and hypersensitivity. J Immunol 1985; 135: 739s-862s.

7.   Jancovic BC, Marcovic BM, Spector NH. Neuroimmune interactions: proceedings of the second international workshop on neuroimmunomodulations. Ann NY Acad Sci 1987; 496: 751.

8.   Pierpaoli W, Spector NV. Neuroimmunomodulation: intervention in aging and cancer. First Stromboli Conference on Aging and cancer. Ann NY Acad Sci 1988; 521: 1-361.

9.   Ader R, Felten DL, Cohen N. Psychoneuroimmunology. 2a ed. San Diego: Academic Press; 1991: 1218.

10.   Kemeny ME et al. Psychoneuroimmunology. En: Nemeroff C. Neuroendocrinology. Telford, NJ: Telford Press; 1992: 563-591.

11.   Lewis CE, O'Sullivan C, Barraclough J. The psychoimmunology of cancer. Mind and body in the fight for survival? Oxford: Oxford University Press; 1994.

12.   Glaser R, Kiecolt-Glaser JK. Handbook of human stress and immunity. San Diego: Academic Press; 1994: 414.

13.   Leonard BE, Miller K. Stress, the immune system and psychiatry. Chichester: John Wiley and Sons; 1995: 238.

14.   Blalock JE. The immune system as a sensory organ. J Immunol 1984; 132: 1067-1070.

15.   Smith EM, Harbour-McMenamin D, Blalock JE. Lymphocyte production of endorphins and endorphin-mediated immunoregulatory activity. J Immunol 1985; 135: 779s-782s.

16. Pert CB, Ruff MR, Weber RJ, Herkenham M. Neuropeptides and their receptors: a psychosomatic network. J Immunol 1985; 135: 820s-826s.

17. Besedovski HO, Del Rey AE, Sorkin E. Immune-neuroendocrine interactions. J Immunol 1985; 135: 760s-764s.

18. Blalock JE, Smith EM. A complete regulatory loop between the immune and neuroendocrine systems. Federation Proc 1985; 44: 108-111.

19. Balkwill FR. Cytokines: a practical approach. Oxford: Oxford University Press; 1995: 417.

20. Ellis RJ. Stress proteins as molecular chaperons. En: Van Enden W, Young DB. Stress proteins in medicine. Nueva York: Marcel Dekker; 1996: 1-26.

21. Giraldo, RA. AIDS and stressors: AIDS is neither an infectious disease nor is it sexually transmitted. It is a toxic-nutritional syndrome caused by the alarming worldwide increment of immunological stressor agents. Medellín, Colombia: Impresos Begon; 1997: 205.

22. Keppe, NR. The origin of illness: psychological, physical and social. Englewood Cliffs, New Jersey: Campbell Hall Press; 2000: 162.

23. Bernhardt-Pacheco C. Healing through consciousness. Theomania: The cause of stress. São Paulo, Brazil: Proton Editora Ltda. 1983:180.

24. Temoshok L, Zich J, Solomon MD, Sites DP. An intensive psychoimmunology study of men with AIDS. (Paper presented at the First Research Workshop on the Psychoneuroimmunology of AIDS). Tiburon, CA 1987.

25. Kiecolt-Glaser JK, Glaser R. Psychological influences on immunity. Implications for AIDS. Amer J Psychol 1988; 43: 892-899.

26. Kemeny ME. Psychoneuroimmunology of HIV infection. En: Zegans LS, Coates TJ. Psychiatric manifestations od HIV disease. Psichiat Clin N Am 1994; 17: 55-68.

27. Perry S. Psychoneuroimmunology and AIDS: Challenger or "challenger"? En: Stein M, Baum A. Perspectives in behavioral medicine: chronic diseases. Mahwah, New Jersey: Lawrence Erlbaum Associated Publishers; 1995: 273-286.

28. Giraldo RA. Role of mental stressors in immunodeficiency. In: AIDS and stressors. Medellín, Colombia: Impresos Begon; 1997: 67-69.

29. Giraldo R, de Harven E. HIV tests cannot diagnose HIV infection. April 2006. www.robertogiraldo.com/eng/papers/Farber

30. Giraldo, RA. Milking the market:.Will mothers dish out the W.H.O. formula? Continuum (London) 1998; 5(3): 8-1

# Introduction

# Virology – the misnamed Science

The word 'virus' comes from the Latin for a poisonous liquid, and before that from the Sanskrit for the same. The hunt for them started when, towards the end of the 19th century, it was suggested that invisible living particles much smaller than bacteria might cause the epidemic illnesses for which no bacterial cause could be found. When the electron microscope found tiny particles in the blood serum of patients entering and leaving human cells, this was a Eureka Moment. The prediction was surely about to be proved true. These particles were assumed to be invading and hijacking our cells in order to reproduce. They were thus all condemned as poisons, as 'viruses.'

As more of these were searched for and found in sick people, many illnesses became blamed on them. They became the invisible enemy, the nano-terrorist we must fear. We were instructed that one of our first duties for our newborn children is to vaccinate them against this dreaded foe. Thus was an ever-growing multibillion-dollar pharmaceutical industry created.

But, as I have travelled through the science that underlies this industry, I have gradually learnt to ask questions. I now realise that there is another way to see this story that fits all the data. I have learnt from biologists that our cells naturally produce viral-like particles without being invaded or infected, both when healthy and sick. Currently such particles are named by asking what illnesses they cause as if this is their raison d'être, their only importance, the sole reason for cells making them.[1] They would be named far more positively and comprehensively by asking what cells produce them and for what purpose.

Scientists like Barbara McClintock, who won a Nobel Prize for finding that cells operate with intelligence and seek to repair themselves, have given us a very different understanding of the particles they make. We now know that our cells create multitudes of tiny transport particles (vesicles) to carry the proteins and genetic codes needed within and between cells. The ones that travel between cells, those our cells use to communicate with each other – are puzzlingly just like those that we have long blamed for illnesses.

It now seems that we may have misconceived the virus; that most of them could well be simply inert messages in envelopes carried from cell to cell. In the last ten years scientists have begun to call them 'exosomes', 'particles that leave the body' of the cell, removing the inference that the wor 'virus carries,' of them being dangerous by nature. Distinguishing the healthy particle from the pathogenic is now an enormous problem for the virologist, for it has been discovered that our cells make them all in the same way, in the very same place. It also seems we cannot stop this process without risking severely damaging our cells.

So, perhaps we need to halt the juggernaut of virology with its virus hunt, and look to see if there is another way of helping us keep healthy. We need to know how we can strengthen the malnourished cell, rather than use the many medicines that try to prevent it

---

[1] For an example of 'infection' used as a criteria, see *Retroelement and Retrovirus Universal Classification* - Pat Heslop-Harrison. http://www.le.ac.uk/bl/phh4/retrocla.htm

from making particles by interfering with its essential processes. We need to know if a poisoned cell may produce unhealthy messengers or viruses. We need to learn far more about cells – for only now are we starting to understand how they communicate and the very important role played in this by the particles we had totally demonised as viruses.

I spent over 4 years in the 1990s researching why the vaccines made to protect our children from viruses sometimes instead did them grievous damage. It then took me over 8 years to travel from accepting without question that one virus causes polio and another causes AIDS to discover that most people, including myself, have been vastly misled.

I now realize that science today is so specialized, that every new generation of scientists has had to trust that those who laid the foundations got things right, for they cannot repeat this earlier work except at great cost. If this trust ever proves to be misplaced, it is absolutely vital to correct this with all speed and courage.

I have been horrified to learn from the highest scientific authorities that this trust has sometimes been very grievously misplaced. For example, high-level US governmental inquiries in the 1990s, guided by eminent scientists, explicitly reported the key foundation HIV research papers were riddled with grave errors and deceptively "fixed." They documented these findings with great care – and I likewise do so here. But when the Republican Party gained control over the US House of Representatives at the end of 1994, it ended this most important investigation, buried its reports and left the scientific papers it found to be erroneous uncorrected. These same papers are thus still frequently used by unsuspecting scientists worldwide, who cite them as proof that HIV causes AIDS. I present clear evidence here that these papers were fixed at the last moment before publication. I also reproduce the original documents so you can judge for yourselves.

When I dug back further, to the origins of virology and the great hunt for the poliovirus, I found the story was scandalously much the same. Powerful evidence was presented to Congress linking the summer polio epidemics to summer-used heavy metal pesticides. These scientists suggested remedies, reported curing polio – and were ignored. Instead parents were told to be scared of a yet undiscovered virus. Today thousands of children are still being identically paralysed in regions where such pesticides are heavily used – but all the World Health Organization (WHO) says is: 'Don't worry; we have nearly exterminated the dreaded poliovirus. We have checked. The paralysed children were not infected by it.'

As for childhood vaccinations, surely they have proved a great benefit? I long thought so, but I have found the government scientists we entrust with our children's lives have admitted, at official vaccine safety meetings reported here for the first time, that they cannot clean these vaccines; that they allowed their use despite knowing that they are scandalously polluted with numerous viruses, viral and genetic code fragments, possibly toxins, prions and oncogenes. The World Health Organization has also disclosed at these meetings that it has long known that the MMR vaccine is contaminated with avian leucosis virus. This is a bird virus linked to leukaemia, but the public have not been told about this. Why most children are not falling ill from this dangerous contamination is, it seems, because most are thankfully gifted by nature with very effective immune systems – and because these viruses are generally not as dangerous as these scientists believe.

As for the great flu' epidemic of 1918, it is used today to spread fear of viruses. Yet, shortly after it occurred, an eminent Yale University professor reported that bacteria primarily caused it, and the flu viruses present were virtually harmless. As far as I can discover, his work remains unquestioned but not mentioned. Accordingly, I report it in this book. As for the recent scare over bird flu – any self-respecting bird would fall ill and create new viruses if subjected to the amounts of pollution now emitted in China. What we need to focus on is the pollution – not to waste a fortune on chasing genetic code fragments in birds that are healthily migrating thousands of miles.

What also of the many eminent scientists who have concluded publicly that the HIV theory of AIDS must be scientifically flawed because their research indicates that it has other causes and is curable? Is it right that their research is being suppressed, ridiculed and not funded – simply because they have not confirmed the establishment's theory for this dreaded epidemic? At the end of this book I list some of their names and positions.

Among these dissenters are at least one Nobel Laureate and many senior professors at major universities. But it seems, no matter how important the academic chairs they hold, they are all mocked for so concluding and are scarcely ever interviewed. Instead they are scandalously called 'Denialists,' as if they had denied the Nazi Holocaust, on the basis that their work dissuades people from taking antiretroviral chemotherapy drugs - which logically cannot be lifesaving, despite all claims, if a retrovirus is not to be blamed.

I have to ask what are the consequences of this uncritical adherence to the theory of HIV? So far this theory has produced no cure and no vaccine despite the spending of some $200 billion on research. So, what if unacknowledged fraud is a major reason for this continual frustration? Is HIV science built upon flawed and fraudulent research? As for Robert Gallo, the first scientist awarded the credit for discovering HIV; it seems he may have only escaped criminal prosecution for fraud in developing the HIV test on a technicality; because it was found by a State Attorney General that too much time had elapsed for his prosecution to be undertaken.

As for AIDS in Africa, journalists rarely check how AIDS is diagnosed in that continent. Most logically presume it is diagnosed the same as in the West. But, if they had checked, they would have learnt that World Health Organization has set very different criteria for an AIDS diagnosis in Africa – explicitly stating that AIDS can be diagnosed solely on the basis of symptoms common to other major diseases! Thus many diseases can be and are diagnosed as AIDS in Africa. I cite these remarkable diagnostic rules in full in this book so you can judge this for yourselves.

If the dissenting scientists were right, if we wrongly fear a sexually transmitted virus, this discovery would have an enormous impact around the world and especially in Africa. It would cause a vast uplifting of the spirits of its people, far greater than anything achieved by "Live AID" concerts. We all know how devastating it is for an individual to be told that they are HIV positive and will inevitably die of AIDS. What then does it do to the morale of the people of a continent to be told that they are not only desperately poor but incurably blighted – due to sex?

We have been taught to greatly fear viruses – and yet scientists have long known that these are fundamental parts of life, made by the millions by all healthy cells. I hope this book will help by combating this fear, this damning of the invisible because we do not understand it. Without this fear, hopefully the focus in medical research will shift to the environmental toxins that really do put us, and our world, gravely at risk.

As for myself, my work as an investigative journalist previously was on relatively safer subjects for one's reputation in the liberal press, such as arms for Iran, Aboriginal land rights, and blood diamonds. I do not expect such a relatively easy ride this time, given the emotion connected to this issue. Indeed, attempts have already been made to prevent this work appearing, by the same academics who have tried to prevent publicity for the works of the 'dissident' scientists. I suppose I should be honoured to be seen so early as a danger by them, even before this book appeared! You can read here verbatim their attacks on my work and judge their validity for yourselves.

But the truth needs to be out. I hope my account will help to lift the fear with which these natural and fascinating tiny particles have been enshrouded for far too long. They are the products of our cells – and they helped make us.

When I began some twelve years ago my journey into medical research, it took me into the grim world of the virus hunters – but then, utterly unexpectedly, it led to me being utterly enthralled by the marvels of the miniscule world of the cell and of its messenger particles or viruses, a world that may well extend across galaxies. I invite you to join me on this journey to meet with our oldest, smallest ancestors, ones whom we are only just now starting to know.

# Contents

# Chapter 1

# First Lessons

Like most of us, I had never thought to question why viruses are such a terrible threat to us – despite friends dying of AIDS in the 1980s. Medical matters were safe in the hands of medical authorities – or so I presumed up until recent years. Viruses I had learnt were horrible germs, invading, hijacking, competing with us for life – but in truth I knew little about them.

Other issues then absorbed me as an investigative journalist. When President Ronald Reagan's Administration announced the discovery of HIV in 1984, calling it a great 'triumph of US science', I was out in the deserts of Australia making a film about the Aboriginal struggle for justice and land. When Oprah Winfrey predicted that a million Americans would soon die of AIDS, I was helping expose secret links between the Reagan Administration and Iran's Ayatollahs. When the US Government failed to keep its promise to soon have a vaccine for HIV, I was making a series for television about the worldwide diamond industry that led to an invitation to testify about blood diamonds at a US Congressional Hearing.

But out of the blue in 1994 I received a phone call from a parent asking for help. Her apparently healthy baby had become severely brain damaged within days of having a Measles, Mumps and Rubella (MMR) injection. She wondered if the vaccine had played a role in this. If it had, I thought it must be a rare side effect. Well, this was not my normal area of expertise, but I had some skills in document retrieval and logical analysis, so I set to work to discover what I could, but with no great expectations. [2]

Shortly after this, the UK government's Department of Health issued a series of terrifying national emergency health warnings, stating there would 'definitely' soon be a deadly measles epidemic infecting between 100,000 and 200,000 British children and that 'around 50 children, mostly of secondary school age, would die' - that is, if all children 'between 5 and 15' were not immediately revaccinated. This panicked both parents and children. Those with children aged 4 or 16 years besieged the Health Services, begging for their children to be also revaccinated lest they might die,

During the following nation-wide vaccination program for measles and rubella, the normal safeguards were suspended. The requirement that only a doctor should give the rubella vaccine was lifted, as also was the requirement to tell girls of childbearing age of the danger the rubella vaccine carries for any unborn child. Not warning them would be faster – and not using doctors cheaper. It was justified because of the predicted oncoming deadly measles epidemic.

I applauded this campaign. It was a sign that our health authorities were ready to nip any danger in the bud. But then I read that a Dr. Richard Nicholson, the Editor of the prestigious *'Bulletin of Medical Ethics'*, was highly critical. He said there was no emergency, and no need to panic families. I went to see him to discover why.

---

[2] The woman who asked for my help was Jackie Fletcher. She went on to found a parents' vaccination support group now known as JABS – and she can now remarkably hold her own in arguments with government regulatory scientists on many a leading BBC news program.

He explained; 'There was no talk of an impending measles epidemic a year ago. On the contrary, the leading UK government scientists reported that measles was practically extinct, that nearly everyone in England was now immune to measles.'

'But,' I asked, 'Why then did they call for this campaign?'

He explained that the World Health Organization (WHO) was trying to drive the measles virus into extinction and that governments were competing for the honour of being the first country to achieve this. This led to UK Government scientists publishing a year ago a paper saying that, to fulfil the WHO target, they must find a way to motivate a population no longer scared of measles into having an extra vaccination. This paper did not predict an epidemic – but the very reverse. It said nearly everyone was already immune.

Dr. Nicholson thus could not find any proof that a major measles epidemic was imminent. He told me that the government's estimate of up to 50 deaths in an impending epidemic was based on an 'improper use of statistics.'

I went out to interview an author of the above paper, a Dr. Elizabeth Miller, at the major Government medical research centre in Colindale, a London suburb, and asked her why was the government predicting that up to 50 might die of measles?

She replied: 'We were faced with an unprecedented crisis. Before the development of vaccines, there was no risk for measles in our schools. All school children were immune to measles for life, but this is no longer true.'

I was perplexed and asked 'Why are these children now more vulnerable?' I had presumed MMR gave our school children a protection they did not have before.

She explained that the vaccine uses a measles virus that is weakened, 'attenuated' so it won't give measles, but this also meant it was too weak to give a guaranteed 'life-long immunity.' In fact, the immunity it gave might not last more than five years. Thus children vaccinated in infancy might no longer be protected when attending school. So it was a trade-off – no measles as infants – and more vulnerability to measles in later life. This seemed reasonable, but I still needed to know how vulnerable this had left our older children. I asked again how they worked out that 50 children might die in the predicted epidemic?

She explained: 'This unprecedented new situation has forced us to adopt a mathematical model with a wide range of variables. This predicts deaths in the range of none to fifty.'

I was astonished. A range of 0 to 50 did not make 50 deaths likely. It was merely one end of a speculative range. Their prediction was based on unproven 'unprecedented' facts. This told us nothing. No wonder Dr. Nicholson had scathingly reported both 'statistical manipulation' and scaremongering.

A World Health Organization 'virus extermination' goal had thus led to UK government virologists organising a fear-based campaign that frightened children and parents to achieve its ends. I hoped similar tactics were not being employed around the world. It also seemed totally unrealistic. The UK might be an island nation – but it has millions of visitors every year, every one of whom could potentially reintroduce the virus.

But why was this campaign also against rubella? Dr. Miller explained that the rubella vaccine component of this campaign was designed to achieve 'the interruption of rubella transmission in the United Kingdom' –that is, also to drive the rubella virus into extinction.

But Dr. Nicholson came to a different conclusion. 'There was no justification for the concomitant rubella immunisation' as the risk from rubella was minimal. The official statistics stated that 99% of teenage girls over 14 years of age were already immune from rubella and therefore not at risk.

Extraordinarily, the scientists working with Miller had themselves reported the statistics he was using. They provided them in the Communicable Disease Report of 24

June 1994. They said all British teenage girls were already probably immune to rubella for life. They thus did not predict a rubella epidemic. They also stated: 'The Department of Health recommends that single antigen rubella vaccine need not be given to girls who have a documented history of MMR vaccination. The administrative cost of checking records may outweigh the cost of extra doses of vaccine especially if the vaccination is performed in schools.'

Because of the risk the vaccine carried to unborn children, the government had previously stipulated that doctors, not nurses, must administer the vaccine and that all the girls had to be asked if they could be pregnant – and be told to avoid pregnancy for 12 weeks after having the vaccine.

But the Chief Medical Officer of the UK, on the 27th September 1994, advised there was no longer any need to pass on any warning to the million teenage girls being vaccinated in this campaign. He stated: 'We do not believe there is justification for counselling all girls to avoid pregnancy for one month following immunisation.' He also advised: 'there was no objective evidence of harm' to pregnant women from vaccination.

Yet when I checked, I found that the latest Government figures reported that every year some 'pregnancy terminations were caused by vaccination.' [3] SmithKline Beecham, a major manufacturer of rubella vaccine, still warned in bold print on the package insert it supplied with the vaccine: 'Never give to pregnant women, or women of child-bearing age not fully aware of the need to avoid pregnancy for one month after vaccination.'

I went to SmithKline Beecham to ask if it had withdrawn this warning. A company spokesman replied that, although the government had cancelled its warning, 'we are keeping the warning in place for the vaccines we sell.'

The UK Department of Health justified the removal of its warning by saying that the evidence was that children born to women immunised in pregnancy were healthy. But it could not have been as convinced of this as it seemed, for, once the campaign was over, it restored the health warning. It knew the principal risk was to the life of the child prior to birth – not after birth. Their reassurance was evidently evasive 'politician's speak.'

The 1989 Report of the U.S. Preventive Services Task Force stated: 'Rubella is generally a minor illness, but it can result in serious foetal complications when women become infected during pregnancy ... When a mother catches rubella in the first 3 months of pregnancy in most cases it causes a miscarriage or still-birth ... Although further evidence is needed regarding the risks of transmitting rubella to breast-fed infants, the virus has been isolated in the breast milk of up to two-thirds of vaccinated women.'

It was not only girls that were put at risk by this rubella vaccination campaign. Boys normally do not have to fear rubella, as it is a mild disease for them. But, by having the vaccine they ran the risk of arthritis - as do girls. The prestigious Institute of Medicine, based at the National Academy of Sciences in Washington DC, reported in 1991 that there was a clear risk of acute arthritis from the rubella vaccine used in the UK (RA 27/3) and manufactured by SmithKline Beecham. The government again did not pass on any warning.

I interviewed parents who believed the rubella vaccine damaged their sons. David, the 5-year-old son of Julia Powell in Wales, became severely arthritic after his vaccination. His mother said: 'He would spend endless nights screaming with the pain. He couldn't run. He walked like a crippled old man. He had splints put on his legs to straighten them at night. He wore a plaster on his arm to straighten it. He is now going into remission but the hospital said the arthritis would never leave him. It can return and cripple him at any time.'

Ashley Wade, the 8-year-old son of Lisa Finley, went down with arthritis soon after being vaccinated in the measles-rubella campaign. He could no longer walk. He also had

---

[3] According to a UK Government report of 11 November 1994, there were in 1991 eight pregnancy terminations caused by vaccination and in 1992 ten.

allergic purpura. His mother said: 'Our son's immune system was seriously damaged. The antibodies in his blood were attacking his organs and blood vessels. ... It is untreatable. I feel terribly guilty for agreeing to his vaccination.'

Allergic Purpura is now known to be 5 times more prevalent as a consequence of vaccination than previously thought. [4] It is also known as idiopathic thrombocytopenic purpura (ITP). "Idiopathic" means simply that its cause is not known. The rest of the name means that its victims bleed easily and suffer from extensive bruising.

Dawn Corrigan is the mother of 1-year-old George, who came down with ITP, She told me: 'On Christmas Day, 10 days after he had the MMR, I found his nappy full of blood. His nose then started bleeding. The roof of his mouth was dark mauve. His skin was covered in spots. It was really frightening. He was 2 weeks in hospital and still is not fully recovered.'

James, the 12-year-old son of a nurse, Susanne Severn, became violently ill four weeks after his vaccination. His joints ached with arthritic damage. 'He went from being a keen football player to being like a cabbage. He could not walk and his knees were very swollen. It was really very frightening. He became virtually lifeless. Eventually he was diagnosed as having 'IgA nephropathy,' meaning the antibodies in his blood were attacking his kidneys, killing them. This disease can be controlled but not cured.

The anti-rubella campaign did not exterminate the virus as planned. Instead the vaccine proved ineffective. In the first 20 weeks of the following year there were 2,461 cases of rubella in England and Wales.

A report in the British Medical Journal recommended that 'antibody status should be checked before immunisation' so that children do not incur unnecessary risks through vaccination. But, no such checks were, or are, carried out. The idea behind vaccines is to expose a person to a measured safe amount of a pathogen, so that our bodies learn to produce antibodies that neutralise it. If a child already has antibodies against a danger, vaccination is pointless.

What were the consequences of this rubella vaccination? We simply do not know how many unborn babies were lost through the withdrawal of the warning. To the best of my knowledge, no checks were ever carried out.

As for the effects of the Measles-Rubella campaign as a whole, many parents told me their children fell seriously ill shortly afterwards and that their doctors reported these cases to the government as possible consequences of vaccination, But when I tried to establish how many such complaints were filed, the Department of Health blithely assured me that no children at all were suffering from such after effects!

I then arranged for questions to be asked in the UK Parliament – hoping this way to get some facts. I asked how many cases of measles the health authorities believed their campaign had averted – and how many cases of illness suspected to result from these vaccinations had been reported by doctors to the government.

I was amazed by the answer.

The Government reported that the campaign had averted an estimated 170 cases of measles; that is, not dangerous cases requiring hospitalisation, just cases of illness. Typically 170 measles cases would include just one or two so serious that they required hospitalisation.

But doctors had reported over 2,500 cases of illness as possibly side effects of this campaign, with over 500 of these so serious that the child had to be admitted to hospital! Since UK government research shows doctors typically only report one in ten cases of possible side effects, since most will presume vaccines to be harmless, these results meant that the MR vaccination campaign had resulted in up to 25,000 cases of illness potentially

---

[4] Reported in the *Lancet* medical journal of June 1995

caused by vaccination, with over 500 in hospital – as against an estimated 170 cases of measles avoided.

I knew the real figures were likely to be much worse, for the government had excluded from these statistics all possible cases where the illness developed slowly and all cases of illness during pregnancy that might have been caused by the rubella vaccine.

I wondered why so many side effects, so went to the manufacturer of the MMR vaccine to see if they had any explanation. They arranged for me to speak on the phone with their top expert in the US, Dr. Maurice Hilleman, the internationally renowned specialist who developed the MMR vaccine.

I said to him 'I understand this vaccine is made up of living viruses that you have so weakened so they will not make the child ill, but not so weakened that they will not give the child immunity. It must be difficult to so exactly weaken viruses?'

'Exactly, you have hit the nail on the head.' he replied.

I then queried, 'Do you have any guidelines for doing this?'

'Yes,' he said, 'Twenty percent.'

I did not understand this very brief answer so asked him to explain.

He replied: 'If only 20% of the children fall ill from the vaccine, that is judged acceptable.'

When I gasped with surprise, he quickly added, 'Oh I don't mean seriously ill. Just lightly ill.'

I next interviewed the top British expert on immunisation at London University, Professor Michael Stewart of the School of Hygiene and Tropical Medicine. I asked him; 'Some parents are telling me they suspect their children have been made ill as a consequence of vaccination. Are their fears groundless?'

I nearly fell off my chair when he replied: 'What else would you expect? We all know the current childhood vaccines containing living viruses are dangerous. That is why I am heading up a team to develop safer vaccines.' He went on to explain that, with living viruses, there was always potential for some to mutate or to be insufficiently attenuated for safe use in the vaccine.

I then interviewed some of the parents who believed their child had been damaged by the MR vaccination campaign in the UK.

Karen is the mother of a large family in Essex in eastern England. She was extremely proud of her 12-year-old son 'Sam.' Before this vaccination campaign he was 'ridiculously healthy. He never had anything wrong with him, apart from some mild asthma, was doing well at school and loved football. He was an avid Spurs fan.'

But, when she received notice of the November inoculation campaign, she wrote asking if it would be safe for him, given his asthma and that another child of hers was epileptic? She was told not to worry. But: 'Four weeks later, coming down the stairs, his knees suddenly gave way and he tumbled down. He kept on falling.'

She continued: 'Sometimes, when I was talking to him, he would suddenly go blank. I accused him of being on drugs. Two months later we were in Great Ormond Street Children's hospital where they tested him for every disease. Then one doctor said to me: "Has he been exposed to measles?" I said; "No, Sam has never had measles." The doctor replied; "No, I meant, has he had a recent measles injection?" Then I clicked. All this had started after the vaccination.'

When I met Sam he was in a wheelchair and had lost the power of speech. Nevertheless his face was bright and attractive. He seemed to be enjoying life. His mother told me: 'On one of our last good days, he went down to see the Tottenham Hotspur players. He had not so far gone then and the players were wonderful with him.' His brain was now seriously deteriorating with the expectation that sooner or later he would slip into a coma and stay in it for years before he dies. His mother's life had been turned into a nightmare. She was constantly exhausted and scarcely had time to care for her youngest.

Their doctor supported her belief that the vaccine was the cause of this disaster. The renowned Great Ormond Street Children's Hospital agreed. Karen found herself uselessly blaming herself for letting him be immunised. She believed she has already lost him.

The other mother I interviewed, Susan Hamlyn, told me her son Francis came down with juvenile arthritis a month after being immunized. This is a known side effect of rubella vaccine. He could now scarcely walk for the pain. He was previously a chorister at Windsor Castle and played the trombone – but now was so weak he could not lift his trombone to play it. His mother told me their hospital consultant suspected the rubella vaccination was to blame

When Susan and her husband contacted the Secretary of State for Health, Virginia Bottomley, they received a reply admitting; 'there have been a small number of late onset and longer lasting suspected adverse reactions that have occurred post MR (Measles and Rubella) vaccination. It is of course of the utmost importance that these be investigated' particularly since 'abnormality of the joints ... is reported after rubella vaccination.' The Health Secretary added that the Medicines Control Agency were; 'following up many of the yellow card reports of suspected adverse reactions.'

Dr. Nicholson, of the Bulletin of Medical Ethics, told me he suspected the Department of Health may have acted illegally in not calling for competitive tenders for the £20 million worth of vaccines used in this campaign. 'The Department told me that normal competitive procedures were followed but government contracting databases clearly record that the procedure followed was "without a call to competition" as legally stipulated. It claimed exemption from this because of "extreme urgency brought about by events unforeseeable".'

'Yet,' he continued: 'This campaign was carefully planned over many weeks. The Department of Health's actions [in not calling for competitive tenders] benefited two drug companies, SmithKline Beecham and Merieux UK. Two years ago these companies withdrew from circulation their measles, rubella and mumps vaccines when the mumps element was associated with meningitis. This contract reopened the market for the left over measles and mumps elements just before the end of their shelf life.' He also noted that a Tory government minister involved in this transaction had subsequently taken up a position on the manufacturer's board.[5]

I have since discovered a frank World Health Organization Report that tells in detail of illnesses to be expected in some children as a consequence of vaccination. It is entitled *Supplementary Information on Vaccine Safety*. Its Part 2 is entitled 'Background rates of adverse events following immunization.' It was published in 2000.[6]

It stated. 'Symptomatic local reactions can be expected in about 10% of vaccine recipients (except for DTP and TT boosters where it affects about 50%). Fever occurs in about 10% or less of vaccine recipients (except for DTP where it is again about 50%).' This was far higher than I had expected – and, I thought, would surely appal many parents. Finally it added: '[After] MMR, 10% have local pain or swelling, fever and rash occur in from 5% to15% up to 10 days after taking the vaccine. Febrile [brain] seizures occur in 333 in every million cases.'

I now felt I was getting somewhere. Could this explain what happened to the brain-damaged son of Jackie and John Fletcher, the case that began my research? The reported incidence rate of 333 cases in a million meant that 2,644 children were expected to have febrile seizures as a result of the UK 1994 MR vaccination of 8 million children – over ten times more than the measles cases this campaign was designed to avert,

The official report also stated: 'Natural measles virus infection causes post-infectious encephalomyelitis (brain damage) in approximately one per 1000 infected

---

[6] http://www.who.int/vaccines-documents/DocsPDF00/www562.pdf

persons. At least 50% of those affected are left with permanent central nervous system impairment.' Just a bit of elementary mathematics here. The MR vaccination campaign targeted 8 million children of which only about 170 were expected to be infected with measles if the campaign did not happen. If the risk of permanent central nervous system damage from the wild virus is in the order of about one in 2000 infections, as this report stated, there was a very small chance of any child getting such damage if the vaccination campaign did not happen.

But the report did not admit, or deny, this consequence of it own statistics: 'While many have been concerned about the attenuated measles vaccine's ability to produce such a syndrome, the United States Institute of Medicine concluded there was not enough evidence to accept or reject a causal relationship.' [7]

The report went on to describe other vaccination side effects: 'Minor local reactions such as pain, oedema [swelling from water retention] and erythema [inflammation] occur in 40% to 80% of cases when DTP vaccine is administered.' I was surprised by how common these were. It also stated: 'Most of the rare vaccine reactions (e.g. seizures, thrombocytopaenia [low blood platelet numbers, often resulting in bleeding], hypotonic hypo-responsive episodes [serious reaction often involving unconsciousness and breathing difficulties], and persistent inconsolable screaming) are self-limiting and do not lead to long-term problems.'

It also warned: 'Generally speaking, live vaccines should not be given to individuals who are pregnant, with immune deficiency diseases or to individuals who are immunosuppressed due to malignant disease, therapy with immunosuppressive agents, or irradiation.' In other words, before having a vaccine, check that the child's immune system is already in good order. Only when it is, should the vaccine be given.

I found this particularly shocking, for this check is scarcely ever done – even by WHO specialists. From all reports, WHO is currently rushing out vaccines as a first measure of help for millions of severely malnourished children, and thus immune system compromised, in Iraq and all the poverty-stricken crisis regions of the world.

A 2007 WHO manual similarly reported: 'of 460 children aged 13-18 months, 32% developed moderate or severe fever after MMR vaccine (vs. 9% with placebo)' – concluding that 'serological techniques cannot distinguish between the immune response to natural infection and immunization.' [8]

Thus I was introduced to the world of medical reporting and was alarmed by what I found. But I still was extraordinarily ignorant. I had no idea how Dr. Hilleman had weakened or 'attenuated' viruses to make them suitable for the MMR vaccine. Had this process forced some of the viruses used to mutate, a danger that had been explained to me by a top UK specialist, Professor Michael Stewart?

Alternatively, were some children reacting to chemicals put in the vaccines as preservatives or adjuvants? One of these was mercury. Could it be to blame? Or were the painful side effects happening because many vaccines were being given to infants at the same time? Was it simply because some children were unsuited to this 'mass' medicine? Were we presuming a few cheap vaccines could suit all?"

And ultimately, were these risks worth taking? This was increasingly a major issue for me. I wanted to find out just what went on within that needle. I was at this point not questioning the role viruses play in causing many illnesses, nor the need for vaccination, the most common medical treatment on the planet, but whether due care was taken in making our vaccines.

---

[7] Stratton et al.1994

[8] WHO *'Manual for the Laboratory diagnosis of measles and rubella infection.'* Second Edition printed August 2007

# Chapter 2

# A Scientific Storm

I write for the pleasure and for the sense that my investigative work is of value, but when an editor of a major UK newspaper told me that, by publishing my work on vaccines prominently, they were paying me with 'prestige', it gave me the impetus to be more ambitious. I soon found the editor was right. On the back of my work for the paper, I was commissioned to produce a film on the fraudulent MR vaccine campaign for the investigative 'Dispatches' television series on the UK's Channel 4.

But the subject of the film changed in January 1997 when we learnt of an emergency international scientific workshop just about to happen, summoned by a major US governmental research institution, the National Institutes for Health. Apparently monkey viruses had contaminated the polio vaccine – and were now turning up in human cancers. This was horrific, for this vaccine has been given to an estimated billion children. Within days my co-producer Rosie Thomas and I were on a plane to Washington.

We soon learnt that laboratories around the world had detected Simian Virus 40 (SV40), a virus from the Indian Rhesus monkey, in many types of human cancers – and learnt, to our astonishment, this was because tens of thousands of this monkey species were killed so their organs could be used in the making of the polio vaccine. These monkey organs had turned out to be infected. How on earth, we asked, could a vaccine be made so carelessly? If millions of doses had been so polluted, this must surely be one of the worst medical disasters of all time? We anticipated it being a colossal news story. It seemed there was solid evidence that this had occurred; otherwise surely it would not be so agitating the top people in the US government's medical establishment – and the British too, as we had learnt they would be at the emergency scientific workshop, as well as representatives from the World Health Organization (WHO).

However, when we checked with WHO, we were told not to be alarmed – for the vaccine was now purified; it had only been contaminated in its early days. We then found the UK Government had admitted to this monkey virus contamination of the vaccine back in 1988, in a long-forgotten statement to Parliament. The Secretary for Health had then assured the House that this contaminating virus had been tested by American scientists and found not to be dangerous. Maybe this story was not going to be so big after all?

In Washington we made our way through a maze of laboratories to the Natcher Auditorium where we found assembled over two hundred scientists from around the world. The media were also present –from France, Canada, the UK and the USA, but when Dr. Kathryn Zoom, the head of the FDA division that licenses vaccines as safe, said she preferred the media to leave its questions to the press conference at the end, most journalists promptly vanished, not to reappear until this press conference. As far as I could see it was only one UK journalist and ourselves who stayed to listen first-hand to what the scientists had found – and to ask our own questions at every drink or meal break.

Consequently, most of the press missed an incredible event. One after another that morning, scientists from around the world got onto the stage to shock us with what they had found. They had discovered this monkey virus, SV40, in children's brain tumours and adults' mesotheliomas – the last being the deadly cancer that starts in the lung-lining that was previously associated solely with asbestos.[9] It seemed the more they looked, the more they found it in other types of human cancers – but not in the surrounding healthy tissues.

And, when we asked from where did they think this virus came, most said it surely had to be from the polio vaccine.

One of the leading speakers, Dr. Michele Carbone, set out their results. 'Sixty-two papers from thirty laboratories from around the world have reported SV40 in human tissues and tumours, ... It is very difficult to believe that all of these papers, all of the techniques used and all of the people around the world are wrong.' After he had finished, I was dismayed to hear scientists from leading laboratories confirm what he had said, by telling how they had found SV40 in over 80% of some childhood brain tumours, in 85% of deadly mesotheliomas, in about 25% of bone cancers – and in 40% of spermal fluid from a small sample of apparently healthy males! [10]

But not all the scientists present were in agreement. Dr. Keerti Shah stood up bravely as the only one who could not find the virus in cancers, no matter how hard he looked. He therefore doubted that it had caused any cancers. He suggested all the others had mistaken laboratory contamination for the virus. Nevertheless he calculated that 98 million Americans had been dosed with the SV40 contaminated vaccines. There followed a spirited discussion about why only he could not find SV40. Some suggested that he had used out-of-date methods. I was told he had never done this kind of work before.

But surprisingly Shah alone had been scheduled in advance to speak twice that first morning, as both the first and the final speaker. The second time he spoke about statistical research undertaken with Drs. Howard Strickler and James Goedert, two government epidemiologists, They reported finding no significant increase in cancers among the vaccinated, as compared to the unvaccinated – but the validity of their research clearly depended upon them having found a population not exposed to SV40. Their assumptions regarding this were dubious, according to their critics, given how widely the vaccine was distributed.

As this controversy continued, I realised that we had plunged unaware into the midst of a scientific tempest. After the SV40 researchers presented their papers, the chairperson summed up the discussion as if between two evenly matched scientific teams. Yet as far as I could see, on one side there was evidence from many – and on the other, only one experimenter plus some inconclusive statistics. But I soon learnt that Shah was not as isolated as he seemed. The medical authorities were backing him, thus allowing him to box above his weight.

Chief among his defenders was Dr. Robin Weiss from London, one of the UK's top HIV experts and a leading light in the UK's virology establishment. It soon emerged that Weiss had taken a major role in organising this meeting along with Drs. Shah, Goedert and Strickler, and they had prepared in advance a proposal they wanted the meeting to endorse.

Strickler was very delicate in making this proposition. He stated: 'my suggestion is that, in the face of the uncertainty of the data, that what we really need is an exquisitely controlled, third-party study.' It was only later that we learnt this key study was to be headed by him; that he would be 'the third party'. It has been arranged that he would be the judge on everyone else's experiments, or so it seemed.

---

[9] Carbone has more recently had this study published: Gazdar AF, Carbone M., Molecular pathogenesis of malignant mesothelioma and its relationship to simian virus 40. Clin Lung Cancer. 2003 Nov;5(3):177-81

[10] One of these reports was by a Dr Butel, who afterwards had published: Butel JS, et al., Molecular evidence of simian virus 40 infections in children. J Infect Dis. 1999 Sep;180(3):884-7. Also
Vilchez RA, Butel JS., SV40. Oncogene. 2003 Aug 11;22(33):5164-72

At the time, I missed much of the 'behind-the-stage' politics. But I was new to this. I could only judge the issues based on the evidence presented – and for me the case was overwhelming.  Multiple well-reputed laboratories had found SV40 in human cancers – and their scientists thought it was a monkey virus that invaded humans through the release of a contaminated polio vaccine.

Then came the final press conference. It was presided over by Dr. Weiss with, to my surprise, scientists who had mostly played a minor role in the workshop. They told the press that there was no reason to have any concern over SV40 infection. They did not stress the dramatic links to cancer reported at the conference. They blithely assured the press that nothing had been reported that they needed to worry about. One even said he would happily ingest SV40, as it was not dangerous. It was a complete misrepresentation, leaving the press with nothing.

That evening when watching the news, I discovered the NIH had issued a press release at the same time on an entirely different matter that boosted its reputation, and it was this that had grabbed the news. There was no mention of the quite terrifying research presented at the NIH emergency workshop – or of the medical negligence in the making the polio vaccine that surely must lie behind this catastrophe. I ruefully thought it a very fine sample of spin.

But for me, the workshop had not been a total disappointment. It had given me the opportunity to meet with the top scientists involved with vaccine safety – and what I learnt from them outside the scheduled sessions was completely fascinating. I also met a lawyer who had spoken briefly at one session, Stanley Kops, who turned out to hold many documents acquired through legal actions that proved SV40 continued to contaminate the polio vaccine well past the date when this was supposed to have stopped.

I met also with Professor John Martin, who held the chair of pathology at the University of Southern California. He told me he was sure other monkey viruses must have been in the vaccine alongside SV40. He had tracked down one of these; it was cytomegalovirus (SCMV) from African Green Monkeys, another species used in making the polio vaccine. He suspected it as having a role in Chronic Fatigue Syndrome. This was getting even more horrifying.  SV40 might only be the tip of the iceberg. If one monkey virus got in, scores of others might have got in too.

How could this happen? Dr. Maurice Hilleman, whom I had interviewed previously about MMR, made a presentation at the workshop on how they had found SV40 in the polio vaccine back in 1961!  He explained our childhood polio vaccine was made of poliovirus grown in incubators in a soup of mashed kidneys taken from thousands of wild-caught monkeys. It was thus very easy for a monkey virus to get into the vaccine. I resolved to investigate why such an obviously hazardous method of making the polio vaccine had been adopted. Was it that there were no alternatives?[11]

Then Professor Martin totally shocked me by saying there was a very real danger that HIV also may have contaminated the polio vaccine, since it too was originally a monkey virus, – and the health authorities had long known of this danger! I was told that in 1988, without telling the public, they had quietly ordered the polio vaccine to be in future screened for HIV contamination  – some 33 years after the vaccine's launch, and after it had been given to millions of children. This was clearly a case of bolting the door far too late. Was this carelessness the reason why the HIV epidemic had spread so fast? The dates seemed to be right. AIDS was first reported in the States in 1981. I started to plan to make a major investigative documentary on the polio vaccine and HIV, as a follow-up for our documentary on SV40.

---

[11]   Also see Hilleman MR. History, precedent, and progress in the development of mammalian cell culture systems for preparing vaccines: safety considerations revisited. J Med Virol 1990 May;31(1):5-12. PMID 2198327.

Despite these reports, Dr. Gerald Quinnan,[12] a major figure at the FDA, had let it be known that WHO had decided not to test the purity of the original vaccine 'seed' stocks used for the Sabin 'sugar-cube' vaccine. He said this was because there were 'only a small number of vials' of the old vaccine and tests 'might use it all up.' [13]

But this was about to change. I happened to meet at the Workshop with an elderly Dr. Herbert Ratner who told me he was working in pubic health when the polio vaccine was launched in 1955. He doubted its safety at the time– and his fridge still contained unopened vials of it.   When I mentioned this to Professor Martin, he became very excited – saying this was just what was needed to check if the early vaccine was contaminated. I took him to meet with Ratner in his hotel room – but more about these vials later.

As for Dr. Michele Carbone, a well-dressed debonair Italian; for most of those attending he was clearly the star of the conference. He told how he had started on SV40 research after coming across 1960 reports of SV40 causing tumours in laboratory animals. He discovered these reports had only led to a check to see if any cancers had developed in the vaccinated within four years of taking the vaccine. But cancers may take over twenty years to develop, and Carbone knew this. He was appalled to discover that no one had checked to see if cancers had appeared later than four years after exposure. In 1994 he tested human cancers and found his fears justified: they contained SV40,

But his superiors wanted no such publicity. He recalls the head of his NIH laboratory saying 'he was worried that the press might exaggerate our findings and alarm the public.' Carbone was warned that he would be 'punished' if he spoke to the media.[14] Shortly after this, he found another laboratory where he could continue his research.

Carbone explained at the workshop what he had since discovered about how SV40 might help cause cancers.   It seemed the virus had two molecules in its 'skin', one its 'large T-antigen' and the other, its 'small t-antigen' (the 'T' standing for tumour), that could disable 'one of our most vital cancer preventive genes, the p53.' Apparently p53 persuaded cells to commit suicide rather than become cancerous. If SV40 switched off p53, as seemed to happen, then these cells might grow into a cancer.[15] Why would SV40 switch it off?  Carbone suggested that it might be to provide the virus with more cells to multiply in. He thus called SV40 'the smallest perfect war machine ever made.'

I listened to him engrossed. I did not know then that scientists had for decades tried to prove cancers were caused by viruses, and had mostly failed. But he did stress that cancers are caused by many factors working together. SV40 was only one such factor – but, from all he said, a very important factor.

One of his Italian colleagues at the workshop, Professor Mauro Tognon, told me he had checked the seminal fluid of nine of his male students for SV40, and four of these had tested positive.  He had also found it in 23% of their donated blood. This was extremely alarming; an incidence rate vastly higher than normally reported for HIV.  I asked myself, could this help explain the vast expansion of cancers in the West in the last few decades? [16]  Could cancers really be a vast viral 'epidemic'?

However, I would later learn that his theory so far could not explain why cancer levels were far lower in India than the West. It should not have been so.  The early polio vaccine was extensively used there, for it was sent from the States as part compensation for the large numbers of monkeys India had supplied for polio vaccine development. I

---

[12] Then the acting director of the US Food and Drug's Administration's (FDA) Center for Biologics Evaluation and Research

[13] Tom Curtis, *Rolling Stone Magazine*, March 19th, 1992.

[14] The Virus and the Vaccine. Pp 161-3

[15] Ibid. Page 204

[16] Martini et al. SV40 Early Region and Large T Antigen in Human Brain Tumors, Peripheral Blood Cells, and Sperm Fluids from Healthy Individuals. Cancer Research 56:  4820-4825, 1996.

wondered; were toxins needed as co-factors with the virus, as with the mesothelioma cancers linked to both SV40 and asbestos? Did the viruses only multiply in such toxin-damaged cells? This was a clue to what I would later discover about viruses – but at that time I did not realise all the implications.

In the West mesothelioma was virtually unheard of prior to 1950, but its incidence has risen steadily since. Currently it kills about 3,000 Americans a year, or about one half of one percent of all cancer deaths. It is highly associated with asbestos exposure, but so is SV40, with its genetic codes found in over 80% of such cases. Is the virus a needed co-factor or an alternative cause – or is its presence a side effect of the poisoning? However, I noted when Carbone injected hamsters with SV40 (and other unspecified elements that would be in the cell culture along with SV40), some 60% developed mesothelioma without any need for asbestos.

As I delved deeper, I learnt that the evidence for SV40's presence in cancers was mostly produced by an extremely delicate laboratory technique called Polymerase Chain Reaction, or PCR for short. I understood that police use this technique with a very high degree of accuracy to discover who were at murder scenes. I thus presumed that this test was just as accurate when used by doctors to identify the presence of species of viruses.

PCR is used to study extremely short lengths of DNA code. It clones one fragment many millions of times to make it easier to study. If this fragment matches exactly a segment of code found only in a known virus, (a segment often obtained from genetic bank libraries) then that virus is deduced to have been present at that time or in the recent past.

But – there is a major difficulty here. When a forensic laboratory uses this technique at the behest of the police, its accuracy is very high, for the laboratory normally can check its sample against a verified blood sample from a suspect, and thus a full genome. It is quite another thing when it comes to identifying the source of a short genetic code sequence found in a cell culture.

Let me explain: this test utilises extremely minute fragments of genetic code (DNA), perhaps a fortieth of the invisibly short code found in a virus. If finding such a tiny fragment is to prove the presence of a viral species, the fragment must be proved identical to a segment that is already proved totally unique to this viral species. A major problem immediately faces us – so far only a small proportion of viral species have been analysed – so how can we prove any segment unique to a particular species? Logically – this is simply impossible. We must therefore make educated guesses – made more difficult if the suspect virus is mutating.

These experiments must also ensure that the unique sequence identified for use in PCR is not one that mutates. If a stable unique segment is identified – it may be used as a 'primer' in the PCR test to reliably find other such segments. Such sequences are typically stored in data banks where they are made available so viral codes can be checked against them.

As a result, the PCR technique is highly limited when it comes to identifying viruses, a job for which it was not originally designed. It is totally dependent on the accuracy of the prior identification of a segment as unique to a species.   Such identification is not easy to do with total accuracy– often perhaps impossible, particularly when a new virus is sought.

But scientists have another technique that they can use in such circumstances. They may rely instead on 'cloning' – assembling a viral genome from many fragments and then testing this to see if it behaves like the wild virus, but this too is also very difficult to achieve. (More about this later.)

However, I was told that the genetic code of SV40 was entirely sequenced in 1978 – and is now reliably used as the reference gold standard [17] against which any segment of genetic code can be checked to see if it is identical – and thus from SV40.

But, at that time all this was a surprise to me. I had imagined that, when doctors say they have found SV40, or any other virus, in a patient, they meant they have found a whole virus, not a tiny fragment of code said to be unique to a viral species. I wondered, somewhat sceptically, how often really was this matching exact and unique? However, I had no reason to presume that these laboratories had not got it right. After all many had indentified SV40's prior presence in human cancers by finding codes they believed unique to this virus.

Nevertheless, from what I was learning, I was starting to understand how difficult it was to prove absolutely such an identification of a viral species, when so many have mutating codes and so many remain to be discovered – experts say we have studied at most 0.4% of those that exist. On top of this, we live within a sea of free particles of genetic codes. Our banks of identified viral codes are accordingly still very limited. How then to we prove a code segment unique to one species of virus?

What I have since learnt is that virologists today rarely attempt the very hard work of identifying the presence of a whole virus. For example, when we hear of the discovery of Bird Flu Virus in a dead bird – we are actually only hearing of the discovery of part of the genetic code of one of the protein molecules making up that virus. If this fragment or protein is not unique to a viral species, then we cannot be sure where it is from.

Thus, when Carbone said he had found SV40 in cancers, I later learnt that what he had actually found was a genetic code fragment that matched a code sequence found in a certain molecule believed to be unique to SV40. This was SV40's most dangerous molecule, 'the large T-antigen.' The fragment he matched was absolutely minute, just 127 base pairs out of the 5,243 base pairs in the genome of SV40.[18] (Genetic code fragments are measured in 'base pairs,' meaning a count of the paired nucleotides that lie along the twinned strands of DNA.[19] )

But even when a segment is reliably proved to be from part of the genetic code of a protein, this only indicates this protein's prior presence, not that of the whole virus. I wondered if these proteins could exist by themselves? Someone must have proved that they could not? Clearly there was earlier experimental work that proved this. I had not read this. I made a note to look for this.

Another scientist at the Emergency Workshop, Joseph Testa, said he had found this DNA sequence in cells with damaged chromosomes. He blamed SV40 and said, 'it looks like somebody set off a bomb inside the cell's nucleus, because of all these chromosome rearrangements.' But I wondered if this was right, for I knew damaged chromosomes are a feature of all cancer cells, and only a few of these showed signs of SV40 infection, i.e. contained this code. Was it possible that something other than SV40 might be doing this damage?

Carbone reassuringly noted that most people with SV40 will not develop cancer, since a healthy immune system destroys dangers – including the large T-antigen of SV40; that is unless, he warned, a person has been exposed to asbestos, a known damager of cells, and thus a suppresser of the human immune system.

The role of such toxins is often overlooked. We have in us countless viruses and bacteria that do us no harm – unless toxins have damaged our cells. For example, nearly all of us have the TB bacteria and the fungi linked to PCP, a deadly pneumonia, but few of

---

[17] The Virus and the Vaccine Page 179

[18] The Virus and the Vaccine. Page 205. Also see in its Appendix D, an extensive collection of related memos and other documents.

[19] There are about 4 million base pairs in a bacteria's genome and 3 billion base pairs in a human cell's genome.

us ever get these diseases. The fact that viruses are found near damaged cells does not prove that they cause this damage. Some scientists argue that some might be there to scavenge and repair the damage. We always have to ask, is the virus there because of the damage, or did the virus cause the damage? But – it took me time to come to this understanding. When I went to the SV40 conference I simply presumed the whole virus had been found in the cancers and was causing the cancers. I did not doubt it.

More of Carbone's research was published six months after the workshop, in the June 1997 issue of *Nature Medicine*. It reported that Carbone and colleagues had arranged for four laboratories to independently check with PCR to see if they could find in human cancers an identified fragment of SV40's genetic code (presumably the sequence previously identified by Carbone). They reported they had succeeded in this quest.

The link with the polio vaccine was now strengthened by another Carbone discovery. He reported that in Finland and Turkey, where the contaminated polio vaccines were not used, there was far less mesothelioma than in the USA or Italy, where the SV40 contaminated vaccines were widely used. He likewise could not find the fragment of SV40 genetic code in clinical samples of mesothelioma from Finland and Turkey but could find it in cases from Italy and the USA. Today Finland has one of the lowest rates of mesothelioma in the Western world. This was powerful evidence of a relationship between the SV40-contaminated polio vaccine and certain cancers – except it did not explain why India has a low cancer rate despite it extensively using the same contaminated vaccine.

What I had learnt at the workshop left me with many questions. Why was this SV40 genetic code only being found in cancer cells? Surely it would need to travel through other cells to get there? Also, why did it sometimes seem to cause cancer without being present? This happened in an experiment on female rats. They all got breast cancer after injection with a filtered laboratory culture containing SV40 – but no SV40 code was found in these cancers. [20]

I returned to the UK at the end of this workshop determined to make a powerful documentary on SV40. Soon after our return, we met with the only British scientists working on SV40. Their laboratory was at the University of Wales in Cardiff where they had analysed biopsy samples of mesothelioma cancers – and found S40 genetic code in about half of those tested. [21]

But I did not realise quite how controversial this research was before I met with doctors at the Maudsley Hospital in London. They were treating patients with the brain tumours in which SV40 might be present. When I told them of the research presented at this Workshop, they were greatly surprised. I was shown the notes they gave their students. These baldly stated 'cancers are not caused by viruses.' I later learnt that this had been the conclusion of many scientists after the failure of President Nixon's 1970s War against Cancer. That 'war' was based on the theory that viruses caused cancers, but it had flopped badly, finding practically no viruses linked to human cancers.

However, the Maudsley specialists were intrigued by what I had shown them from the Workshop and said they would set up PCR experiments to see if they too could find SV40 in cancer biopsies – but they later phoned to say they failed to find it. Clearly the PCR test for SV40 was difficult. Carbone had told them that there was a particular method to use for finding it.

---

[20] A December 1996 paper in Oncogene by a German team headed by Roberta Santarelli, reporting research partly carried out by them at the US National Institutes of Health, stated that "SV40 T-antigen induces breast cancer formation with a high efficiency" in 100% of lactating and 70% of virgin animals. They further noted that it was indicated that "immortalisation of mammary cells by SV40 T-antigen is a hit and run mechanism" in that not all the cells affected by SV40 remain SV40 positive.

[21] Bharat Jasani, et al., Association of SV40 with human tumours, Semin Cancer Biol. 2001 Feb;11(1):49-61.

It was not going to be easy for us either, for Channel 4 Television then decided it wanted more from us. They asked if we could find SV40 in British cancer patients and document this in our film! No one had ever checked living UK cancer patients for SV40. All the cases discussed at the workshop were found in the US, Europe and Japan. We were not scientists, but were told, if we did not succeed, our documentary might not be broadcast. We searched but found no laboratory in the UK that was equipped and ready to undertake this work. Eventually we found a laboratory in Italy that would do the analysis for us. We then had to persuade UK patients and their doctors to give us access to their biopsy tissue. It took time, but we secured about 11 samples – and SV40 genetic code was found in two of them – one from a patient dying from mesothelioma, the other from a recovered patient who had cancer in a leg bone. Our documentary, *Monkey Business,* was soon completed and broadcast immediately before Christmas 1997, very frustratingly far too close to the festive season to make the huge media impact we had anticipated.

But by the time it was completed, the film did not reflect all I had learnt. A documentary is effectively a short story. It can only include so much. In the last days of making the film I had learnt that the polio vaccine might well be still contaminated with SV40 – but was told it was too late to change the film to include this. It also left out the possibility that HIV might have spread in the vaccine, but I hoped to research and use this for a subsequent film on HIV and the polio vaccine – if the commissioning editor at Channel 4 agreed.

Meanwhile in America, Carbone was locked in fierce science wars as the staff of the NIH tried to water down his findings, in fear that these might scare people off from having their children vaccinated.

But Carbone did meet with Ratner. He picked up some of the 1955 polio vaccine stored in the latter's freezer and tested them. He found they contained SV40 of the same type as had been found in bone cancers. He also noted that it was a slow growing type that took some 19 days to develop – so would not have been removed from the vaccine, as the manufactures were only told to observe the vaccine culture for 14 days to make sure that SV40 was not present. [22]

I would later discover to my disgust that the US health authorities in 1961 deliberately limited the period of safety surveillance to 14 days, after discovering that, if they watched the polio vaccine cultures for longer, it became evident that many more cultures were contaminated with SV40 viruses, enough perhaps to put a halt on all vaccine production. [23]

The authorities had found by studying 120 monkey kidney cell cultures, that, if the cultures were observed for from 4 to 8 weeks, ten times more SV40 would be detected than could be found if they had only studied them for 2 weeks. 'The percentage of viruses increased ten-fold. The longer the cultures were kept, the higher the percentage of virus isolations obtained.'

They produced a table that showed, after 2 weeks, only 3 cultures of the 120 revealed signs of SV40 contamination. After monitoring for 3-4 weeks, some 16 cultures manifested the signs of SV40 contamination. After 4-8 weeks SV40 was revealed in 36 cultures, or 30% of them all. So, by only asking for the vaccine lots to be monitored for 14 days, the vaccine safety authorities had knowingly missing nearly all the SV40. They then had shockingly released this vaccine as guaranteed 'SV40-free'.

The same study stated the cultures came from the kidneys of apparently healthy animals, but the scientists involved had reported 'much to our surprise an unusually high

---

[22] Rizzo P, Di Resta I, Powers A, Ratner H, Carbone M; Unique Strains of SV40 in Commercial Poliovaccines from 1955 Not Readily Identifiable with Current Testing for SV40 Infection, CANCER RESEARCH 59, 6103-6108, December 15, 1999.

[23] Lederle corporate memo dated 1973. See further discussion below.

percentage of cultures that were considered "normal" showed virus infection.' It seemed SV40 did not cause any illness in its natural host and thus was not detected in them.

Meanwhile in Washington, Strickler and Shah pressed ahead with their 'confirmatory' project as presented at the workshop. They invited Carbone to participate, saying they planned to have many laboratories independently examine 95 samples of mesothelioma tissues to see if they could find SV40 in them. But when he looked at their proposal, Carbone was furious. He wrote back saying he had already published in *Cancer Research* the results from a nearly identical experiment carried out in four independent laboratories and asked, who would finance looking unnecessarily at 95 more samples? It was expensive work, finding and matching DNA. He added angrily: 'The first two pages of this draft ... contains gratuitous and unnecessary biased comments.'

Carbone's critique of their scientific methods had an unexpected result: Strickler and his colleagues promptly removed him from the study with a letter expressing regrets that their experiments were too expensive for him; but once he left the team, they immediately reorganised the experiment to make it far cheaper, by cutting it to 25 samples, not 95.

When Jasani in Wales looked at the first draft of the proposed experiment, he concluded its 'scientific methods were extremely loaded against getting a positive result' – in other words against finding SV40. Then, when Strickler in 1999 sent him a 'final draft' of a scientific paper reporting that they did not find SV40, Jasani exploded.

He replied, jointly with his laboratory boss, Alan Gibbs, to say this was 'a studied effort to ... sidestep the many flaws in this study rather than engage in meaningful, good-faith exchange of legitimate scientific issues ... flaws and unresolved scientific issues have become so cumulative as to outweigh any positive scientific benefit which might be derived from the publication of this study ... It cannot be that all these [SV40 finding] laboratories are contaminated and that contamination always happens in mesotheliomas, osteosarcomas and brain tumours, while the negative controls are always negative. Contamination is a random event... We strongly feel that the scientific integrity of this study (by 9 labs) has been seriously undermined and is in need of evaluation by a neutral third party.'

Strickler's reaction was to send off his paper without Jasani's endorsement to *Cancer Research* for publication– but much to his surprise the editor rejected it. This greatly embarrassed the NIH as they employed Strickler. A climb-down resulted. Jasani and his colleagues were asked to help rewrite the paper. It was their version that was published in May 2001.

But meanwhile the old guard fighting to protect the reputation of the polio vaccine had no intention of giving way. The FDA said it could not find SV40 in old samples of polio vaccine made by Lederle. It had tested them with PCR, by trying to match 564 base pairs of SV40's genome, about a fifth of the virus's whole genome. It reported it was unable to find a match.

Carbone counter-attacked, saying, among other things, that only short lengths of viral genetic code would survive in the vaccines, so the FDA were wrong in looking for longer sections.[24]

On the face of it, it seemed to me that using a larger part of SV40's genome should be more reliable than Carbone's match of less than half as much – but I was no expert on PCR, and on whether the use of longer sequences of DNA were better. I could not judge this argument – I would have to learn more.

But one thing did occur to me. If only such tiny fragments of the genetic code of SV40, a 30th of the whole, were being found by Carbone and his fellow-scientists, then the mystery was, why wasn't the whole virus being found?

---

[24] *The Virus and the Vaccine.* Page 264

I later learnt more about the difficulties that are involved in using PCR to identify a virus.  Professor Martin has recorded in a paper the difficulties he faced when using PCR to identify genetic codes found in humans suffering from Chronic Fatigue Syndrome. He used an electron microscope to examine his patients' brain cells and reported: 'Typically one may merely see accumulations of viral-like components, possibly with incomplete virus-like structures, in a cell which displays intense cytopathic effects.' He noted some of these were 'herpesvirus-like … [thus] suggestive of human cytomegalovirus (HCMV).' This similarity gave him a clue as to what he should to look for.

He then compared genetic codes he found with PCR to see if they were identical with sequences known to be from HCMV, but could find no identical matches.  As the study progressed, 'sequences were identified' that revealed 'a greater relatedness [similarity] … to the Colburn strain of simian CMV (SCMV)' rather than to the human or Rhesus version of CMV. However, all he had found was a similarity. The sequences were not identical.

Forgive me, but to explain this I have to be a bit technical. It is important to understand why PCR. a tool that is widely used to study viruses. often is unable to reliably identify them.  The importance of this will come plain later.

Professor Martin explained that the major problem he faced was that 'only a small amount of genetic information is available for cytomegaloviruses or other primates. Five sequences [only] are recorded in GenBank for the Colburn strain of African green monkey simian cytomegalovirus (SCMV).' (The Genbank is a widely used database of identified genetic sequences that can be computer matched.) Five sequences made up 'only a small amount of genetic information.' This made it very hard for him to identify the segments he found as from a primate, let alone from a specific species.

He also reported other difficulties.  He had 'assumed that the genome consists of multiple fragments, rather than as an entire full-length cytomegaloviral genome. As shown in the accompanying papers, the situation is even more complex, since many of the clones contain sequences that cannot be aligned to [that of] a conventional cytomegalovirus.'

So what he had found did not fit in anywhere. It was as if one were doing an enormous jigsaw puzzle and the final piece only resembled the remaining hole. He also was trying to match these with the wild virus, but with a 'clone' – an artificially made virus assembled from fragments. These are supposed to be identical to a wild virus – but clearly in this case he could not prove this.  He was saying  the cloned virus had a genetic code that 'cannot be aligned' with that of the wild virus.

He also reported: 'Although the PCR findings distinguished CFS (Chronic Fatigue Syndrome) patients as a group from normal individuals, and possibly distinguished some CFS patients from others, the data were difficult to interpret. If the detectable sequences are of CMV, EBV or HHV6 origin [from 3 different viruses], the data would suggest that the virus is incomplete and only partially represented.' He also noted 'the patterns of PCR responses … can vary over time (unpublished data) and this may reflect ongoing cellular and/or viral changes. ' He further noted 'apparent genetic instability' and 'recombination.'

He finally suggested, since he could not match his fragments, that his genetic code might be from a new recombinant mutant virus.  He continued: 'More likely, the data reflect a new virus with partial DNA sequence homology with herpes viruses.' But, it was only an inspired guess.

As I have said, PCR can only identify a genetic code fragment as definitely from a particular virus, or human, if that fragment is shown to be identical to code already proved unique to that virus or human.  But, as Dr. Martin now explained, the accuracy of PCR has to be deliberately compromised when looking for an unknown virus. 'The stringency, and therefore, the specificity of the assay, has to be compromised when one is searching for an unknown virus using primer sets [genetic code sequences] matched for a known virus.' He said this could lead to 'cross-priming to distantly related viral and even normal cellular

DNA sequences.' In other words, the decline in accuracy was so severe that the sequences found might be from a normal cell, not from a virus.

This was a revelation to me. None of the papers I had read previously had admitted to these difficulties with such honesty. It seems the identification of a virus through PCR is a complex process full of uncertainties. I subsequently learnt that scientists frequently 'contract out' PCR work to technicians, so many may not be aware of all these problems.

But despite all his difficulties, I must report that Professor Martin remained enthusiastic about PCR. He wrote: 'PCR can be applied to the detection of virtually any pathogen for which even limited DNA (or RNA) sequence information is known and in which a specimen of infected tissue can be readily obtained.' 'The PCR technology represents a major breakthrough in efforts to detect persistent viral infections. Highly specific assays can be performed providing the exact DNA or RNA sequence is known.' [25]

Again, one has to note, only if the 'exact DNA or RNA sequence is known.'

He noted that, to be really accurate, the sequences searched for with PCR had to be identical to 'conserved regions of bacterial, viral or fungal genomes' – in other words to parts of their genomes that do not change or mutate. But he also noted; 'It has generally been assumed, however, that both viral and cellular genomes were relatively stable. Stealth viruses [like the one he was investigating] appear to be an exception.' The fact that varying genetic code sequences may be present, makes using PCR much less reliable. One day there would be a match; the next day there might be none.

He concluded that to use PCR to identify a virus, the test 'may need to be run at a lower than normal stringency.' In other words, PCR lost its accuracy.

This Workshop, and the reading I had to do to understand its papers, had been a revelation to me. When I wrote previously of virus contamination in vaccines, I had not checked to see how its presence was proved. If I read that the presence of viruses was detected by PCR, I had simply presumed, along with most of the public, that whole viruses were proved present. I had now discovered that modern techniques often provide far less certainty; however, this did not mean that whole viruses were not present – or that the fragments found could not be dangerous.

Indeed, I trusted that they did detect identifiable fragments of SV40; no matter how difficult this was, given how many laboratories had confirmed this. I had no reason to question that they had found SV40.

For me, the issue now was urgent. I wanted to know how long was the polio vaccine contaminated with dangerous monkey viruses? How on earth could this happen? Where did the blame lie for this  – with the government or the manufacturers – or with both? Or, is a certain amount of contamination the inevitable price we have to pay for our children's protection from greater dangers?

Above all else, I needed to know the consequence of this to human health. What had we been giving our children for the past fifty years? Could we possibly have been feeding them, not just SV40, but also HIV?

---

[25]   Martin. Stealth Adaptation of an African Green *Experimental and Molecular Pathology*, April, 1999

# Chapter 3

# Monkey Viruses in the Vaccine

*'The discovery in 1960 that a DNA tumour virus, designated simian virus 40 (SV40), was an inadvertent contaminant of rhesus monkey cells, and consequently of the poliovirus and adenovirus vaccines made in these cells, was a watershed event in vaccine development...'* **FDA 1997**

All that I learnt about the contamination of the polio vaccine at the SV40 Workshop, that had so shocked me, became no surprise when I learnt how the polio vaccines were manufactured. What I now discovered was a miserable story of negligent science, with risks to children knowingly ignored for commercial gain and to boost the reputations of governments.

It had all started, I learnt, when scientists decided in the early 1950s that they could take the risk of growing the virus needed for our polio and adenovirus vaccines on the extracted kidneys and testicles of tens of thousands of Indian, S.E. Asian, and African wild-caught monkeys even while knowing that they were full of monkey viruses.

The problem with vaccines is that they require the production of enormous numbers of viruses – and these are exclusively a product of cells. The poliovirus is naturally a product of human cells, but for vaccines monkey cells produce it. Likewise the 'wild' measles virus is also a product solely of human cells but the vaccine usually contains a product of chicken cells. Any virus thus produced for a vaccine is very unlikely to be identical to that produced naturally by human cells.

The manufacturers did not need to use wild-caught monkeys for the polio vaccine. The risk of monkey virus contamination of the vaccine was well known – and leading scientists warned at the time that it would be far safer to produce the polio vaccine virus from fertilised chicken eggs or human cells. In fact, Lederle, a major pharmaceutical company, originally produced the poliovirus for their vaccine from bird embryos, thinking a safer method would give them a commercial advantage.

But other pharmaceutical companies were allied with scientists who preferred to use monkeys, since polio is a human disease and monkeys are the species most like us; despite the risk that monkeys might have viruses that could adapt to live in us. As far as I can judge, the 1950s decision to authorise only polio vaccines grown on monkey cells for the US and UK was made partly because they feared that using human cells might pass on human cancers.

Since then, many tens of thousands of monkeys have been trapped in Africa, Asia and the Caribbean, transported, anaesthetised, operated on to remove their organs and then 'sacrificed' (the vaccine industry's euphemism for 'killed'). Their kidneys and testicles are then mashed to make a 'substrate' of separated cells that can be persuaded to produce the needed virus. These particular monkey organs were selected because they are easy for amateur surgeons to find and remove.[26]

The minced organs are then 'seeded' by being mixed with a poliovirus-rich fluid from an earlier culture (much more about this in next chapter). The seeded monkey meat is then kept for 3 days in 'incubators' before fluid is filtered out to be used as a vaccine.

For the first polio vaccine, the one invented by Dr. Jonas Salk and commercially released in 1955, to be withdrawn in 1961, and re-introduced recently in a new version as the polio vaccine for the UK and USA, the polioviruses are 'killed' with formaldehyde before being injected into children. Salk admitted to 'sacrificing' 17,000 monkeys and chimpanzees in the course of developing this vaccine.

His principal rival in the race to develop a commercial polio vaccine was the white-bearded Albert Sabin. They both knew using monkeys might be dangerous. In 1932 a monkey had bitten a colleague of Sabin's at New York's Bellevue Hospital. He had developed paralysis and died. Sabin later reported: 'At the autopsy I collected specimens and isolated a virus.' This would be labelled as the 'Monkey B' virus. He admitted that 'often [safety] procedures were not followed.' In fact, there was a great deal of carelessness.'

The Sabin vaccine nevertheless would be approved and released in 1960. In this vaccine the polioviruses are not killed nor administered by injection, as with the Salk vaccine, but weakened ('attenuated') before being administered on a sugar cube. Both Salk and Sabin expected their killed or weakened monkey polioviruses would stimulate the immune systems of

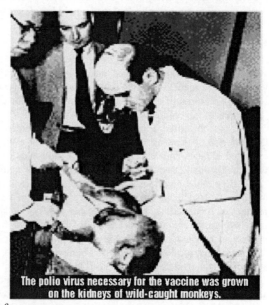

The polio virus necessary for the vaccine was grown on the kidneys of wild-caught monkeys.

children into producing protective antibodies against human poliovirus. Neither of them looked to see if children were already immune – it was later found that most children were and thus did not need the vaccine.

Sabin set out to weaken his poliovirus to make it safe to use by forcing it to mutate. He passaged the fluid containing it rapidly though 51 cultures of mashed monkey kidneys. He tried to weaken it further by growing it on kidneys from two different species of monkeys, Indian Rhesus and African Greens. He surely must have realised that he had thus exposed his vaccine to contamination with incompatible viruses and cellular fragments from three continents, including America. But he bottled filtered fluid from his final cultures and patented this as the commercial 'Sabin Original Merck' poliovirus seed lot. In this process he admitted to 'sacrificing' 9,000 monkeys, plus chimpanzees.

Why chimpanzees? Because, as a species, they are the most alike to humans. They are thus used to safety-test vaccines. Sabin tested his 'Original Merck' polio seed by

---

[26] *Lancet* (1 8 April 1953; page 777) stated that monkeys' testicles as well as their kidneys were used as sources of the cells that form the culture-medium for the polio virus.

injecting it into the brains of living chimpanzees, and then by giving it to 133 young human inmates of an Ohio prison – and then to some tens of millions of Russian children. Sabin enjoyed during this the support of the pharmaceutical giant Merck, Sharp and Dohme, which produced for his Russian trials some 25 million doses of vaccine.

Most AIDS experts today say HIV-1 evolved from a mutated chimpanzee virus from Central Africa, and HIV-2 from the Sooty Mangabey monkey of West Africa. Originally, in the 1980s, HIV was thought to be from the African Green Monkey. Each of these is said to have a similar virus to HIV, called an SIV, but one that contradictorily does not damage their immune system. The similarity to HIV seems mostly to lie in their genetic codes.

It is thought that these SIVs evolved during the early 20$^{th}$ century into a form that can infect humans and which we now know of as HIV. Well, from what I was reading, there was at that time ample opportunity for any Chimpanzee virus to get into the polio vaccines. These animals were kept next to each other in small cages at the laboratories, with their carers using little hygiene.

One could say, with hindsight, that this process could not have been better designed to produce HIV! Passing a fluid processed through monkeys and chimps into humans would surely provide the monkey viruses present with all the challenge they required to persuade them to mutate into forms that could replicate in humans?

In October 1967 Joshua Lederberg of the Department of Genetics, Stanford University School of Medicine, warned in a letter to the editor of *Science* about the lack of safety involved in using live-virus vaccines; 'In point of fact, we [are practicing] biological engineering on a rather large scale by use of live viruses in mass immunization campaigns...Crude virus preparations, such as some in common use at the present time, are also vulnerable to frightful mishaps of contamination and misidentification.'

When I read this warning, it sharply reminded me of what I was told in 1996 by Professor Michael Stewart, London University's top vaccine expert. 'We know living virus vaccines are dangerous. That is why we are developing alternatives.' Had so little changed in all these years?

The experiments of Hilary Koprowski, another polio vaccine pioneer, were even more liable to create HIV. He was developing his vaccine along the same lines as Sabin. His experiments allegedly included passaging poliovirus vaccine through chimpanzee brains, meaning that he injected it into the living brain, left it there for some time, extracted some of the contaminated virus fluid from this brain and passed this into other living chimpanzee brains. He similarly injected it into the brains of other species– and it is entirely possible that other scientists did the same. Similar experiments were then commonly performed with chimps to safety test vaccines.

If HIV had come from an SIV found in chimpanzees, as is widely held today, surely such experiments must have provided an excellent opportunity for a chimpanzee SIV to contaminate the polio vaccine? [27]

Koprowski based his vaccine on a sample of 'poliovirus' – which in fact was a 'suspension of [ground up] backbone' from a polio victim. He presumed this would contain the virus. This sample is now known as the 'Brockman poliovirus isolate' although it is anything but an isolate. He injected this backbone mash into the living brain of an albino mouse, waited some days, then took fluid from its brain and injected this into the living brain of another albino mouse. He repeated this until seven mice were 'infected.' Then fluid taken from the final mouse was injected into the brains of monkeys. When these monkeys survived without apparent harm, he injected the mouse brain extract into a series of three cotton rats. The fluid extracted from the final rat brain was deemed to

---

[27] A later book *'The River'* by Edward Hooper (Allen Lane, Penguin 1999) focussed on the possibility that Congo polio vaccine laboratories run by Hilary Koprowski were implicated. What I have found is that there were ample other earlier opportunities for a chimp virus to get into the polio vaccine.

contain 'attenuated poliovirus' safe enough to inject into humans. He named this vaccine 'TN', and it was most probably then safety tested by being 'passaged' through the brains of chimpanzees, as this was the common procedure.

The process of 'attenuation,' of the weakening of a virus to make it suitable for a vaccine, made me uneasily wonder if a monkey virus contaminating a vaccine thus evolved into an HIV that can infect us? 'Attenuation' is really induced mutation. The monkey cells in the culture are subjected to enormous stresses in order to make them produce weakened viruses. What if the viruses they produced became more virulent, not less? If HIV evolved though these highly unnatural transplantations, it would not have been detected, for in those days HIV could not be tested for, as it was still unknown. The same must be true for the many other viruses present during this highly impure laboratory process.

On February 27, 1950, Koprowski tested his experimental polio vaccine on an eight year-old boy from Letchworth Village, New York. When he suffered no apparent ill effects, Koprowski enlarged his experiment to include 19 more children. He then decided to weaken his poliovirus some more by 'passaging' it through 20 living mouse brains. In 1951 he safety-tested the result on 61 'mentally retarded' children in the Sonoma State Home. It was apparently considered ethically acceptable to experiment on children.

Sabin and Koprowski, must have known of the risks they were taking, and exposing others to, by making and so testing "living virus' vaccines. They were all virologists, men who saw viruses as dangerous and as the cause of terrible epidemics. They believed monkey viruses had killed several scientists during these vaccine experiments.

The danger was acknowledged in the UK Parliament. On April 24th 1955 the UK Minister of Health, Mr Iain Macleod, told the House, as thousands of monkeys arrived from India at Heathrow Airport: *'Perhaps it is as well to put the facts in plain words to the House. This new vaccine involves inoculating our children at repeated intervals with a preparation derived from the kidneys of dead monkeys. The House and the country will surely agree that we must carry out intensive tests as to the exact effects of this so we can eliminate any possible dangers from it.'*

But despite the Health Minister's firm words, such intensive tests were not carried out before millions of UK children were injected with the vaccine. As I discovered when I made my film on SV40 – the government did not even charge a UK laboratory with the responsibility of monitoring the future health of these children for any slow-developing cancers or other ill effects.

But some scientists were very worried. They pointed out how unwise it was to use monkey kidneys, since this organ naturally collects toxins, and presumably viruses. Kidneys remove these by putting them into urine. They said this urine is certain to have gone with the kidneys into the vaccine cultures and thus into the unpurified vaccine doses.

But the release of the first of the polio vaccines, the Salk, might have been completely derailed – if a 1954 report by the scientist in charge of the US government safety-testing laboratory, Dr. Bernice Eddy, had not been ignored.

While Salk was 'safety trialling' his 'killed virus' polio vaccine in 1954, by testing it on 2 million American children, with parents volunteering their children, so eager were they for their children to be protected; Eddy was still carrying out the required polio vaccine safety tests in her laboratory. This work should have been done beforehand, but the rush to get the vaccine out had left her behind. She was thus horrified when she discovered that monkeys were paralysed when she injected them with the polio vaccine. It was far too late to discover this. It had already been injected into hundreds of thousands of American children.

Dr. Edward Shorter reported what happened in his 1987 work, *The Health Century*: 'In 1954 the rush was on. Her lab had gotten samples of the inactivated polio vaccine to certify on a 'due-yesterday' basis. This was a product that had never been made before and they were going to use it right away.' She and her staff worked around the clock. 'We had eighteen monkeys. We inoculated these eighteen monkeys with each vaccine that came in. And we started getting paralyzed monkeys.'[28]

She photographed the diseased monkeys and took these photos to her boss – but astonishingly he sharply reprimanded her for being alarmist. He ordered her to cease these tests –and to work instead on flu. No criticism of the polio vaccine was to be tolerated, for it was about to be endorsed as utterly 'safe,' without further tests, in a major 1955 event organised by President Eisenhower's Administration.

She reported she was not sure what caused the paralysis. Something deadly was clearly in the vaccine culture. It was not necessarily a virus. She called it a toxic 'substance.' Now at that time a cosmetic or a food would have been immediately withdrawn if just one or two hamsters died in such tests – so it was utterly outrageous that the polio vaccine was not then immediately withdrawn.

Incredibly William Sebrell, her boss and the director of the NIH, later certified all brands of Salk vaccines as safe as though Eddy's research had never happened. He even stopped by the animal house where she was working, not to query her, but to ask if she and her co-workers wanted their children immunized, as 'the vaccine was in short supply.'

Yet at that very same time, Robert Hull, a scientist employed by vaccine manufacturer Eli Lilly, was finding so many monkey viruses in the polio vaccine, and in other medical preparations, that he had started to number them. So far he had found eleven species. These he had called SV (Simian Virus) 1 to 11. He had identified the first, SV1, in fact a year earlier in early February 1954, in some 17% of the polio vaccine cultures at Lilly. Then SV2 was found in the cultures in August and so it went on. This was before and during the so-called Salk 'safety trials' involving 2 million American children. We still use the numbers Hull gave these viruses – hence SV40.[29]

To put it bluntly, Dr. Jonas Salk had lied to the public to alleviate their safety concerns. On the CBS News on the 12th February 1955, when the interviewer asked him: 'The only thing I know about this vaccine is that it starts with a monkey kidney and finishes going into a child's arm, so can you explain some of the process in between?' Salk responded by producing a dish containing a monkey kidney and a kitchen blender. He put the kidney through the blender while reassuringly saying: 'One of the reasons this method of growing virus for vaccine is most satisfactory is that it is possible with a microscope to examine the cells to be sure that there are no other agents, either viruses or other harmful influences, present.'[30]

In fact Salk knew this experiment was a farce. He was secretly relying on the formaldehyde he was adding to the vaccine to destroy all the monkey viruses he knew to be in his vaccine. He instructed that formaldehyde must be added shortly before use – and the poison then neutralized with a chemical (sodium bisulphite). He hoped that the corpses of the poliovirus would stimulate the children's immune system to give them protection from polio, if they did not already have it.

But in the UK he did not get such an easy ride. *The Manchester Guardian* reported on April 15, 1955: 'One of Britain's greatest physiologists said today that if it means that a child should be re-inoculated at frequent intervals with a preparation derived from monkey kidney "it is terrifying in its possibilities".' The government was also concerned. Mr. Iain Macleod, the Minister of Health, mentioned the same risk in the House of Commons in April. Dr. G. Humble, of the Westminster School of Medicine, asked in the

---

[28] Edward Shorter, Ph.D., The Health Century, Doubleday, New York, 1987, p. 67.

[29] Robert N. Hull, et al., New Viral Agents Recovered From Tissue Cultures of Monkey Kidney Cells, American Journal of Hygiene, 1956, Vol. 63, pp. 204-215. Also 1958,Vol. 68, pp. 31-44.

[30] Bookchin and Shumacher *The Virus and the Vaccine* St Martins Press. 2004. Pages 43-44. When they surveyed Salk's papers held at the Mandeville Special Collections, they found 'few references to the issue of extraneous viruses in his (or other) vaccines.' P 345.

*Lancet* of May 7th 1953: 'is it certain that injection of this preparation will not produce Rhesus [monkey] antibodies when injected into susceptible human subjects?' And on June 11th 1955 the editor of the *Lancet* wrote: 'In addition to the possibility of producing the very disease the vaccine is used to prevent, there is a risk, of unknown dimensions, that repeated injections of a vaccine prepared from monkey kidney may eventually sensitize the child in some harmful way.'

But in the US the production of the vaccine rolled on. In the UK this eventually forced Wellcome to abandon its attenuated polio vaccine grown on chicken eggs, despite its belief that this was safer. The *Beckenham Journal* of June 11th, 1955, reported the company as saying they had neither the staff nor facilities to carry out their own ideas, thus they had no choice but to contract to manufacture the Salk vaccine on monkey cells like the Americans.

An emergency importation service was set up to provide the vaccine manufacturers with all the monkeys they needed. Dr. C. L. Greening of the UK reported: 'In the early days of large scale vaccine production from monkey kidney tissue culture, increasing worldwide demands for monkeys resulted in indiscriminate purchase from uninspected and other totally unsuitable animal centres. Minimum attention was given to transport conditions in aircraft or ships, and it was common practice to house stock monkeys at laboratories or animal farms ... in large cages holding upwards of 150 animals.' In such conditions bacteria and viruses were sure to spread. [31]

The trade was highly profitable. Indians were paid around £1 each for the monkeys and the traders sold them for £7 in London. But President Nehru of India stopped the trade in 1955 when over 390 monkeys were found dead from suffocation at London Airport, while transiting on the way to New York. The Indian government wanted no publicity about this since the monkey is sacred to Hindus and it feared mass protests. [32] However, exports were resumed when it was agreed that India would receive priority supplies of the vaccine.

It was calculated that the kidneys from one monkey would produce enough poliovirus to provide for 6,000 vaccine injections; that is for 2,000 children, assuming 3 inoculations for each. But this proved over optimistic. Three times more monkeys were needed. In 1955 alone some 47,710 wild monkeys were imported into the USA, and another 8,000 into the UK – nearly all to be slaughtered for the polio vaccine. [33]

Between 1955 and 1976 some two million monkeys were consumed to make the polio vaccine. Nearly as many were said to die en route. The monkey species then most used was the Rhesus, the one commonly found in the Hindu temples of India.

Every Western government required its own monkey supply. The *Manchester Guardian* on April 27, 1955 published a letter complaining of the 'serious shortage of monkeys'. It concluded: 'If mass inoculation is to become a fact the demand for more monkeys will be great. It is estimated that between Messrs. Glaxo and Burroughs Wellcome about 8,000 animals would be required in the first year, and then probably more later if the results were satisfactory.'

However, back in Washington, Vaccine Safety Officer Eddy remained extremely worried. When she heard, within weeks of the launch of polio vaccination, that over 200 vaccinated children had fallen seriously ill, she must have feared that this was the terrible consequence of her warnings being ignored. When the government explained away these cases, saying it was due to one laboratory, the Cutter, ineffectively poisoning the

---

[31] C. L. Greening; 'The Controlled Collection, Holding, Transport and Stock Housing of Monkeys Intended for Tissue Culture Production,' in *Proceedings of 7th International Congress for Microbiological Standardization.'* Cited in *The River* by Edward Hooper; Page 813; reference footnote18

[32] *News Chronicle,* Delhi July 4, 1955

[33] *Manchester Guardian* April 27, 1955.

poliovirus due to a faulty laboratory procedure now put right, she knew there was still very much more to fear; for human cancers might take years to appear.

She teamed up with a colleague, Sarah Stewart, who also wanted to discover if viruses could cause cancers. They tried injecting extracts of mouse tumours from one infant mouse to another to see if this would 'transmit' cancers. When these mice did get cancers, they concluded that they had injected a virus that caused cancers. They named their suspected virus 'polyoma' and suddenly gained international fame through coverage in *Time* magazine.

However, we know today that it was not only viruses they were injecting into these animals. In the unpurified fluid they used, there would have been many things smaller than viruses, such as toxins, bits of DNA and proteins – as well as different viruses. They did not have the technology necessary to remove them; indeed, most were not then detectable. Thus any of these contaminants might have caused the cancers they observed.

Nevertheless Drs. Salk, Sabin and Hilary Koprowski continued to insist that it was safe to use monkey cultures to produce human vaccines. Koprowski had originally produced his own trial vaccine on monkey cells, and had secretly continued to do so even after his boss, John Cox of Lederle, ordered him not to, because of the danger from monkey viruses. Cox wanted him to use instead rat brains and chicken eggs.[34]

Koprowski then left Lederle and went to the Wistar Institute where he openly used monkeys and chimpanzees. Around 1957 he tested his experimental polio vaccines first on people in Belfast, Northern Ireland, where they caused severe reactions, then on a quarter of a million Africans living along the Congo River – as well as on many in Poland. Some scientists suspect this is when HIV was spread into the Africans and I also thought this very likely. Surely the presence of both monkeys and chimps in his vaccine labs, alongside human researchers, could have provided the perfect opportunity for their viruses to mingle and spread?

In 1959 Bernice Eddy secretly began to re-examine the Salk vaccine cultures made from virus-seeded monkey kidneys. She froze a sample with dry ice, ground it up, thawed it and filtered out cellular debris. The resulting fluid she injected into 154 hamsters. 70% got cancers within 18 months.[35]

She also prepared kidney extracts from 8 to 10 rhesus monkeys, and injected tiny amounts of this under the skin of 23 newborn hamsters. Within 9 months, she observed that 'large malignant, subcutaneous tumors' had appeared on 20 of them. She injected other hamsters with minced cat and human cancer tissues. These did not get cancers. She deduced that something particularly dangerous must be in the monkey kidney cultures.

But, as she was unable to prove it was a virus, grow it in a culture or isolate it, she could only label it as a dangerous 'substance,' although she suspected it was something like the 'polyoma' virus she had named earlier. But when she reported this to her laboratory boss, he again sharply rebuked her for doing 'unauthorised' research. He suggested the hamsters might have developed the tumours spontaneously.

Stubbornly she carried on, checking the adenovirus vaccine culture, for it was also grown on monkey kidneys. She found it too was dangerous. Again her supervisor scornfully rejected her finding.

Eventually, without asking permission, she accepted an invitation to address a New York Cancer Society meeting on polyoma virus. Towards the end of this talk, on 11

---

[34] It has been argued by Leonard Haylick that the earlier reports of successful passages of poliovirus in rodent and chick embryo cells were probably mistaken, and were merely recording the progressive dilution of the virus with each passage.

[35] Bernice E. Eddy, Tumors Produced in Hamsters by SV40, 21 Fed'n Proc 930, 930–35 (1962); Bernice E. Eddy et al., Identification of the Oncogenic Substance in Rhesus Monkey Kidney Cell Cultures as Simian Virus 40, 17 Virology 65–75 (1962)

October 1960, she quietly added that there was something like polyoma in the monkey kidneys used to make the polio vaccine. This caused an immediate sensation.

Eddy recalled her boss's reaction: 'Smadel called me up, and if there was anything in the English language ... that he could call me, he did.' The NIH then took her lab away from her, prevented her attending professional meetings and delayed the publication of her scientific papers. [36]

Maurice Hilleman was asked years later why on earth was the discovery of monkey viruses in the vaccine kept secret? His answer was: 'Because you could start a panic! They had already had production problems with [vaccinated] people getting polio. If you added to that the fact that they found live [monkey] virus in the vaccine, there would have been hysteria.'

But, while the NIH seemingly ignored Eddy's findings, Hilleman had not. He had just been put in charge of the vaccine department of the pharmaceutical company Merck. One of the first tasks he was given was to develop and market a hopefully more effective version of the Salk polio vaccine, one called 'Purifax.'

His job was to ensure that Purifax prevailed over its rival vaccine, the Sabin. The latter was then being safety tested in Russia and was said to be more effective than the Salk, possibly cheaper, and thus a very serious rival. A forthcoming conference on the polio vaccine was expected to endorse it.

But Hilleman thought the Salk vaccine had a key competitive edge – in now being safer. When he tested its latest version, the formaldehyde used seemed to remove Eddy's toxic substance, now said to be a virus called SV40. He suspected the rival Sabin vaccine remained contaminated with SV40 since it was not protected with formaldehyde. He ordered his researcher, Ben Sweet, to test the Sabin vaccine.

The only way they had to diagnose SV40 infection was by examining cells for signs of damage. If empty spaces had developed between cells, then SV40 was presumed to be the cause. It was thus initially called the 'Vacuolating Virus.' However, it remained an assumption that this damage was done by a virus. It could have been caused by exposure to toxins and cellular fragments in the vaccine culture. (Such methods are still used. Professor John Martin showed me micrographs of similar damage to brain cells that he believed to indicate the presence of the virus SCMV.) But whatever caused this damage, it meant that the vaccine was much too risky to use.

Sweet reported back to Hilleman that the same cellular damage was found after exposure to the Sabin vaccine. They surmised that this meant the virus was present there too. In June 1960 Hilleman announced the presence of SV40 in the Sabin vaccine at the Second International Conference on the Polio Vaccine, the one expected to endorse this vaccine. The meeting was held at Georgetown University and sponsored by the World Health Organization.

Hilleman stated: 'All three types of Sabin's live polio virus vaccine were found contaminated' with Simian Virus 40 (SV40). This 'raises the important question of the existence of other such viruses [in the vaccine].' [37] Hilleman also said this contamination was limited to the Sabin. He had tested the latest version of the Salk vaccine, as sold by his employer, Merck, and it was apparently not contaminated.

Hilleman added that SV40 was 'essentially ubiquitous ' in rhesus monkey cultures – and 'all the Sabin seed vaccine lots were found to be contaminated.' This was a most serious accusation. It meant every dose of the Sabin sugar-cube vaccine given to several million Russians might have been dangerously contaminated.

---

[36] Edward Shorter, The Health Century 195–199, 200 (1987)

[37]   Second International Conference on Live Poliovirus Vaccines, Pan American Health Organization and the World Health Organization, Washington, DC 6-7 June, 1960, pp 79-85. Also see B.H. Sweet and M. R. Hilleman, The Vacuolating Virus, SV40, Proceedings of the Society for Experimental Biology and Medicine, Oct.-Dec. 1960, vol 105, pp. 420-427

But Hilleman's warning backfired. Soon afterwards Hull announced finding that SV40 survived 30 days of formaldehyde treatment – meaning the same cellular damage was found afterwards. This meant the Salk vaccine was also likely to be contaminated, as it was not treated with formaldehyde for anything like as long.

Both Salk and Sabin continued to insult each other's vaccine, ignoring that the authorities knew both were likely to be SV40 contaminated. In fact, at this stage, both men privately thought this an insufficient reason to ban a vaccine because SV40 had not been yet proved to cause 'human' cancers. Others, however, disagreed, saying contamination should not be tolerated – especially when it had caused cancer in rodents.

But, would the work required to remove the SV40 contamination make the vaccine too expensive to market? Sweet warned: 'if insistence will be made on eliminating the vacuolating agent (SV40), then it may not be possible to produce live poliovirus vaccine.' This was a warning the US Administration had to take seriously. It was very important that they had a poliovirus vaccine. President Eisenhower had staked his reputation on it.

The Administration was thus totally dismayed when the Merck Corporation, where Hilleman and Sweet both worked, informed the US Surgeon General in 1960 that both the Salk and the Sabin vaccines were so contaminated with monkey viruses, that it was far too dangerous for them to manufacture them at all. (None of this was made public.)

The Surgeon General replied, begging Merck to make the vaccines, saying they were vital to the fight against polio. But Merck again declined in December 1960, saying they had: 'again reviewed our decision in the light of your letter ... Our scientific staff have emphasized to us that there are a number of serious scientific and technical problems that must be solved before we could engage in large-scale production of live poliovirus vaccine. Most important among these is the problem of extraneous contaminating simian viruses that may be extremely difficult to eliminate and which may be difficult if not impossible to detect at the present stage of the technology.' [38]

But the government safety regulators instead accepted arguments similar to those put forward by Koprowski. They decided that, since neither contaminated vaccine had been proven to cause harm in humans, there was no reason to ban them. (This was despite knowing that human cancers can take 20 years to develop.)

But under pressure from Merck, the public health regulators eventually decided they must act. They decided that all vaccines had in future to be free of virus contamination that is both 'demonstrable' and 'viable'. It was hoped that this decision would put to an end the dispute.

But this regulation was not enforced and the safety of the Sabin vaccine continued to be contested. The leading UK medical journal, *Lancet*, editorialised on 11th March 1961 that the discovery of SV40 'in many seed lots of the vaccine raises doubts about its long term safety ... [and] suggests it is unwise to use to use a possibly virus-contaminated living vaccine when there is an inactivated alternative [the Salk],'

But in the very next issue of *Lancet*, a scientist responded to say that the UK's Wellcome pharmaceutical company had also found SV40 in the Salk vaccine, so both were contaminated. Then a Scottish doctor reported in *Lancet* that half of the children he had just vaccinated with Salk were now positive to SV40 – meaning at least half the doses he used were contaminated.

The pharmaceutical company Merck by now had repeated Eddy's experiments – and confirmed her results. It found cancers were produced when the Salk vaccine culture was injected into hamsters. Some 80% got tumours - many at the sites of injection. Sweet

---

[38] Letter from John T. Conner of Merck & Co. to Dr. Leroy Burney, Surgeon General of the United States, dated 12/16/60 - Plaintiff's Exhibit No. 54 - In Re Sabin Polio Vaccine Litigation, MDL 780, U.S.D.C., MD - Baltimore, Maryland. Also see related official memos that document how Eddy's research was suppressed and her laboratory taken from her p.344 *The Virus and the Vaccine.*

at Merck commented: 'I tell you we were scared of SV40. If it could produce tumours in hamsters, it could produce tumours in man'.

In June 1961 Hilleman grimly told the government's Safety Technical Committee that it should immediately withdraw the Salk polio vaccine, including Merck's own, as this contamination was a 'fearful thing'. He hoped in six months time they might be able to market a far cleaner vaccine. But the committee refused to withdraw it. It said that: 'it is too early to draw a conclusion.' Doctors thus continued to use the polluted vaccine.

But then Sweet discovered that if he injected the vaccine 'substrate' [culture] of rhesus monkey kidneys and testicles into rhesus monkeys, there was no sign of cancers; but if it were injected it into African Green Monkeys they did develop cancers. Now one would have thought he might have concluded from this that the African Greens did not like having cells from another species injected into them, but he concluded that the test revealed Rhesus monkeys were the natural hosts for SV40, since viruses do not hurt their natural host (presumably not knowing that humans are the natural host of the poliovirus).

He further deduced that SV40 was not naturally present in African Greens – on the basis that it made them ill.  Thus, he concluded, it would be safe to use them for the vaccine. The director of Washington Zoo confirmed his deduction, saying: 'Get your monkeys out of West Africa. Get the African Green, as this species is not infected with SV40.' The vaccine regulators were persuaded. They would in future change to making the polio vaccine on kidneys from African Greens.

It occurs to me, with hindsight, that they could have come to a different conclusion; that a species cannot be injected with tissues from another species without a severe risk of provoking cancers.

Hilary Koprowski powerfully defended the polio vaccines. He observed that viruses are everywhere and viral contaminants had to be in all vaccines – but this did not prove them dangerous.  Somewhat heretically, he pointed out that humans consume viruses all the time in their food with no ill effect. There was no proof, he said, that SV40 caused cancers in humans, for no ill effects were observed when millions of Russians were dosed with the Sabin vaccine. But Hilleman replied, in a paper co-authored with Sweet, that 'raw monkey kidney is not an ordinary part of human diet.'

But in 1961 the decision was made – quietly without telling the public, without withdrawing already distributed batches of vaccines, to move production of the Sabin polio vaccine over to African Green Monkeys – but only after the existing two-year supply of contaminated stocks was sold out.

Sweet, Hilleman and the others then joked that the Russians would be unable to compete in the oncoming Olympics, as they would be riddled with cancers from the earlier contaminated version of the Sabin vaccine!

But their theory that SV40 was not in African Green Monkeys soon proved ill founded.  A 1991 review of monkey viruses found 'SV40 had been isolated from the kidney tissues of African Green Monkeys ... obtained directly from the field.'  The authors noted this meant that SV40 might be indigenous to African Green as well as to the Rhesus. [39] Nevertheless, the USA and UK governments continued to swop over to using African Green monkey kidneys for making the polio vaccine.

As for the Salk vaccine, the health authorities of the US and UK decided in 1961 that they would not purchase any further supplies of it.  It was decided that, not only was the Sabin safer; it was easier and cheaper to give a vaccine on a sugar-cube than by injection. They pointed out that the Sabin vaccine would not just immunize the vaccinated. It would vaccinate even the unwilling, for the vaccinated child would pass on the living vaccine virus to others by infecting them.

---

[39] G. D. Hsiung; Bacteriological Reviews, Sept., 1968, p. 185-205 Latent Virus Infections in Primate Tissues with Special Reference to Simian Viruses

Merck on safety grounds stopped making its Salk vaccine in May 1961. This was tardily reported in the *New York Times* two months later, on July 26th, in a story relegated to page 33. It said that Merck and other manufacturers had halted production until they could get a 'monkey virus' out of the Salk vaccine. This was all the media publicity this sensational discovery received. The public scarcely noticed and were not alarmed.

Wellcome in 1961 also stopped making the Salk vaccine – but, as they had six million doses already manufactured, they decided to carry on selling these until all stocks were gone. It thus distributed known contaminated stock until mid-1963.

Sweet now discovered that if he injected cell culture containing SV40 into human cells, they turned cancerous – suggesting that this culture was not dangerous just to rodents and monkeys but also to humans.[40] In May 1961, Eddy's long delayed research was at last published. It was in this that she concluded that the toxic 'substance' she found earlier was in fact SV40.

The anti-monkey vaccine campaign now won a most surprising recruit. It was Hilary Koprowski, the scientist who had earlier scornfully dismissed these SV40 findings. In 1960, just 2 years after trialing his own monkey-kidney polio vaccine in the Congo, Koprowski, with Stanley Plotkin, a colleague at Wistar, contacted the World Health Organization (WHO) to tell them that it was time to stop growing polio vaccine on 'fresh-removed monkey kidneys' as the risk of spreading monkey viruses was far too great!

Koprowski also warned a US Congressional Committee: 'As monkey kidney culture is host to innumerable simian viruses, the number found varying in relation to the amount of work expended to find them, the problem presented to the manufacturer is considerable, if not insuperable,' He added 'As our technical methods improve we may find fewer and fewer lots of vaccine which can be called free from simian virus.' [41]

He now recommended moving all vaccine production over to a system developed at the Wistar Laboratory by Dr. Leonard Hayflick. This involved growing the poliovirus, not on monkeys, but on healthy human cells in a laboratory culture called WI-38. He thought this shift of production methods was essential, if the vaccine were to be made safe. Koprowski moved his own vaccine production over to the new system. He warned doctors that the next batch of killed monkeys might contain other 'virus surprises.' It was, he said, time to end the 'obsolete practice of slaughtering thousands of monkeys for their kidneys' but nonetheless this practice would continued for the rest of the century in the US and UK.

However, Sweden had avoided the monkey virus danger. According to the *Lancet* by May 1955 the Swedes had made enough vaccine on human tissues to immunise 120,000 children. They used human foetal tissue taken from abortions, then killed the poliovirus grown on it with formaldehyde. The Swedes supplied in 1958 this foetal tissue for Hayflick to use for his own vaccine substrate. He was following their lead.

Hayflick stated: 'Monkey kidneys were notorious for their content of unwanted viruses – potentially dangerous viruses, maybe even [the precursor for] HIV, who knows?' [42] He said of the Sabin polio vaccine as used in the US and UK 'the final substrate was constantly contaminated monkey kidneys.' [43] He claimed his human-cell substrate could safely grow every virus that attacked humans – while being guaranteed 'absolutely clean' of contaminating active viruses. It would also grow far more virus than any other method, since the poliovirus is indigenous to humans and thus replicates best in human cells.

The *Lancet* reported that some scientists were now growing the poliovirus on human placenta tissue, claiming: 'a vaccine prepared in this way would be free from one

---

[40] Bookchin and Shumacher *The Virus and the Vaccin.e* St Martins Press. 2004. Page 105

[41] Quoted by Tom Curtis in a major article in Rolling Stone reproduced at http://whale.to/vaccines/curtis.htm#Monkey_Virus_==_Human_Virus_

[42] Cited in *The River*, Page 487

[43] *The River* footnote 15 page 486 – also page 100

of the possible disadvantages of the Salk vaccine—namely, the risk of sensitivity induced by monkey-kidney tissue.' [44] They reported that only a tiny proportion of monkey viruses have so far been identified, and the non-identified could not be screened out. Thus if monkeys are used one can guarantee that their viruses will be in the vaccine.

Hilleman now joined Koprowski in endorsing a shift away from monkeys. He strongly recommended that all polio vaccine manufacturing should be on human tissues. He issued a warning; '[The] use of tissues of wild-caught animals is just asking for trouble because of the lack of control and the known high probability for viral contamination.'

But Sabin fought back, fiercely defending the comparative safety of his vaccine, He alleged Hayflick's human-cell substrate was not as safe as claimed– for it might be found one day to contain an unknown human cancer virus.

With this vague allegation, he succeeded in retaining the US and UK markets for his contaminated polio vaccine. In vain Hayflick argued back that no human virus had ever been found to cause cancer – and Sabin's vaccine was contaminated with SV40 that provably had a link to cancer. The UK and US health authorities continued to blindly put their trust in Sabin and the contract they had with him. They continued to use monkeys – and are still using them today for vaccine tests.

But at that time Merck still held out. It had stopped making the Salk and was now refusing to make the Sabin, saying the use of monkey kidneys made it too dangerous for them to take the risk. But the US government now sought out other companies that might be prepared to take the risk. The temptation was too much for Lederle. It dropped its attempt to make vaccines by safer methods, took up the government offer and obtained in 1981 a license to make the Sabin polio vaccine on meat from monkeys.

This was a great surprise. Lederle's John Cox had been the first to refuse to use monkeys because of the danger of viral contamination.[45] He had corresponded in January 1961with Bernice Eddy on the dangers of using monkeys. But Lederle now decided that profits came first. It dropped its health reservations, its own vaccine and its principles, in order to pick up the contract that Merck had refused. In future Lederle would supply a known dangerous vaccine for use on countess millions of children – and lucratively keep on doing so, despite the health authorities reporting a great increase in cancer cases.

Sabin supplied Lederle in October 1962 with 5 millilitres of his 'Type III master virus strain' filtered from his cultures; enough to seed their monkey kidneys and to start the production of his polio vaccine. But to evade legal risk, he simultaneously warned Lederle that he could not guarantee the safety of this master virus strain! He told it that Merck, the maker of his vaccine seed strain, had refused to guarantee its purity. Hilleman of Merck had insisted that it might still be contaminated with SV40. [46]

These warnings nearly put a stop to Lederle's plans. In March 1961, Lederle was instructed, by the Food and Drug Administration (FDA) that; 'Each seed virus used in the manufacture shall be demonstrated to be free of extraneous microbial agents.' [47] Lederle would need to test the master strain mercilessly – and watch the vaccine lots like a hawk for signs of SV40 contamination.

But despite these instructions, the vaccine remained contaminated, for Lederle now was not bothering to check its safety, despite this being legally required. The US government knew this and was complicit in it, according to its own records, as unearthed and alleged by the lawyer Stan Kops with whom I had spoken at the 1997 SV40 Workshop. He obtained these records while engaged in courtroom battles over vaccine

[44] *Lancet* July 9.1955, p. 88

[45] Herald R. Cox, Viral Vaccines and Human Welfare, The Lancet July-December 1953, pp 1-5

[46] Federal Register, Saturday, March 25, 1961 at page 2565-2568, Sec. 73.110, et seq

[47] Federal Register, Saturday, March 25, 1961 at page 2565-2568, Sec. 73.110, et seq

safety. In September 10th 2003 he presented these documents to Congress when he testified before the House Subcommittee on Human Rights and Wellness.

A 1961 Lederle 'interoffice' memo he obtained reveals that the doctor the US national authorities put in charge of vaccine safety in 1961, a Dr. Robert Murray, not only knew Lederle's production of the Sabin polio vaccine was contaminated with SV40 but had decided to permit this. 'The decision by Dr. Murray to allow SV40 to be present ... was the basis for us allowing these lots to pass.' As a result, SV40 had been allowed to contaminate at least a fifth of the company's production.[48]

On top of this, the same memo revealed that the company was 'harvesting kidneys' from a monkey species from the Philippines, the cercopithecus, which also carried SV40.[49] In other words, it was crassly ignoring many warnings in the pursuit of profit.

A Lederle corporate memo dated 1973 revealed it was told at a key 1961 FDA meeting why the government had laid down that vaccine cultures should be monitored for 14 days for signs of contamination. It was that, if they watched for longer than 14 days, they would find all the vaccine contaminated and thus would have to destroy it. Clearly this would cause great financial loss!

This memo incredibly stated: 'Manufacturing regulations limited the observation of tissue culture control bottles (containing 25% of the monkey tissue used to manufacture polio vaccine) to 14 days - a time period chosen for the specific purpose of passing vaccine lots made in tissue harbouring extraneous viruses in 'eclipse' [not significantly multiplying]. Longer observation periods (21 or 28 days) were rejected because the expected appearance of contaminants might require rejection of a monopool of the vaccine. The NIH adopted the 14-day time period and manufacturers switched to the untested African green monkey kidney tissue in which SV-40 was not indigenous. Everyone at the meeting agreed that the potential for the presence of a then undetectable virus in African green monkey tissue was great, but since nothing could be detected [at 14 days], the material would pass regulations for production as drawn.'

This cynicism totally shocked me. I wondered if Dr. Carbone had read this memo. He had reported years later that he had found some SV40 took more than 14 days to appear and warned this meant SV40 contamination might evade the 14-day watching period. But this memo reveals that the authorities knew of this danger for many years before Carbone discovered it. They had knowingly put the health of children at risk for commercial reasons, for else there might be no profits in vaccine manufacturing!

I have also learnt that in 1962 scientists reported that not two weeks but five weeks of monitoring were required if SV40 contaminated vaccine lots were to be detected![50] This was making it even more scandalous. Their warning also was ignored. Countless millions of children were needlessly exposed.

Despite this, Lederle would continue to cynically assure the public that its vaccines were pure and safe and US vaccine safety regulatory authorities would continue to hide their knowledge that the polio vaccine remained contaminated. A US government memo sent to an Australian health authority in 1979 betrayed their knowledge. It stated: 'It should be made clear that Lederle did not test the original Sabin seeds for extraneous agents or neurovirulence.'[51]

Other Lederle memos also document this negligence. A memo dated August 23rd, 1968, refers to Dr. Robert Murray of Biological Standards, the Federal officer responsible for vaccine safety. Infectious contaminants had again been detected in vaccine cultures

---

[48] Lederle Interoffice Memo, *Re Presence of SV40 in vaccine lots* 8 November 1961

[49] Cell and molecular biology of Simian Virus 40: implications for human infections and diseases. Butel J, Lednicky JA. J at Cancer Inst 1999; 91 (2) 119-134

[50] Meyer HM, Hopps HE, Rogers NG, Brooks BE, Bernehim BC, Jones WP, Nisalak A, Douglas RD (1962) Studies on Simian Virus 40. Journal of Immunology Vol 88:796-805.

[51] Lederle internal memo, 14 March 1979 *Re Request of information for Australian Bureau of Health.*

made from the kidneys of African green monkeys and the company feared their use of these monkeys would now be banned. But Dr. Murray told them not to worry, as the discovery was of 'little consequence' as no illness had been linked to this contamination.[52]

The memo reads: 'I told Dr. Murray that there was some concern at Lederle about a possible requirement barring the use of African green monkey kidney as the substrate for the growth of attenuated polioviruses.' However, the doctor reassured Lederle that this would not happen. It continued: 'Dr. Murray has stated that the adventitious agents that Dr. Kendall Smith is presumably detecting by his techniques are of little consequence for an oral preparation in that such a large experience exists with the use of oral polio vaccine without any evidence of trouble relating to these agents.'

Two years after this memo, the first human casualties of SV40 were discovered. One of the first was Mark Moreno. He had a large brain tumour removed in 1970, and has since had further operations. His tumour was riddled with SV40. Many similar cases have since been found.

Drs. Leonard Hayflick and Bernice Eddy testified before the US Congress in 1972. Hayflick reported that the monkey kidneys used were *'a veritable storehouse for the most dangerous kinds of contaminating viruses ... the 'dirtiest' organs known,'* Eddy warned: *'If you continue to allow these contaminated vaccines to go out, I guarantee you that over the next 20 years you will have epidemics of cancer unlike the world has ever seen'.*

But Congress ignored their warnings and cancer rates continued to soar. No one seemed to check if these events were related – not until Carbone came along in the 1990s.

## Did other monkey viruses contaminate the polio vaccine?

In 1972, Lederle and the US government's FDA Bureau of Biologics completed a 'Joint Study into Polio Vaccine Safety.' They tested 11 monkeys imported for polio vaccine production – and found all were positive for yet another monkey virus, Simian Cytomegalovirus (SCMV, a Herpes virus). It was only detected because the test was done more rigorously than required. 'All eleven monkeys studied demonstrated the presence of CMV-like agents. These monkeys all originated from Kenya over a short period of time. Seven of these monkeys would have passed our existing test standards ... We plan to continue to process monkeys at the rate of five per week, probably through October 1972, to provide us with thirty million doses of trivalent poliovirus vaccine...'

This contamination was allowed to continue because 'unless and until Pfizer's Diplovax [a polio vaccine] is in abundant supply, the BB [Bureau of Biologics] cannot risk Lederle being off the market.' Thus controversially the priority of the government was to keep the vaccine in production, not to keep it safe.

Instead of cleaning up its vaccine, or checking the health of the children given polluted vaccine, Lederle worried that rival pharmaceutical companies, such as Pfizer, might use this contamination as a weapon against it, as revealed in a memo sent to the President of American Cyanamid in 1973. (In 1968 Lederle became a subdivision of American Cyanamid – in 2008 owned by Wyeth.)

'I do not believe our problem with the slow release of specific lots of Orimune(R) [vaccine] are a result of a Pfizer influence... Furthermore, if the Bureau wanted to restrict us they could bring up the subject of CMV (Cytomegalovirus) in our substrate [i.e. in African green monkey kidney cells in the vaccine culture] which they have not done, even though they have told us the monkeys in the collaborative study performed in 1972 were all positive for this agent.'

In 1976 yet more SV40-linked human cancers were detected and *'researchers at the US bureau of Biologics found that polio vaccine lots made by Lederle contained between*

---

[52] 1992 Lederle internal memo, 14 March 1979 Re Request of information for Australian Bureau of Health.

*1,000 and 100,000 simian viruses per ml. of vaccine;'* that is, **every dose of vaccine given to a child contained 100 to 10,000 monkey viruses** – and, according to WHO regulations, was permitted to contain five times more than this! [53] This was 16 years after SV40 was supposedly eliminated from the vaccine.' [54] With the withdrawal of Pfizer that year, Lederle became the only manufacturer of the Sabin polio vaccine in the US.

In 1978, John Martin, the Professor of Pathology I mentioned meeting at the 1997 workshop, examined a bulk shipment of polio vaccine. He reported: 'I worked at the time as Director of the Viral Oncology Laboratory at the Bureau of Biologics... There was a lot of extraneous DNA in the vaccine. I sent electron micrographs to three outside experts to ascertain if these were the dreaded Type C retroviruses or not. The answers came back no, but there was so much debris and DNA in the vaccine that it was impossible essentially to do a nice clean prep of the viral vaccines, of the viruses. That was my first indication that, in fact, the vaccines were rather crude.'

But when he reported this vaccine contamination, he was most surprised to be told by his employer that 'vaccine manufacturing was an essential component of industry, this country's protection against potential biological warfare. A number of companies had given up making vaccines. It's an economically risky business. If one criticizes, in this case, Lederle, too much and they stop production, then all the production will go to Switzerland. The Swiss would then be bought out by the Russians, and then there will be biological warfare.'

He now believes what he saw might have been simian cytomegalovirus. What he did not then know was that the authorities already knew it was present. It was very hard to remove –as admitted in a memo sent by R J Vallencourt of Lederle on 31st January 1972: 'Cytomegalovirus (CMV) is a recent example of an adventitious agent which, although it exists in cell cultures, is not being tested for at this time. ... Since 100% of the monkeys are serologically positive for CMV [antibody], no testing of monkeys prior to production can take place. We do not know which monkeys are suitable for production until kidneys are processed. Our data shows that 50% of today's 'clean' monkeys would be disqualified for production needs' if the new regulations were put into effect. [55]

In an internal 1983 report, Lederle reported a 13-year study of 2,239 'harvests' of poliovirus fluid for vaccines, taken from incubators within 72 hours of inoculation ['seeding'] with poliovirus. It stated almost half of the harvests had to be scrapped because of contamination... and that Simian cytomegalovirus, SCMV, was the leading cause of rejection, amounting to 38% of rejections ...but there were also some for measles virus, foamy virus, and occasionally SV40 contamination. [56]

As I have mentioned, Martin told me he suspected that Simian Cytomegalovirus (SCMV) causes Chronic Fatigue Syndrome in humans by damaging brain cells. He showed me slides of damage he thought done by the virus.

So, SCMV and SV40 were known for decades to be in our polio vaccine. Nothing was done about this and no parents informed. What other monkey viruses might also be present? It appears that little research on this has been done. Yet in 1960 Dr. Robert Murray, director of the Federal Division of Biological Standards, admitted that 'killed polio vaccine must have contained simian agents undetected at the time of preparation and undetected and undetectable after inactivation.'

---

[53] WHO regulations stipulate that an oral dose of Sabin polio vaccine contains from 0.1 to 0.3 ml. http://whqlibdoc.who.int/hq/1999/WHO_V&B_99.12_(p406-p506).pdf

[54] Kyle, 1992

[55] Bookchin and Shumacher *The Virus and the Vaccine* St Martins Press. 2004. Cited on page 328

[56] Lederle memo...referred to in Footnotes of above, p328 all polio vaccines may contain SCMV.–

A 1968 study by Dr. G. D. Hsiung noted: '47 strains of viruses [had been] isolated from a total of 9 chimpanzees.' [57] Another study revealed 'a great number of simian viruses have been recovered from a variety of monkeys, baboons and marmosets. These indigenous viruses have caused considerable frustration and economic loss to workers in terms of contaminated virus stocks and rejected cultures ... in many instances the information is rather limited regarding latent virus infections in primate tissues, with special reference to viruses isolated from the monkey kidney tissues of apparently healthy animals.' [58]

SV40 rather scarily seemed to be combining with other viruses. This study reported finding cells 'doubly infected with SV40 and measles virus' and 'mixed infections with SV40 and foamy agents.' Similarly, another monkey virus, SV5, had combined in infections with foamy agents and with the measles virus. But oddly, it had also found SV5 and measles virus seemingly vanished when monkeys were kept in isolation for over 30 days. This suggested the cells simply stopped making them, – in other words, they were possibly curing themselves?

The study noted that Hull had so far found and named 18 monkey adenoviruses, most from Rhesus and Cynomolgus monkeys, and that the former were also infected with Herpes virus and Reoviruses. Another virus called SA3 had been found in African Green Monkeys. The study further noted: 'It has become evident that many factors may influence the recognition of indigenous viruses,' including environmental factors and the nature of the research. Some viruses seemed only to appear in captivity. Another study found that: 'Salmonella carriers in newly imported Rhesus and Cynomolgus monkeys exceeded 20% in some shipments.' [59]

In recent years the UK has made its polio vaccine on kidneys from African Green Monkeys captured from the wild in Barbados, despite many 'pathological agents' being reported as found in these animals. [60]

After such research findings, I found particularly interesting a report from Dr. S. Kalter and others in 1991 about the 100,000 monkeys then imported annually into the USA. In their *'Comparative Virology of Primates'* they state it was difficult to work out from whence came the viruses found, because of the 'practice of intermingling species after their capture.' They concluded: 'Thus in many instances the true origin of many simian viruses is questionable or has been misdirected.'

They reported that experimental results were compromised because of: 'the obscure background of many animals' due to 'the failure of investigators to take into account the amount of contact the animal under study has had with other animals, including man, prior to capture. It is well known that many of the monkeys and apes now in the laboratory have come from places where they have lived in close proximity with man, often sharing the same food and water source as well as deposition of body wastes.'

'Review of the literature emphasizes that most investigators employing these animals in their research still lack understanding of the magnitude of this problem. Little recognition is given to the potential danger ... most laboratories make no provision to protect their personnel or to provide suitable quarters to minimalise the problem. Very

---

[57] G. D. Hsiung Bacteriological Reviews, Sept., 1968, p. 185-205 Latent Virus Infections in Primate Tissues with Special Reference to Simian Viruses.

58 Latent viruses from tissues of chimpanzees affected with experimental Kuru. NY. Acad. Sci. Gajousek D.C., Rogers M. Bessaigh and Gibs.Jrn.

59 Significant Zoonotic Disease of Non-human primates, Division of Veterinary Medicine, Walter Reed Army Institute, Washington DC, November 1988. http://netvet.wustl.edu/species/primates/primzoon.txt

[60] Jean Baulu, Graham Evans, and Carlisle Sutton Pathogenic Agents Found in Barbados *Chlorocebus aethiops sabaeus* and in Old World and New World Monkeys Commonly Used in Biomedical Research;, Barbados Primate Research Center and Wildlife Reserve

little is done to obtain the animals properly in order to maintain healthy stock and prevent the spread of viruses…'

### CHIMPANZEES AND HIV

HIV is said to come from chimpanzees - so how could chimp viruses have come to infect humans? It seems medical research techniques provided ample opportunity. Dr. Patrick Meenan, bacteriologist at St. Vincent's Hospital, Dublin, stated in *Lancet,* on April 18, 1953 that; 'most of the recent work on poliomyelitis has been done on chimpanzees, which seem to react to infection much as man does.'

Similarly Elliot Dick in 1963, after searching for the best animal to use for vaccine cultures, reported in his paper *Chimpanzee Kidney Tissue Cultures for Growth and Isolation of Viruses*: 'apart from the cost … chimp kidney tissue cultures may well be the perfect substrate … simply because it's the closest to us genetically.' He also noted that its kidneys seemed to have viruses in them but this did not change his mind about their suitability. Viruses were found in all kidneys apparently.[61]

It seems the virologists of that time thought little of using chimpanzees for such experiments. These animals were not then regarded as romantically as they are now. They were even favoured because they were more alike to humans, so hopefully suffered from the same diseases. They were a bit more costly than Rhesus, but nevertheless their brains, their kidneys, and presumably their testicles, were all extracted and used – just as happened with the African Greens and Rhesus monkeys.

There was also clearly every opportunity for viruses to evolve or change in the process of making the vaccines. In 1960, Dr. Sweet had reported: 'we found that it [SV40] hybridised [combined] with certain DNA viruses –the adenovirus had SV40 genes attached to it. We couldn't clean up the adenovirus vaccine lots grown in monkey kidney cells.' It seemed that the monkey cells in the cultures were starting to mutate and to produce new types of virus.

These reports were beginning to convince me that HIV might have come from chimps and been spread via the polio vaccine. I had been told at the 1997 NIH workshop that HIV could possibly have been a contaminant in the polio vaccine. Now I discovered that this danger had been known for over thirty years!

I found evidence for this in a history of medicine commissioned by the NIH, *The Health Century* by Dr. Edward Shorter, in which there are interviews with key scientists. I found riveting the transcript of his interview with Maurice Hilleman, the scientist with whom I had spoken on MMR.[62] Hilleman said he had come to the terrifying conclusion that, when they changed to using African Green monkeys to avoid SV40, inadvertently they probably introduced HIV; for these monkeys carried SIV, a simian virus said to be a precursor of HIV. Hilleman concluded: *'I brought African greens in. I didn't know we were importing AIDS virus at the time.'*

His colleague Sweet added that, by the time they realised just how dangerous these contaminants were: *'it was too late to switch gears and start using raccoon or chicken systems, because then you would be dealing with another whole set of viruses. Now with the theoretical links to HIV and cancer, it just blows my mind.'*

They said this *'raises the important question of the existence of other such viruses* [in the vaccine].' Sweet later added; *'It was a frightening discovery because, back then, it was not possible to detect the virus with the testing procedures we had. … We had no idea what this virus would do thirty years later'* although we *'knew SV40 had oncogenic [cancer-causing] properties in hamsters which was bad news.'*

---

[61] 'Chimpanzee Kidney Tissue Cultures for Growth and Isolation of Viruses, ' J Bacteriol. 1963,86, 573-576

[62] Much of this transcript is quoted by Leonid Horowitz in his work 'Emerging Viruses' Tetrahedron 1996, pages 483-486

There was practically no attempt to assess the 39 types of monkey virus found prior to SV40 to see if any of these might also be dangerous – apart from SV20. It was researched in the late 1960s and reported to be an 'oncogenic (cancer-causing) adenovirus'. Since then this virus appears to have been little researched.[63]

I was appalled by what I had learnt about polio vaccine research. I was shocked to realise that most of what had been revealed at the 1997 Workshop was not new to the regulatory authorities; that they had known for decades about this contamination and done nothing. I was forced to conclude that the officials responsible had knowingly contaminated our children.

In the USA, between 1955 and 1963, contaminated polio vaccine was given to 90% of all children and 60% of adults. It has since been given to hundreds of millions more. If one monkey virus could thus spread – could the AIDS epidemic have also spread in the same way? It seemed that I had stumbled on a terrifying can of worms.

---

[63] CK Fong and GD Hsiung *Productive and abortive growth of an oncogenic simian adenovirus SV30 in cultured cells.* Cancer Research 1970 30: 855-862.

# Chapter 4

# The Hunt for the Poliovirus

'At the heart of science lies discovery which involves a change in worldview. Discovery in science is possible only in societies which accord their citizens the freedom to pursue the truth where it may lead and which therefore have respect for different paths to that truth,'
John Polanyi, Canadian Nobel Laureate (Chemistry); Commencement Address, McGill University, Montreal, Canada, June 1990

The hunt for a virus that causes polio began in the first years of the 20th Century as an emergency response to the horrifying onset of major epidemics of paralytic polio in Sweden and the United States. It was guided by a new scientific hypothesis then gathering strength that we now know of as the *Germ Theory of Disease.*

These polio epidemics were new – and yet poliomyelitis, to give it its full name, was not a new disease. It had been around for centuries and was long associated with metalworking. But the virus we now blame for polio is a common human gut virus with no obvious connection to metalworking. This virus is produced solely by human cells, and spreads from us to be common in soil. Human infants acquire lifelong immunity to it as soon as they go into the garden and put a grubby hand in their mouth, as stated in a paper published on the website of the Centers for Disease Control (CDC) in the US.[64]

So – how did this virus come to cause these crippling and deadly epidemics? Sit back comfortably and read on, for this is also the story of the birth of modern virology and much of modern medicine. It took me some time to untangle it – but I think I can now explain it quite straightforwardly.

Polio at its worst causes paralysis of the chest muscles of children, thus suffocating its victims. It was formerly known as Infantile Paralysis. The critical damage is to the motor neuron cells inside the backbone that control the chest muscles. Some children were so crippled by it that they could only breathe through being put into 'iron lungs.' Many died – but fortunately these were only a small proportion of those afflicted. In most cases the paralysis was only temporary and minor, some victims scarcely felt paralysed at all – but nevertheless these epidemics were unpredictable and thus totally terrifying. They hit at kids and they struck in the manner of bushfires in summer, sometimes destroying a whole neighbourhood but then not returning for years.

'Poliomyelitis' comes from the Greek for 'inflammation of the grey spinal cord;' the grey marrow of our backbone where live the motor neuron cells that control our muscles. Damage to these cells can cause paralysis. Going by skeletons and paintings of victims, it has been around from the time of ancient Egypt. What was new, when the polio epidemics started at the end of the 19th century, was that it had never before struck at so many at once and never before had been epidemic.

These epidemics grew to a climax in 1952 when some 3,000 Americans died – but one should put this in context. In 1957 an influenza epidemic reportedly killed 62,000 in the US and in 1950 34,000 died of tuberculosis.

---

[64] See Dr. John H. Lienhard of the University of Houston, author of *Polio and Clean Water* on the CDC website

But polio was considered worse because it mostly targeted children – and inexplicably children not living in poverty. It mostly struck at middleclass children who presumably had good sanitary conditions at home. Also, winter is normally the time when infections kill, when cold and damp affect immune systems, so why were these 'Summer Plagues?'

The *British Medical Journal* currently reports on its website for students: 'Polio was never a big killer, but the evil of this disease was its ability to reappear and disappear every summer and autumn.' [65]   Why was the virus only active around harvest time? This is still an enigma for virology although, as you will find, the toxicologists had an explanation.

During the latter part of the 19th century, the great epidemics that once plagued the industrialised cities in Europe, with their overcrowded slums and open cesspits, were mostly defeated by the provision of clean water, sanitation and better nutrition, as well as by quarantining the ill away from the healthy. So – why was polio so frighteningly different? Why did these measures not work with polio?

When the polio epidemics struck, there was no cure or effective medical treatment. All preventive measures failed. Middleclass parents made sure their children had healthy diets, including much fruit – but the same children were among polio's first victims – as reported by the health inspectors of New England.

Among polio's victims was also an American President, Franklin D. Roosevelt. He was paralysed after swimming in polluted seawater. This virtually guaranteed that the fight against polio would be funded vastly better than any other medical research. Many medical theorists thought that epidemics were caused by minute filterable particles, like bacteria but so small that they could scarcely be seen. These were called viruses and an unknown one was suspected to cause polio. Roosevelt thus organised a 'war' against it. He set up the 'March of Dimes' to raise funds, pumping these into hunting this putative virus, warning people that in the interim they must kill any flies they saw as they might be spreading polio. Thus this 'fly' poster was produced.

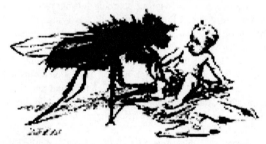

With the middle classes so targeted, laboratories around the US became absorbed in a race to discover this still unidentified virus – the first step before any vaccine could be developed. Enormous rewards and high prestige awaited any scientists who succeeded. This well-funded campaign would effectively establish a whole new class of scientists, the 'virologists' who have ever since dedicated themselves to a war against viruses.

However, the same level of panic did not affect the British. In 1953 the Glasgow Public Health Department declined the offer of a supply of anti-polio serum made by the trustees of the United States Roosevelt Memorial Fund. The reason given was that, with the comparatively small incidence of poliomyelitis in that

---

[65] http://www.studentbmj.com/issues/04/11/education/399.php

city, it would have required the inoculation of 1,250,000 people to prevent an epidemic that might affect at most only 250, according to the *Weekly Scotsman* of January 22nd 1953.

The scientists on the hunt conceived of viruses a priori as dangerous parasitic rivals to humans in the competition for life. The electron microscope had not yet been invented, so for them these were invisible disease agents. Most viral 'isolates' were little more than filtered cell cultures in which viruses were presumed present. They were thus named 'virus' since this word means 'poisonous liquid' in Latin.

Ever since, viruses have been regarded with fear, as if intelligent nano-terrorists that 'invade' our cells, hijack them and outwit our defences. Viruses are feared as the ultimate mass destruction enemy, invisible agents able to kill millions in inevitable epidemics; mutant creatures that we must spend billions fighting.

This is still the common view of viruses. We all had thoroughly drummed into us since we were children the need to exterminate, as far as possible, all of them. Disinfectant advertisements preach the same sermon. The health institutions charged with defending us constantly tell us the same; while they monitor for unknown viral genetic codes, ready to pounce on any new danger.

But I was surprised to discover that during the major US polio epidemics in the first half of the 20th century, some scientists did not agree that a virus were to blame. Doctors who were treating polio victims sometimes blamed the new powerful pesticides, particularly those sprayed repeatedly on crops during the summer months. These were neurotoxins that killed insects by paralysing them. Were they doing the same to humans? These doctors presented evidence supporting their diagnosis to the US Congress, but they did not win much media or political support. The virology specialists at that time, and ever since, have firmly dominated our major health institutions, such as the Centers for Disease Research, and persuasively held that epidemics must be caused by infectious agents, either bacteria or viruses.

I long believed the same. It seemed self-evident. In any case, as far as I then could judge, the very fact that polio vaccines now protect us from polio is sufficient proof that polio is caused by a virus.

Still, I would not be a reasonable investigative journalist if I did not read all sides of arguments. I have often found that the vital clues lie in minutia, in details often overlooked. I was intrigued by learning polio was associated with metal working prior to the beginning of the epidemics. Why would a virus linger around metal forges? And what would make it suddenly start to spread so widely? Something must have happened.

When I read the related research, I was surprised to discover how little we know of how the poliovirus causes polio. Professor Akio Nomoto of Tokyo University stated in 1996, 'little is known about the mechanisms by which the poliovirus causes paralysis ... it is not known how the virus moves into the blood from the primary multiplication site [the guts], how the virus invades the CNS [Central Nervous System] ... Humans are simply lucky that the polio vaccines worked.' He also noted the only way 'polio can be shown to damage brain cells is to directly inject it across the barrier into monkey brains.'[66] This was a very major surprise; if this virus could not naturally get to these cells, how could it cause polio?

But I knew that toxins make their way with relative ease across the blood brain barrier. The scientific papers of toxicology are full of documented cases. For example, *The Journal of Immunology* reported: 'Neurotoxins are known to directly damage or kill neurons, including: lead, mercury.'

---

[66] '*Molecular Mechanism of Poliovirus Replication - Control of Poliomyelitis*' Akio Nomoto (Professor, The Institute of Medical Science, The University of Tokyo, Japan) 1996

This made me pause, for both lead and mercury are found in metalworking. If they damaged neurons, could this explain the paralytic illness that once plagued metal workers? Also, lead arsenate was widely introduced as a summer-sprayed pesticide at the end of the 19th century, both in the US and parts of Europe. This was immediately before the polio epidemics started! It was then used intensively for about fifty years.

The same paper went on to say: 'Some organophosphate chemicals (including some pesticides) can cause death or loss of a portion [of a nerve cell.]'.[67] Organophosphates were introduced in the States just before the major polio epidemics of 1950 – 1952.

Could these pesticides then be co-factors, alongside the poliovirus, in causing the dreadful polio epidemics? But, before I went into this, I needed to know how the poliovirus was proved to cause this paralysis. It was not hard to discover who had established this. The World Health Organization (WHO) credits the discovery of this virus, and of the infectious nature of polio, to a very famous experiment performed in Vienna in 1908 by Drs. Carl Landsteiner and Erwin Popper.[68]

We presume today that everyone knows that viruses cause major illnesses, but back in 1908, when the polio epidemics were starting to terrorise, viruses were not yet proved to cause illnesses; in fact they had not even been proved to exist! Initially it was speculated that viruses were smaller invisible versions of the barely visible single-celled bacteria that were already known to be able to reproduce and spread illnesses.

One of the first advocates of this 'Germ theory' of illness was a Venetian called Girolamo Fracastoro, who in 1546 blamed diseases on rapidly multiplying minute infectious bacteria-like organisms in his book *De Contagione et Contagiosis Morbis*. His theory then fell into disuse – perhaps because it neglected toxins and other causes of disease, perhaps because it was before its time. He had no means of substantiating his theory, for there were then no microscopes or other suitable scientific tools. [69]

In the 17th century, the minute world revealed by the newly invented microscope totally fascinated the Dutch scientist Antony van Leeuwenhoek and the English scientist Robert Hooke. The former became the first to describe bacteria; the latter the first to describe and name the 'cell'. But viruses still were not seen.

The earliest mention of 'viruses' and vaccination I can find was by a famous 18th Century British scientist called Edward Jenner. He is widely credited with inventing 'vaccination' as a protection from smallpox. Cows (vacca in Latin – thus vaccination) suffer from a very mild form of smallpox called cowpox. He had heard of a country belief that people who got cowpox never seem to be affected by the much more serious smallpox.

Jenner did his first 'vaccination' by taking pus from an open sore on the hand of a milkmaid Sarah Nelmes whose cow "Daisy" had cowpox, and injecting this into the son of his gardener in the expectation that it would protect him from smallpox. He called the pus his 'virus.' We now know this would contain many kinds of microbes and toxins, but he claimed it was 'pure'. Thus, when in 1800 a Dr. Woodville attacked his method, citing its failures, Jenner replied that a 'contamination' must have entered the needle along with his 'pure uncontaminated cow-pox virus.'

He won £30,000 for inventing vaccination, then a great fortune, and in 1853 the government made his smallpox vaccination compulsory.[70] But many parents went to prison rather than give his pus vaccination to their children, because it frequently seemed to produce illness, not protection. In one English city it was reported that 'over 6,000 summonses had been issued against parents, who were brought before the Magistrates;

---

[67] *The Journal of Immunology*, vol.140, p.564

[68] http://americanhistory.si.edu/polio/virusvaccine/livingchem.htm

[69] http://www.britannica.com/eb/article-9035082/Girolamo-Fracastoro

[70] The 1853 Compulsory Vaccination Act

and there had been 64 commitments to prison, including three mothers, all of whom were put in gaol; nearly 200 homes having been sold up under distress warrants, and between £2,000 and £3,000 being paid in fines and costs.' [71]

But when I dug deeper, I found Jenner did not invent vaccination. He learnt of it from a milkmaid. Also, a Dorset farmer named Benjamin Jesty had published 20 years earlier an account of how he thus protected his wife and family, as well as others who came to him. His account had attracted much attention – and ridicule.[72] But, we now know the Chinese practiced something very similar for 3000 years. They recommended sniffing powdered smallpox scabs to induce immunity to smallpox.

During the 19th century Louis Pasteur (1822–95) further developed the 'germ theory.' His description of microorganisms in milk led to the 'pasteurization' process named after him. He is also given credit for developing anthrax, cholera and rabies vaccines, although it now turns out that other scientists may have been ahead of him.

Pasteur observed that old samples of serum seemed to be less dangerous than new samples – and if the old samples were used as a vaccine, they protected against the newer samples. He postulated from this that exposure to oxygen weakened the bacteria, making them safe to use as a vaccine.

In 1881, in a controlled experiment in front of witnesses at Pouilly-le-Fort, Pasteur claimed to prove his theory. He did so by vaccinating 25 sheep with five drops of what he said was an old oxygen-attenuated sample of anthrax bacilli. But, after his death it came out that this was fraudulent. His private notebooks record that instead he had secretly used a method developed by the scientists Charles Chamberland and Emile Roux of weakening anthrax bacteria by poisoning with the antiseptic potassium dichromate, then serial passaging the sample through 3 mice, as he had not yet resolved problems associated with his oxygen theory but had boasted that he had.[73]

When he then exposed these sheep and 25 unvaccinated sheep to a non-poisoned sample; 'the entire unvaccinated control group died, whereas those vaccinated survived. [All but one.] Within several months, anthrax vaccination was widespread in France. From this point on, his research focused on limiting the virulence of 'germs' to provide a medium for vaccination.' [74]

His later experiments included recovering saliva from a rabbit with anthrax and dosing this into a series of 39 rabbit brains aged in glass jars – but there were frequent disastrous failures in using this 'aged' anthrax as a vaccine.

The *Lancet* described the first use on a human of Pasteur's rabies vaccine: 'On July 6, 1885, a 9-year-old boy, Joseph Meister, became the first person to be vaccinated against rabies, two days after he was bitten by a rabid dog. Pasteur prepared the vaccine from the spinal cord of a rabid rabbit. Having used potash to desiccate the tissue, he recovered fluid from it and inoculated the preparation into another rabbit. Pasteur repeated the process many times on rabbits to hopefully weaken it before using it. Joseph survived and the news spread rapidly, with a rush that overtook Pasteur's desire to test the vaccine scientifically.'[75] For this he gained from a grateful French people his own Institute – the Pasteur; still one of the world's foremost scientific institutions.

---

[71] *The Case Against Vaccination.* AN ADDRESS By WALTER HADWEN J.P., M.D., L.R.C.P., M.R.C.S., L.S.A., Etc (Gold Medalist in Medicine and in Surgery) At GODDARD'S ASSEMBLY ROOMS, GLOUCESTER. On Saturday, January 25th, 1896 (During the Gloucester Smallpox Epidemic)

[72] . http://www.thedorsetpage.com/History/Smallpox

[73] Geison, Gerald: 'The Private Science of Louis Pasteur". It's account is based on the private notebooks of Pasteur that apparently only became available after the death of his last male heir..

[74] As above.

[75] The Lancet 2002; 360:93 http://www.thelancet.com/journals/lancet/article/PIIS0140673602093637/fulltext

As you will observe, this process is extraordinarily similar to how Sabin and Koprowski made the polio vaccines some seventy years later. The main difference is that he used rabbits while they used monkeys.

However, his work was also tainted by charges of plagiarism made by an eminent fellow member of the French Academy of Science, Professor Antoine Béchamp (1816-1908), who had published, six years before Pasteur, a paper stating: 'It thus appears evident that airborne germs found the sugared solution a favourable medium for their development, and it must be admitted that the ferment is here produced by the generation of fungi.' He thus discovered before Pasteur that airborne microorganisms caused fermentation in wine and milk.

But Béchamp saw these organisms very differently from how they are generally seen today. He did not see them primarily as pathogenic, or even as invaders. He stressed their emergence from within us, as born of our cells – and stressed their value to us. He described them as 'a scavenging form of the microzymas (minute fermenting living particles), developed when death, decay, or disease causes an extraordinary amount of cell life either to need repair or be broken up.' Their presence was thus not the reason for a disease but the consequence of disease, as well as of the normal process of cell deaths.[76]

Pasteur emphasized more their possible role in illnesses – and thus received the credit for establishing the germ theory, but he too depicted bacteria as primarily useful. The French scientists also suggested that microbes might be able to change their nature, turning from one type into another.

So, from where came our ideas of bacteria as bad creatures we can kill without compunction, that we need to wipe out with high-tech hygiene in an endless war to remain healthy? Indeed, from where came my own negative view of these creatures, the way I had seen them most of my life?

From what I have read, these views originated more from the work of another great scientist of that time, someone severely critical of Pasteur, a man who would highly influence the hunt for the poliovirus begun a few years later by Landsteiner and Popper. He was Dr. Robert Koch, the head of the Institute for Infectious Illnesses (now the Robert Koch Institute) in Berlin.

I had not realised that politics would come so much into science, but at that time their nations had just fought the Franco-Prussian War. Both Koch and Pasteur had volunteered to fight. Highly competitive governments later promoted the prestige of each other's scientific institutes, seeking to turn the scientific discoveries of each to political advantage.

The Pasteur and the Koch Institutes advocated fundamentally different 'cultures of bacteriology.' The French, according to Andrew Mendelsohn, were more agricultural and positive, seeing bacteria as essential for life; while the German institute grew out of Koch's experiences as a surgeon during the Franco-Prussian war. For him microbes were enemies worse than the French. They were pathogens, to be killed if at all possible.[77]

For Koch, there was normally one causative type of bacteria per disease – with no room for the co-factors or mutations that the French scientists had observed.   He was nothing if not a Prussian in how he militarily organised the bacteria he detected, assigning each to one illness, as far as he was able. In 1905 when he won a Nobel Prize for linking TB to a mycobacteria, Prussia celebrated this as a national triumph.

---

[76] Bechamp wrote thus in 1869 of their role in disease: 'In typhoid fever, gangrene and anthrax, the existence has been found of bacteria in the tissues and blood, and one was very much disposed to take them for granted as cases of ordinary parasitism. It is evident, after what we have said, that instead of maintaining that the affection has had as its origin and cause the introduction into the organism of foreign germs with their consequent action, one should affirm that one only has to deal with an alteration of the function of microzymas.'

[77] Andrew Mendelsohn, Princeton dissertation.
http://www3.imperial.ac.uk/historyofscience/aboutthecentre/staff/drandrewmendelsohn

Thus started a split in biology theory that has persisted until today.

But Koch also contributed greatly by being a very methodical biologist. He invented ways of staining and storing bacteria samples. He was scathingly critical of Pasteur's work, which he saw as lacking the necessary precision. He rejected with derision Pasteur's liquid samples or 'isolates,' for he rightly said these could not possibly contain only one kind of pathogen.

He wrote of the Pasteur rabies vaccine: 'Pasteur is content to inoculate with slime taken from the nose of the dead animal, which, exactly like saliva, was certainly contaminated with many other bacteria.' He also noted that 'there are various different pathogenic bacteria that attack specific animal species and cause fatal diseases with the symptoms of septicaemia' – and that it is thus difficult to link one bacteria to one illness – meaning that bacteriologists had to be very careful. [78]

But Koch gained his fame initially for the way he tackled a terrible cholera epidemic in Hamburg.

At that time in Germany and Britain many public health authorities thought the best way to stop epidemics was not by vaccination but the removal of foul living conditions. The eminent pathologist Rudolph Virchow taught that the most effective way to stop the epidemics was by a dramatic improvement in living conditions, better nutrition, sanitation and the provision of clean drinking water.

This was a change, for earlier the hope had been more in smallpox vaccination. By 1871 some 97% of the population of the UK were vaccinated or immune from already having suffered smallpox, according to evidence given to a Parliamentary Select Committee.[79] But, just as this report was published, a major Europe-wide smallpox epidemic spread, killing some 22,062 in England and Wales and over 124,900 in Germany. Shockingly, this epidemic seemed to mostly target the vaccinated. Other steps clearly had to be taken. This led in the UK to a Public Health Act ordering the cleaning of the cities, vast improvements in water supplies and public hygiene.

The public authorities of Leicester in the UK uniquely combined greatly improving hygiene, water and food supplies with lessons learnt from the Germ Theory, the latter imposing a citywide program of strict quarantine and disinfection. This had startling success. 'The family and inmates of the house are placed in quarantine in comfortable quarters, and the house thoroughly disinfected. The result is that in every instance the disease has been promptly and completely stamped out at a paltry expense.' It was not only smallpox that this stopped. They also eliminated most cases of measles and other infectious diseases.

Leicester had remarkably achieved this while discarding vaccination completely, for the city authorities said they had found it hazardous and no help. Their results seemed to bear this out. 'Our small-pox death-rate was only 89 per million in 1893, with little vaccination; while [nationwide, with vaccination] it was 3,523 per million in 1872.'

A writer of the time reported: 'Thus, from being branded by the Registrar-General in his Annual Reports as one of the most unhealthy of England's large towns, Leicester— by no means advantageously situated geographically, and seriously handicapped by the large proportion of the artisan classes amongst its population—has become the healthiest of the principal manufacturing centres (even competing closely and successfully with health resorts).'

Koch followed the Leicester lead when he tackled the Hamburg cholera epidemic. This city had improved living conditions – but not instituted any measures of quarantine or filtered its water supplies. Since the city's port was full of Eastern European migrants

---

[78] On the Anthrax Inoculation [1872] by Robert Koch from Professor K. Codell's book *'Essays of Robert Koch'*, Greenwood Press, N.Y., 1987.
[79] Evidence given by Sir John Simon, chief medical officer to the Privy Council,

travelling on to America. Koch suspected it was they who were bringing the cholera into the city. When the city agreed to his strict quarantine measures, together with the filtering of the water supply, the epidemic ended after taking nearly 10,000 lives. It is uncertain which of these measures was the more important, but water filtration has since been credited with saving more lives than immunization and chemotherapy combined.[80]

Koch seems primarily to have credited his quarantine measures. On this success he built his theory that a bacteria he detected in cholera cases was the sole cause of this illness, by this contradicting such scientists as Max Von Pettenkoffer, who held that the bacteria were only one of the ingredients needed to produce this disease.

The increasing growth and prestige of the Koch and Pasteur 'germ theory,' each endorsed by their rival states, brought about fundamental changes in medical science. According to sceptical scientists of the time, they dethroned social reform and public hygiene as the primary weapons against epidemics, replacing these with vaccines and other products of the laboratory.[81]

Andrew Mendelsohn commented: 'Virchow and his supporters would always be highly suspicious of germs as any kind of true causative agents, recognizing that the easiest way for a conservative government to avoid expensive and democratizing social reforms (such as the government of Prussia) was to blame epidemics entirely upon a germ from without. Thus they would avoid issues of poverty and inequality and insist that nothing more was needed than quarantine and disinfection.'[82]

Meanwhile soil scientists were coming up with their own ideas of a 'virus.' Martinus Beijerinck coined the term contagium vivum fluidum [contagious living fluid] in 1898 to describe filtered juice from a plant with Tobacco Mosaic disease. He thought the juice was itself alive, saying 'the criteria of life ... are also compatible with the fluid state.' He called this a 'virus'. Dmitrii Iwanowski disagreed. In 1892 and 1902 he suggested the cause of this illness was 'a toxin secreted by bacteria.'

By now many saw the Germ Theory as a route to finding quick simple cures. Dr. Leslie E. Keeley scornfully rejected other theories, stating in 1893: 'Until within fifteen years the medical profession did not know the cause of disease... Within that time Pasteur, Koch, Steinberg, and many other workers in the field of microscopic research demonstrated that the microbe causes disease. ... A remedy that can reach and entirely destroy the microbe of disease will cure a disease. When such discovery is made it is found that a single remedy is a cure. The cause of each special disease is always a specific cause.'[83]

He thus placed no faith in fighting illnesses by improving sanitation and water supplies. Find the germ – and kill it. This stops the disease, or so he was convinced. This was the new solution and message. Today it is much the same. Fighting viruses rather than removing poverty and providing pure water have become the major emphasis of our international health institutions. Perhaps this is inevitable – the alternative demands a much greater investment and does not benefit the influential pharmaceutical industry.

Koch went on to develop rules for finding the cause of an illness. These are now known as the four 'Koch Postulates' and are still taught as fundamental in virology. They embody his theory that there is one microbe per disease and they are:
  # The agent must be present in every case of the disease.
  # The agent must be isolated from the host & grown in vitro [in the laboratory].

---

[80] Preface to Brock's *Robert Koch: A Life in Medicine and Bacteriology* by James Strick, Program in Biology and Society, Arizona State University, Tempe, AZ 85287-1501
[81] JSTOR Isis. Vol 86 no 2 (june 1995) pp 268-277. *Typhoid Mary stirkes back* by Andrew Mendelsohn.
[82] Cited above.
[83] *Chicago Tribune*, November 23, 1893

\# The disease must be reproduced when a pure culture of the agent is inoculated into a healthy susceptible host.

\# The same agent must be recovered from the experimentally infected diseased host.

But for Koch, in practice these rules were not set in stone. He found he could not always fulfil his own first postulate –and was unhappy with his formulation of the 3rd, for he was often unable to infect animals with his suspected bacilli and cause the same disease. He failed particularly with TB. We now know many microbes are harmless in their natural host – and thus their presence does not equate with illness. As mentioned; the bacteria that Koch identified as causing TB are now known to live harmlessly in most human adults.

But Koch and Pasteur inspired Landsteiner and Popper to begin their 1909 hunt for a virus causing polio. They hoped to link a microbe to polio by employing both the Koch postulates and Pasteur's methods. As they couldn't find a bacterium to blame for polio – they guessed there must exist minute invisible forms of bacteria able to pass through all available filters and still cause disease. They called these mini-bacteria 'viruses.' We now know that their filters would not have stopped many other particles, including DNA fragments, proteins, prions, toxins and much more. There were thus other 'invisible' non-viral agents that might cause the disease they observed.

Landsteiner and Popper first looked for suitable animals to use, in accordance with the 3$^{rd}$ of the Koch postulates, and selected two monkeys that were made available by Sigmund Freud in Vienna, who had been testing their intelligence against that of humans. The experiment they then carried out is today celebrated by the World Health Organization, and by other authorities, as being the first to isolate the poliovirus and prove it causes polio.

It is still praised by our universities. For example Leicester University on their website states the theory that polio is not caused by an infection 'was finally dispelled by Landsteiner & Popper (1909), who showed that poliomyelitis was caused by a "filterable agent" – the first human disease to be recognized as having a viral cause.' [84]

But when I read the details of their experiment, I was shocked by its crudeness and the questions it left unanswered. The experiment involved taking the spinal cord from a 9-year-old victim of polio, mincing this and mixing it with water. They then injected a cup of the resulting suspension of human cell debris, blood, DNA, RNA, proteins and enzymes – together with any viruses or toxins present – directly into the brains of these two living monkeys, as well as into other animals.

This toxic mix killed one of the monkeys immediately. The other was slowly paralysed – and later found to have 'similar' damage to its motor neurone cells as found in human polio cases. Landsteiner concluded the paralysis must be caused by an 'invisible' microbe present in the injected material. He wrote: 'The supposition is hence, that a so-called invisible virus or a virus belonging to the class of protozoa causes the disease.' [85] (Protozoa are living single-celled entities, as are bacteria, and can reproduce independently. They are thus very different from what we call viruses.)

Landsteiner and Popper did not stop there. They wanted to prove their virus was infectious. They acquired more monkeys and tried to 'transmit paralysis' between them by grinding up the spinal cords from the sick monkeys and injecting these into the brains of other monkeys, as they had with the child's spinal cords – a process that is still used in vaccine research and technically called 'passaging.' But, they were disappointed. They failed to pass on paralysis.

The following year Simon Flexner and Paul Lewis of the illustrious Rockefeller Institute for Medical Research 'proved' a similarly made noxious soup was 'infectious' by

---

[84] http://www-micro.msb.le.ac.uk/109/introduction.html Leicester University – notes for undergraduates reading microbiology.

[85] Landsteiner K, Popper E. Übertragung der poliomyelitis acuta auf affen. *Z Immunitätsforsch* 1909;2:377-390.

succeeding where the above experiment had failed – by apparently passing paralysis from one monkey to another.   What they did was to similarly prepare a suspension of ground up human backbone and inject this into the living brain of a monkey. They then extracted some fluid from its brain, injected this into another monkey's brain, and so on through a series of monkeys, but this time succeeding in paralysing all of them in the process.

Flexner and Lewis recorded their experiment in the pages of the *Journal of the American Medical Association*. Their conclusion was: 'We failed utterly to discover bacteria, either in film preparations or in cultures, that could account for the disease,' They then went on to say the cause must then be the mysterious virus: 'The infecting agent of epidemic poliomyelitis belongs to the class of the minute and filterable viruses that have not thus far been demonstrated with certainty under the microscope.'[86] Toxic causes were not even considered – let alone the multitude of other things that could well have been in this toxic stew injected directly into the monkeys' brains, thus completely bypassing their immune systems.

Such a soup cannot possibly be considered an 'isolate' of the tiny particle we now call a virus – despite this being claimed. It also proved strangely non-infectious for a virus, for Flexner and Lewis found that the monkeys were not paralysed when made to drink it or when one of their limbs was injected with it, nor did they infect other monkeys. It had to be injected into their brains to have any effect.

The procedures of Flexner and Lewis were just as dubious as their conclusions. They took no account of the contaminants in their mashed-up soup and presumed what happened in monkeys would be replicated in humans. Their experiment thus shed no light on what element had paralysed the monkeys, and for that matter, what had paralysed the children with polio.

Yet these experiments are today celebrated in virology as of great historical importance, as being the first time a virus was proved to cause a human disease and a major epidemic.   But – how could these experiments be so celebrated? How could a scientist credibly claim that injecting cellular debris into the skull of a monkey proves a virus to cause polio?

The more I read of what are supposed to be the victories of polio research, the more I have been, quite frankly, appalled. During the 1920s and 1930s all kinds of biological materials—spinal cord, brain, faecal matter, even flies—were ground up and injected into living monkey brains to induce paralysis, causing great harm to many animals – all in the hope that such experiments would explain why humans were getting summer polio.[87]

The method they used to exclude bacteria from their injected sample of backbone was also quite extraordinary. They put some of the backbone suspension into a dish and watched to see what happened.  They reported: 'If there was no [bacterial] growth after approximately 22 hours of incubation at 37 C., the specimen was considered suitable for inoculation into monkeys. This was not a sterility test, since growth would usually occur on longer incubation; it was rather an indication of the amount of bacterial contamination in the specimen.' Slow growing bacteria were thus deliberately not removed – and no toxin was looked for – yet they knew these might well be present.[88]

From all I read, I was forced to conclude that these 'scientists' shared a doctrinal conviction that the cause of polio must be a particular virus and could be nothing else. They routinely described as 'isolated virus' what was nothing much more than fluid from a cell culture contaminated with many diverse particles and possibly toxins. What else but an irrational belief in a theory could so blind these scientists?

Yet, for a long time they admitted that they could not actually locate a particular particle within these various ground up suspensions called 'viruses' – let alone separate it

[86] S Flexner and PA Lewis; The Journal of the American Medical Association; 33: 639; 13 November 1909

[87] S Flexner; [Trans M Rec]; 78:924-926; 19 November 1910. Also R Scobey; 'Is the public health law responsible for the poliomyelitis mystery?' Archive Of Pediatrics; May 1951

[88] F.B. Gordon and colleagues in the *Journal of Infectious Diseases*,

out so it could be identified. Their practical concept of a virus thus seemed not to differ to any significant degree from the cowpox pus that Jenner had first named as a virus over a hundred years earlier.

The search for the poliovirus led to the invention of the electron microscope in 1932 by Ruska and Knoll, but the epidemics continued unchecked.[89] This made the public extremely impatient with the health authorities, for all they had been told during the first half of the 20th century was that a mysterious invisible virus caused polio and was public enemy Number One – despite it not having been identified.

It was not only polio research that was so blighted. Dr. Max Theiler of the Rockefeller Institute claimed he had invented a vaccine against yellow fever. He had made it by taking serum samples from sick patients and 'passaging' these repeatedly by growing them in mice tissues. He took fluid from the final mouse in the series and injected this into fertilized chicken eggs. After a week of incubation, the chick-embryos were removed from the eggs and finely minced. Human blood serum was then added to 'stabilize' the viruses, although this may give the bird and mouse viruses the chance to mutate into forms that might infect humans. The resulting fluid was his yellow fever vaccine. In 1938 more than one million Brazilians were inoculated with this vaccine before it was discovered that it was contaminated with hepatitis B. [90]

Another example: Harris in 1913 injected filtered tissue material from pellagra victims into monkeys and observed a similar disease developing in these animals. He concluded a virus must be present and be the cause of pellagra. But it was then discovered that this disease is not caused by a virus but by vitamin deficiency. Dr. R. Scobey scathingly commented in 1952: 'It is obvious that if the investigations of pellagra had been restricted to the virus theory, it would still be a mystery.'

It was only in the late 1940s that the scientists researching polio came to identify a particular virus with polio. It was through what is now another famous experiment. In 1948 Gilbert Dalldorf and Grace M. Sickles of the New York State Department of Health claimed to have 'isolated' in the faeces of paralyzed children an 'unidentified, filterable agent' or 'virus' that might be the cause of polio.[91]

They had done so by diluting the excrement of polio-victims. They said they took a '20% faecal suspension, prepared by ether treatment and centrifugation.' (Ether to kill bacteria and centrifugation to remove large particles.) This they had injected 'intracerebrally into mice'– meaning into the living brains of mice. The result was 'suckling mice, 3-7 days of age, became paralyzed...'

So what had they proved with this experiment? Surely, only that paralysis could be induced in young mice by injecting diseased human excrement into their young brains? I was utterly shocked that serious scientists could get away with describing this as the successful 'isolation' of a virus that they had thus proved to cause polio in humans.

They claimed to have proved it was the same as the cause of human polio by injecting the mice with blood serum from paralysed children at the same time as they injected the diluted human excrement. They reported not so many were paralysed. But surely this proved no more that human antibodies might protect from human excrement?

The highly respected bacteriologist Claus Jungeblut critically stated that such 'viral isolates,' including those developed by Salk and other vaccine scientists, had not been

---

[89] Personal communication in 2007 to author from Professor Etienne De Harven.

[90] Polio Vaccines and the Origin of AIDS  B. F. Elswood and R. B. Strickler
*Medical Hypotheses*, vol. 42, 1994, pp. 347-354

[91] G Dalldorf and GM Sickles; 'An unidentified, filterable agent isolated from the faeces of children with paralysis'; Science; 108: 61; 1948

proved to cause polio – as they had not been shown to give monkeys the disease found in human cases of infantile paralysis – and thus had failed to meet the Koch Postulates.[92]

In fact quite the contrary had been demonstrated. Jungeblut said the virus would be so changed or mutated by the way these vaccine scientists passaged it through monkey cells that it would be quite unlike the wild virus by the time it was used for a vaccine. He concluded: 'The highly specialized ... virus which has been maintained in the past by intra-cerebral passage in rhesus monkeys is more likely a laboratory artefact than the agent which causes the natural disease in man.'

It also might not be the only agent at work. Daldorf and Sickle thought at one point that they had detected an agent at work alongside the 'poliovirus,' helping to cause polio. 'The patients we studied may possibly have been coincidentally infected with the new agent and classical poliomyelitis virus.' They tried to test the putative 'new agent' but it was 'not successful in [causing disease in] the rhesus monkey.'

A year later a team lead by Harvard's John F. Enders claimed they could produce this virus from human embryonic cells, thus making it far easier to make a vaccine. For this achievement they were awarded a Nobel Prize in 1954, despite still not having demonstrated that a virus caused polio. They had only shown that their suspension of human cellular material caused illness in laboratory animals.[93]

This 1949 experiment became the scientific basis for the development of the polio vaccines. All this was for me a rude awakening. I never expected to read such crude science.  But, I clung to a last hope  – surely it could not have been dangerous, for if it were then surely many thousands of vaccinated children would be falling ill? Somehow or other, it must have been purified?

Dulbecco and Margaret Vogt in 1954 set out another way to produce virus for the polio vaccine. They used 'virus supplied as a 20% suspension of spinal cord of rhesus monkeys in distilled water.' This was a strange definition for a virus. None in fact was isolated. They said their suspension caused polio but in fact only showed it killed cells in 'plaque assay' tests and could paralyse monkeys. They also claimed that their plaque assay showed a 'single virus' had caused paralysis when at no stage had they produced pure virus. [94]

Up until around the time of these experiments, scientists had logically sought to find the suspect poliovirus in the diseased spinal cords and nerves of polio victims, where it should be found if it caused the illness. That was why they had focused on similar nerve tissue in monkeys. But by 1945 they had searched for over 30 years – and no virus had yet been identified in these tissues as responsible for this damage.

Monkeys were expensive to acquire, but nevertheless many thousands were bought and 'sacrificed' in this hunt. Sabin exposed hundreds of monkeys to cellular material from his polio patients and then watched the monkeys for a month to see if weakness or paralysis developed. If it did, then he performed autopsies to see if the monkeys had suffered the damage to the spinal cord found in human polio victims.  But for him these studies failed, for he could not find in the damaged tissues the virus he was convinced must cause this damage.

---

[92] CW Jungeblut; Journal of Pediatrics; 37: 109; July 1950. R Scobey; Archives of Pediatrics; April 1952

[93] Enders, J.F., T.H. Weller, and F.C. Robbins. 1949. Cultivation of the Lansing strain of poliomyelitis virus in cultures of various human embryonic tissues. Science 109:85.

[94] Dulbecco, R. and M. Vogt. 1954. Plaque formation and isolation of pure lines with poliomyelitis viruses. J. Exp. Med. 99:167-182. I would also like to thank Neenyah Ostrom for her outstanding analysis in 2001 of these experiments. http://www.chronicillnet.org/articles/paralyticpolio.html

Prior to Daldorf and Sickle's experiment many scientists had similarly hopefully named their filtered fluid samples from monkey brains as the 'poliovirus' – but in each case had failed to prove it caused polio. But, if they had succeeded, then growing enough of this to make the vaccine would have proved extremely expensive. The National Foundation for Infantile Paralysis estimated in 1948 that to grow enough poliovirus to inoculate all Americans would need the 'sacrifice' of 50,000 monkeys.

Thus Daldorf and Sickle's 'findings' were most welcome to Sabin and other polio vaccine developers, No longer would they need to try to find the poliovirus in expensive monkeys. No longer would they have to search for it in the nerve cells it reputedly damaged, for Daldorf and Sickle had found it in easily procured human excrement. Under the electron microscope, a small ball-like particle was located in diluted excrement and named as the poliovirus. It was logically classified as 'enterovirus,' a gut virus - not a nerve virus at all, but in their elation, they left aside the issue of how a virus in the gut could cause polio in backbone and brain nerve tissues.

This tiny particle, some 24-30 nm (thousand millionths of a meter) in width, isolated from excrement, thus became the basis of our polio vaccine. Dr. Salk developed the first commercial polio vaccine with virus found in 'the pooled faeces of three healthy children in Cleveland.'[95] It was not found in the victims of polio. That was said to be not necessary! It was undoubtedly safer coming from a healthy child's excrement!

Gut enteroviruses (EV) are very common in humans. Mostly they are linked to mild illnesses such as the common cold. They are reportedly hard to work with in the laboratory. Poliovirus was recently reclassified as a HEV – meaning an enterovirus produced only by human gut cells, therefore not an invader at all. Typically human viruses will not cause disease in humans – meaning this one must be highly unusual – if it is the real cause of polio.

Then the vaccine developers found there were three variants of this gut virus, all naturally in excrement from polio victims. This was bad news for the manufacturers. It meant, they thought, that all three were needed for an effective polio vaccine.

Given how many millions of humans were to be dosed with this vaccine, an incredible number of viruses now had to be produced for it. But the scientists fortuitously now discovered a cheap way of doing this that did not require the purchase of monkeys. They would grow poliovirus on the prolifically multiplying cervical cancer cells of a woman called Henrietta Lacks who died in 1951. These cell cultures are now known as 'HeLa' after her. [96] In 1953, the National Foundation for Infantile Paralysis (NFIP) established facilities at the Tuskegee Institute for the mass production and distribution of HeLa cells, shipping some 600,000 cultures around the country, initially for safety testing the polio vaccine but soon also for multitudes of other scientific experiments.

But, without anyone noticing, HeLa cells grew so fast that unnoticed they contaminated vast numbers of 'viral samples' around the world, a disaster for thousands of experiments – and one that did not say much for laboratory sterility practices. [97]

Major polio vaccine scientists, such as Koprowski, thought they were growing poliovirus on monkey cells, only to be horrified to discover that they were inadvertently using human cancer cells. After this, HeLa, and all other human tissues, were banned in

---

[95] A.B. Sabin, A.B. & L. Boulger, History of Sabin Attenuated Poliovirus Oral Live Vaccine Strains. 1 J. BIOL. STAND. 115, 115–18 (1973).

[96] 'Studies on the Propagation In Vitro of Poliomyelitis Viruses,' J. Exp. Med., 97: 695-715, 1953

[97] In 1974 Walter Nelson-Rees would devastatingly report that HeLa cells had infiltrated the entire world's stock of cell cultures, and that for decades scientists had been doing experiments on what they thought were breast cells, or prostrate or placental cells, for example, when in fact they were using HeLa cells.

1954 for vaccine manufacturing in the States. The health authorities feared that they might introduce cancer-causing elements into the vaccines.[98]

However, Sabin had not been affected. He was using monkey cells rather than cancerous human cells to grow the poliovirus found in human excrement. He was financed to do so by an $8.1 million grant from the National Foundation for Infantile Paralysis (NFIP). He took as his raw material the 'Mahoney poliovirus isolate' filtered from the diluted excrement of polio patients by 2 scientists, Francis and Mack.

But Dr. Jonas Salk had to admit to an appalled audience of cell biologists and vaccine makers that HeLa cancer cells had also contaminated his cell lines on at least one occasion. [99] He confessed he had thought he was injecting a culture of monkey cells into 30 or more elderly cancer patients to see if these would stimulate their immune systems into fighting their cancers. But he had inadvertently injected them with cancerous human HeLa cells, about the worse thing possible. He discovered this when abscesses developed at the injection sites.

In 1954 Salk safety tested his 'polio vaccine' on more than 400,000 US children. It was reported afterwards that 'only' 112 of the children who received three jabs of his vaccine contracted polio within the next few months. Salk counted this as a great success.[100]

But Salk had manipulated these vaccine safety trial figures. From his own reports, he had not removed from his vaccine the host of monkey particles, proteins, DNA, other viruses and prions that such a crudely designed vaccine contained. It was also likely to contain some of the toxin formaldehyde (as has since been verified. The polio vaccine used (2008) in the US still contains formaldehyde.)

Although Salk claimed his polio vaccine was a great success, his official safety report states that that it only proved to protect '30 to 90 per cent' of recipients, a remarkably vague statistic. However, with a highly lucrative 300% mark-up, manufacturers were keen to make the vaccine even if it were often ineffective.[101]

Salk had also failed to make an allowance for the many children who did not need his vaccine because they were already totally immune to the poliovirus. One report stated that, in households with poor cleanliness, over 80% of the unvaccinated children already possessed protective antibodies against the poliovirus. [102]

Salk marketed his patented vaccine 'seed' to manufacturers who sprinkled it onto vast quantities of minced monkey kidney to make the invisible virus multiply a million-fold – before destroying it with formaldehyde. Six US manufacturers thus made 27 million doses in 1955 under their own brands, in absolute confidence that it would subsequently be approved as safe by the National Foundation for Infantile Paralysis, a powerful lobby group that was desperate, as was the public, for a remedy for polio.

Despite these many problems, the Foundation declared on April 12th 1955 that Salk's polio vaccine was totally safe and gave complete protection from polio. It launched it that same day before an invited audience of 500 doctors and 200 journalists, plus some 54,000 doctors linked by closed-circuit television in cities throughout North America.

---

[98] In 1974 Walter Nelson-Rees would devastatingly report that HeLa cells had infiltrated the entire world's stock of cell cultures, and that for decades scientists had been doing experiments on what they thought were breast cells, or prostrate or placental cells, for example, when in fact they were using HeLa cells.

[99] A detailed account of this medical catastrophe is given in Michael Gold's 'A Conspiracy of Cells: One Woman's Immortal Legacy and the Medical Scandal It Caused.'

[100] T Francis Jr; 'An evaluation of the 1954 poliomyelitis vaccine trials summary report'; American Journal of Public Health; 45: 1-63; 1955

[101] Bookchin and Shumacher *The Virus and the Vaccine* St Martins Press. 2004. Page 37

[102] Melnick JL, Paul JR, Walton M. Serologic epidemiology of Poliomyelitis. Am J Public Health 1955; 45:429-37. http://epirev.oxfordjournals.org/cgi/reprint/21/1/7

President Dwight Eisenhower awarded Salk the Congressional Medal while declaring the vaccine a great victory for American science. In *The Manchester Guardian* Alistair Cooke wrote: 'Nothing short of the overthrow of the Communist regime in the Soviet Union could bring such rejoicing to the hearts and homes in America as the historic announcement last Tuesday that the 166-year war against poliomyelitis is almost certainly at an end.'

But within two weeks of being vaccinated, over 260 children fell ill with polio, of which nearly 200 were paralyzed and 11 died. In the resulting urgent inquiry, the pharmaceutical company Lilly let it be known to the authorities that they knew several monkey viruses were contaminating the vaccines. They said the presence of these monkey viruses might mask that of live poliovirus. [103] But the public were told there was nothing to worry about – for the President's grandson had the vaccine with no ill effects!

The result was that the Cutter laboratory was scapegoated, accused of not properly mixing in the formaldehyde, although the evidence was that other laboratories were also producing flawed vaccines.

Cutter had its production temporarily shut down. But more cases of polio among the vaccinated were then reported. On May 6th 1955 it was reported that in 9 out of 10 cases the paralysis occurred in the arms in which the vaccine had been injected – suggesting that the vaccine itself was causing polio. [104] Thus on May 8th all the US polio vaccine-manufacturing plants were shut pending safety tests. The difficulties proved to be so serious that Sabin proposed over a month later, on June 23,[rd] that the entire nation's polio vaccine production should be suspended immediately.

However, Salk's people held key positions on the relevant vaccine safety committee and they disregarded Sabin's reservations completely, rejecting them as those of a commercial rival, and voted to continue production.[105] It was simply ordered that, in future, the vaccine should be mixed and filtered better – and no lumps allowed in it.

In June 1955, an article authored by the Nobel Laureate, John Enders of Harvard, appeared in the University of Michigan Medical Bulletin. He had won his Nobel Prize for his work on polio vaccines and he now declared that the current technique was flawed. He warned that, beyond the risk of failing to kill the poliovirus, the defective technique also raised 'the risk of including other agents whose presence may or may not be recognized.'

But Enders' cautionary words had no effect. Instead scientists fought to have their polio vaccines replace Salk's in the market place. Hilary Koprowski in 1956 gave his experimental vaccine a field trial in Belfast in Northern Ireland, but this was discontinued when virus found in the stools of the vaccinated was reported to paralyse monkeys. Koprowski then modified his vaccine and tested the new version on a quarter of a million Congolese – despite them never having suffered from a polio outbreak, and despite it being known that nearly all of them were already immune to the virus through normal infanthood exposure.

Sabin headed to Russia, where he tested his polio vaccine on 4 million of their children, despite Professor Konstantine Vinokouroff of the Institute of Neurology, part of the Russian Academy of Medical Science, having told the Americans in 1952, to their disbelief, that the Soviet Union had never had an outbreak of polio.[106] Cox of Lederle conducted his trials in Florida and Berlin, Germany, but these led to a high rate of paralysis said to be due to vaccine-derived strains reverting to virulence.

---

[103] Bookchin and Shumacher *The Virus and the Vaccine* St Martins Press. 2004. Page 52

[104] News Chronicle. May 6, 1955. This is now known as 'Provocation POLIO,; apparently produced by the arm muscle injected being poisoned by the vaccine. It is still common, especially in over vaccinated children in developing nations.

[105] Bookchin and Shumacher *The Virus and the Vaccine* St Martins Press. 2004. Page 295

[106] This was at the Second International Congress on Poliomyelitis, held in 1952

In 1958, the National Institutes of Health created a special committee on live polio vaccines to supervise tests on the strains of virus 'isolates' authorized for the oral vaccine. The Koprowski and Cox strains were eliminated, as were those of Yale University, in favour of three 'sugar-cube' strains produced by Sabin. These would from 1961 rapidly replace the Salk and become the only strains used worldwide until recent years. The Salk vaccine had proven to be so ineffective at stopping polio that the Journal of the American Medical Association said of it on February 25, 1961: 'It is now generally recognized that much of the Salk vaccine used in the U.S. has been worthless.' [107]

There was another problem perplexing the polio scientists. It was difficult to explain why it was mostly the middle-class children that got polio. In other epidemics, the children most likely to fall ill were those living in poverty, with poor water supplies and little hygiene. So, why were the polio epidemics so very different?

But this riddle has since been solved, or so it seems. The Centers for Disease Control (CDC), the foremost US institution in the hunt for viruses, has published a surprising explanation. On its website Dr. John H. Lienhard of the University of Houston explains in *Polio and Clean Water*: 'The cause of the epidemics turns out to have been, of all things, improved hygiene. There was a time when everyone got polio. It was in everyone's drinking water. When it struck a very young child, the child would suffer a little diarrhoea, bounce back, and then be immune. Polio was rarely severe enough at that age to cause severe damage, so we were hardly aware of it. Like measles, mumps, and chicken pox, the disease simply immunized the child.'

But this hygiene had proved dangerous! Lienhard explained it made children from middle class households more susceptible to polio because they were cleaner than working class children, and thus less exposed to garden dirt. The poliovirus lives in garden soil but can only reproduce in the human gut. It is thus dependent on being eaten by infants who are not yet immune to it. As working class children are more exposed to dirt, or so goes this theory, they eat more of these viruses, and these kick-start their immune systems – making them immune to polio for life. Thus when a polio epidemic strikes, it hits the middle class children who do not eat garden dirt – or so goes this CDC endorsed theory. [108]

The American Food and Drug Administration (FDA) had reported much the same: 'In less hygienic times … there was plenty of opportunity to contract polio. Polioviruses infected each new generation of babies, who were protected in part by antibodies passed on to them by their mothers. These infections early in life were usually mild and non-paralytic, sometimes appearing with cold-like symptoms, sometimes with no symptoms at all. They were often indistinguishable from a host of other childhood diseases, and were rarely diagnosed as polio. With better hygiene, there was less chance for babies and young children to contact the mild form of the disease and acquire immunity. When the disease struck older children or adults, it was more likely to take the paralytic form.'

I thought this at first a brilliant theory. I learnt from it how nature has equipped us with incredibly efficient immune systems. But I then thought, surely middle-class children go out in the garden to play? Surely they would be exposed to the same dirt? I mischievously thought for a moment, why not expose them to dirt – wouldn't this be more effective and cheaper than vaccination?

But seriously, if the cause of polio was not a gut virus found in excrement, then do we have any likely alternatives?

---

[107] Journal of the American Medical Association February 25, 1961

[108] GN Callahan; 'Eating dirt'; Emerging Infectious Diseases; August 2003; www.cdc.gov/ncidod/EID/vol9no8/03-0033.htm

# Chapter 5

# What could cause polio, if not a virus?

Robert Koch taught that there was one causative germ per disease. His doctrine has ever since dominated much of virology.

But, in 1951 the vaccine scientists reported that to their surprise they could not find the designated poliovirus, the gut virus, in many polio victims! This should have stopped the vaccine trials dead. If the virus were not there, the vaccine would be useless. Even worse was to come. They found a different virus might be present, such as the Coxsackie, and speculated this also might cause polio. This news was grimly received. The Koch Postulates state that an agent could not be claimed to cause an illness if it is not present in all cases.

Salk and Sabin could not stomach the idea that they might have got the wrong cause. They were still wed to the idea that the cause had to be a virus - but if other viruses could cause polio, this was disastrous to their hopes of success with their vaccine. It meant that their vaccines would not give the protection promised against all forms of polio. AL Hoynel reported in the journal *The Medical Clinics of North America* that there was 'some feeling of dismay ... [it] added one more problem to the nebulous conditions surrounding poliomyelitis... the more we learn about poliomyelitis, the less we know,' An editorial in the *Lancet* stated this discovery brought 'a crop of new snags' to developing a vaccine. If other viruses were involved, the vaccines in development would at best diminish, not stop, the polio epidemics

But, from all that I have read, that the health authorities then promptly resolved this dilemma by forgetting about it, for I could find no trace of any subsequent attempts to develop vaccines for these other polio-causing viruses. It must have been hoped that no one would notice. This was indeed likely. At that time polio cases were diagnosed by clinical symptoms, as with other diseases. This meant in diagnosis the poliovirus was presumed to be present and not actually looked for.

With the other viruses seemingly obliterated from memory, from now on finding the poliovirus in the excrement of victims became essential to diagnosing polio, This diagnostic rule still applies and is on the World Health Organization's website. They demand that samples of two turds from each victim of infantile paralysis be sent to their laboratories. If no poliovirus is found in these, the cases are declared not to be polio, even if these children are suffering from the same severe paralysis, symptoms and pain, that would have been diagnosed as the gravest form of polio during the American epidemics.

When I discovered this, I thought this was an insane way to prove the illness was caused by the poliovirus. They were excluding by fiat all cases where another virus is present! Also, surely the absence of the poliovirus in such cases suggests that it may be misidentified as a major cause of this disease?

All this made me sit back and think. If the nominated viruses were not present in all polio cases – could the disease be caused by a toxin or environmental factor that worked with several viruses? I went back to reading the accounts of the doctors who treated the polio cases during the great epidemics, hoping that their research might shed some light on this.

I soon found that, outside the hothouse of virological research, there were doctors treating the casualties of the polio epidemics who had very different ideas about what caused polio, based on their observations during clinical diagnosis.  I found they were inclined, from the evidence they observed, to blame the polio epidemics on toxins rather than on viruses.

The germ theory is so well established that I did not feel I had any right to reject it – but I now wondered if there might be a compromise? Even if one accepted that poliovirus had a major role in causing polio, could some other factor be needed to make this virus dangerous?  Could an environmental factor affect the victims' immune systems,' making children susceptible to this virus? Might bacteria also be involved? Could toxins produced by bacteria or coming from other sources make the suspected viruses more virulent, and thus help create these epidemics?

I soon found that the doctors who blamed toxins had precedents to draw on. It is now mostly forgotten that environmental factors were frequently blamed for causing epidemics before the 20th century.  Several epidemics were successfully brought to an end simply by the provision of clean water and better sanitation.

Most of us are thus unaware of the historical importance of the hunt for the poliovirus during the first half of the 20th Century.  It was the decades-long 'Manhattan' project of virology; the project that established this science in the pattern that it has followed until today.  It set out to prove a virus caused a major disease and took forty years to do so. It effectively removed from consideration all other possible causes of epidemics. It made vaccine provision a prime responsibility of governments, given this priority in practice over the provision of good water supplies and adequate nutrition.

Before this it had been bacteria that featured in the 'germ theory' of disease. A virus was then either Jenner's cowpox pus or a theoretical entity, a liquid containing invisibly small bacteria that might explain the spread of disease when no bacterial agent could be found.

But this 'Manhattan project' was slow to bring results. It commenced in the 1890s and by 1950 little had been achieved. The most famed of the poliovirus experiments reveal, when read in detail, that sixty years of this hunt failed to isolate any virus proved to cause polio.  What were being experimented with, and named as polioviruses, were fluids from cultures, filtered extracts from diseased tissues and even from the excrement of sick children. In other words, they were still working with toxic fluids they called viruses and it was these that they were testing to see if they caused polio.

Before the invention of the electron microscope, the identifying characteristics of a virus, according to published research, was to be invisibly present in finely filtered fluid taken from laboratory cell cultures, or sick humans. They were thus identified as 'filterable agents.' It was presumed that invisibly small mini-bacteria had gone through the anti-bacteria filter – as the resulting fluid was still pathogenic.  Their final defining feature was that these particles could 'replicate'. This meant in practice that cells made ill with this noxious brew, seemed to produce more of this brew.

But we now know there are many things smaller than viruses that might pass through the same filter and be potentially hazardous – such as DNA and RNA fragments, proteins, prions, enzymes – and chemical toxins. There was also the 'alien' factor. Human material was being put into monkeys or other animals, and since this was alien to them, this might be what was poisoning them.

Scientists tried to exclude these possibilities by 'passaging' samples of their culture from one animal to another to another, as in the monkey experiments described above. They mostly picked monkeys, as these were most alike to humans.  They hoped the repeated 'passaging' though monkey tissues would remove anything in their fluid that was not being reproduced, or 'replicated.'

In the early stages of polio research they had no idea how their postulated viruses might be reproducing themselves. As the poisonous liquids seemed to be passed from one individual to another without losing virulence, they presumed these must contain dangerous mini-bacteria, able to divide and reproduce themselves.

It was not until the 1930s that electron microscopes made it possible to see tiny particles that might be the sought after viruses. These were apparently too simple in construction to be able to reproduce themselves, but since they were observed to be produced by cells and to be going into cells, it was postulated that the cells' massive reproductive chemistry must be 'hijacked' by them in order to preserve their viral species.

These viruses were presumed nearly equal to bacterial cells in aggressive ability, but we now know that the genetic codes of viruses are vastly smaller than that of bacteria. The former averages around 500 million base pairs long, while that of a typical virus is around ten thousand long.

The scientists engaged on this hunt had to establish that these particles caused the illness in question. This in itself was a long and difficult process. According to Koch, they should be given to an animal, to see if they caused the same illness. Logically they should have been given to a human. This was rarely done. It was clearly unethical without informed consent.

To help in this work, they developed a technique called 'plaque purification.' A sample of their culture was filtered to remove bacteria and particles larger than viruses. It was then added to a dish containing a one-cell thick layer of cells. If cleared spaces or 'plaques' appeared in this layer, these were counted to measure the virulence of the virus presumed responsible for clearing these spaces by killing cells. The sample was then diluted to the point where diluting it further stopped plaque formation. It was hoped this meant it contained a 'purified' virus. But, what if many things contributed to the cells' deaths – as Koch himself said of septicaemia? Further tests were still required.

What of toxins? Could they be present in these cultures? What also of cellular waste products – could these pass on illnesses? Comparatively little scientific work seems to have been done to exclude this possibility. Also, could viruses be a natural product of poisoned cells? Again I could find little research on this possibility. But, I thought it was unlikely that toxins were involved, for how could toxins have caused the massive summertime polio plagues? Surely the cause had to be something infective?

I went back to the first medical reports on the polio outbreaks. They were from Vermont in New England and issued by the Government Inspector, Dr. Charles Caverly. He noted the families affected did not know each other, so his report explicitly ruled out it being a 'contagious' disease (much to my surprise). He also noted without comment that some parents told him their children fell ill after eating fruit.[109]

His official report surprisingly stated that the outbreaks of infantile paralysis 'usually occurred in [a single child from] families of more than one child, and as no efforts were made at isolation it was very certain it was non-contagious.' He thus concluded the paralytic outbreak was probably caused by a toxin, and not by a microorganism. Reading this, I wondered if the vaccine scientists had ever bothered to consult with him?

What toxin could it be? There was an outstanding candidate. Jim West has noted, on his well-documented website, that this report was dated 1892, just two years after lead arsenate pesticide started to be sprayed many times every summer to kill the codling moth on apple crops. Vermont was a major apple-growing region – and its polio epidemics started shortly after this pesticide came into widespread summer use.

---

[109] CS Caverly; Yale Med J.; 1:1; 1894. I obtained this report from Mr Jim West, a researcher who maintained an extensive online library on the relationship between polio and pesticides - and on the West Nile Virus – at a website *Images of Poliomyelitis*. This is not currently online (September 2008) but his highly recommendable work is now available at http://www.wellwithin1.com/PolioJimWest.htm

It seems Caverly's report had rung alarm bells among doctors other than virologists. Some remembered that metal workers had suffered for centuries from a seemingly identical paralysis caused by the lead and arsenic in metals they were processing – the very same 'heavy metals' that were sprayed up to 12 times a summer over apple orchards. The pesticide was made of neurotoxins that paralysed – for that was how they killed the moths. The toxins suffocate the moths by attacking the nerves that go to the muscles that enable them to breathe – the very same nerves that are damaged in humans in the worse cases of polio, that forced patients to use iron-lungs to breathe! Seemingly, no one seemed to have thought that what was done to insects might also affect humans.

The paralytic effect of these metals had been observed as far back as 1824, when the English scientist John Cooke observed: 'The fumes of these metals, or the receptance of them in solution into the stomach, often cause paralysis.'[110] The common name for this illness then was 'palsy,' short for paralysis. This was an ancient disease  - there is evidence that the ancient Egyptians suffered from it  (see leg in picture) – but I do not know if there it were among their metal workers.

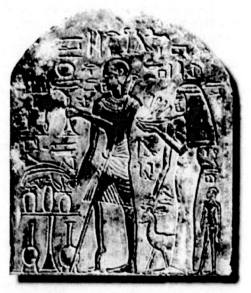

In 1878 Alfred Vulpian had experimentally established that lead damages the motor-neuron cells of dogs.[111] This is the same damage that is found in children with infantile paralysis. Then in 1883 the Russian Popow discovered the same damage could be done with arsenic.

They had completed their research while Koch was developing the germ theory, but his focus was on epidemics. These heavy metal poisoning cases involved no general epidemic. They were only then among metal workers.

Perhaps if their work had been better known in the West, lead arsenate would never have been used as a pesticide? The spraying was in summer and autumn – so this would explain why polio epidemics struck in summer and autumn. It would also explain why the first of these epidemics occurred in orchard-rich New England – for that is where lead arsenate was widely introduced from 1892. It would also explain why some New England children went down immediately after eating fresh fruit. This was making much sense. None of these observations were explained by the poliovirus theory.

Lead arsenate was not the only new pesticide then coming into wide use. In 1907 calcium arsenate was introduced primarily for use on cotton crops and in cotton mills. A year later in a Massachusetts town with three cotton mills and apple orchards 69 children suddenly fell ill with infantile paralysis.[112] This was apparently the world's second outbreak of epidemic polio.

Other cases were linked to milk supplies.  At that time formaldehyde was added to milk to prolong its 'shelf life.' This might also have been responsible for some cases of

---

[110] Cooke, John: Treatise of Nervous Diseases, 1824

[111] Vulpian, A.: Quoted by R. W. Lovett, Ref below.

[112] CS Caverly; Yale Med J.; 1:1; 1894.  Also CK Mills; [Boston M & S J]; 108: 248-250; 15 March 1883

polio. In 1897 The *Australian Medical Gazette* reported that formaldehyde in milk had caused several cases of paralysis.[113] Lead arsenate was also used in cow dips.

The UK banned apple imports from the States because they were so heavily polluted with lead arsenate. Today many former US apple orchard sites are listed as heath hazards, on which no building can take place without the total removal of poisoned soil.

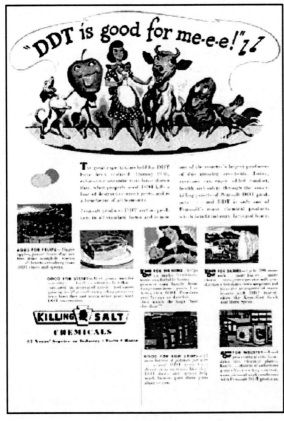

A toxic cause for polio would crucially explain why farmyard chickens and animals were reported as suffering paralysis at the same time as the children. This should not have happened, according to the virologists, for their poliovirus can only infect humans.

I had never before questioned if the poliovirus were responsible for polio. I had taken it as a given fact – so I was extremely surprised at finding this research. It was fascinating to find evidence that so challenged established theories. It stretched my mind, helped me think laterally. But I said to myself, none of this explained why a polio vaccine stopped the epidemics. Surely this by itself finally proves the poliovirus causes the illness, that the vaccine scientists, despite many blunders, had eventually got things right? If they had not – why were there now no polio epidemics?

The answer was none too clear to me. Again I thought, perhaps it was that the virus and the toxins were co-factors; that the toxins weakened the immune systems to allow the virus to attack?

I read how Dr. D. Bodian of Baltimore found in 1954 that injecting a 'poliovirus sample' into the hearts of monkeys made half of them paralysed. But he had then found, if he injected them first with toxins or irritants, including penicillin or DPT vaccine, the number paralysed went up to 80 per cent and the paralysis frequently occurred in the limb injected![114]

This raised the issue for me of whether the DPT vaccine could also be a factor. I knew that UK doctors had observed paralysis occurring in some of the arms vaccinated. This vaccine was also introduced around the time of the polio epidemics.

[113] *Australian Medical Gazette; 24 August 1897*

[114] Bodian D. (1934) .*Amer. Jour. Hygiene.* 60, 339.

Once I started on this line of inquiry, the evidence poured in like a flood. I learnt other pesticides could also cause paralysis. In the mid 1940s powerful neurotoxin pesticides were introduced, including the organochlorine DDT. A local polio epidemic in the UK town of Broadstairs, Kent, was linked to a dairy where the cows were washed down with DDT. It ended when the dairy was stopped from supplying milk. Apparently local doctors discovered this toxin link.

Albert Sabin, a major developer of polio vaccines, had earlier reported some crucial evidence, the significance of which he did not seem to fully appreciate. He discovered that poliomyelitis was the major cause of sickness and death among the American troops based in the Philippines at the end of the Second World War, while the neighbouring Philippines settlements were not affected.[115] US military camps in the Philippines were sprayed daily with DDT to kill mosquitoes.

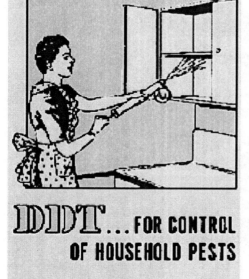

**DDT ... FOR CONTROL OF HOUSEHOLD PESTS**

But stronger evidence came, to my surprise, from the great American national laboratories. The National Institutes of Health reported in 1944 that DDT damaged the same anterior horn cells that are damaged in infantile paralysis.

However, these reports did not prevent DDT from making its way into shops to be sold as a common household pesticide – or from being advertised as 'good for you.' DDT after the Second World War rapidly replaced lead arsenate as the pesticide of choice. By 1950 the number of cases of infantile paralysis had increased nearly threefold over those of 1930. **On the right: an advertisement of the time.**[116]

Endocrinologist Dr. Morton Biskind found in 1949 that DDT causes 'lesions in the spinal cord resembling those in human polio.' In Germany in that same year, Daniel Dresden found acute DDT poisoning produced 'degeneration in the central nervous system' seemingly identical to that found in severe cases of infantile paralysis.[117] Both DDT and the new more powerful organochlorine pesticide DDE were found to penetrate the blood-brain barrier that protected the central nervous system.

Then two years later in 1951 the US Public Health Service reported: 'DDT is a delayed-action poison. Due the fact that it accumulates in the body tissues, especially in females, the repeated inhalation or ingestion of DDT constitutes a distinct health hazard. The deleterious effects are manifested principally in the liver, spleen, kidneys and spinal cord.' Again, I noted that the spinal cord was where the damage was done that caused polio paralysis.

---

[115] Albert Sabin in *The Journal of the American Medical Association*. June 1947.

[116] I am grateful to Jim West's website, 'Images of Poliomyelitis' for unearthing these posters.

[117] D Dresden; Physiological Investigations into the Action Of DDT; GW Van Der Wiel & Co; Arnhem; 1949

Dr. Biskind, a practitioner and medical researcher, also came to the conclusion that pesticides were the major cause of the polio epidemics. He presented the evidence to the US Congress, but the medical establishment ignored it. The germ theory of polio had captured its attention – and nearly all the available funding. He lamented: 'Despite the fact that DDT is a highly lethal poison for all species of animals, the myth has become prevalent among the general population that it is safe for man in virtually any quantity. Not only is it used in households with reckless abandon so that sprays and aerosols are inhaled, the solutions are permitted to contaminate skin, bedding and other textiles.'[118] Children's bedrooms were 'protected' against the suspected poliovirus by having their walls covered with wallpaper pre-soaked in DDT.

His words made me stop and think. Surely it was mostly the middle-class households that used pesticide sprays with such abandon? Working-class households had less money to spray – and would instead have clouted flies with rolled up newspapers – or so I surmised. Could this be why the middle classes suffered from polio so much more?

They sprayed because they were terrified of the widely reported, but scientifically still undiscovered, poliovirus. Posters everywhere asked parents to stop the virus by keeping their kids clean. No medical help was available. They begged and begged the authorities to find a cure. Yet for decades the only advice the health authorities had for these distraught parents was to wash hands, disinfect doorknobs, keep the children clean, indoors and away from public swimming pools – all for fear of the unknown poliovirus.

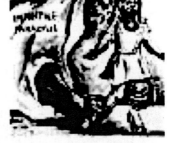

These scary posters were distributed by the 1938-founded National Foundation for Infant Paralysis, and designed, not just to educate, but to motivate people to fund the hunt for the poliovirus – which in the 1950s consumed \$200 million dollars raised in the 'March of Dimes.' Other medical research was neglected

Many middle class parents went further to protect their children. They feared the invisible virus as if it were hunting their children. They turned their homes into sterile zones by constantly spraying insecticides and washing down the walls with disinfectants. Their fear became contagious and their zeal fanatic, encouraged by health authority posters showing giant flies attacking children. Parents literally hid their children from all strangers lest they might infect them.

Their excessive use of household pesticides made the argument that pesticides were to blame for these epidemics seem ever more plausible – but I still thought, if pesticides were involved, how then could the success of the polio vaccines be explained?

Biskind of course was doing his research before a vaccine was released and so was not affected by such doubts. He was not primarily a laboratory scientist but a doctor treating the victims of polio. He thought pesticides caused their illness so treated them as victims of poisoning. The first step in such a treatment is to remove the toxin from their food and environment. He did so and found many recovered, especially when contaminated milk products were also stopped. He tested butter purchased in New York and found high concentrations of DDT. The government ignored his important discovery, so he wrote in anger: 'Although young animals are much more susceptible to the effects of

---

[118] MS Biskind and I Bieber; 'DDT poisoning: a new syndrome with neuropsychiatric manifestations'; American Journal Of Psychotherapy; page 261; 1949

DDT than adults, so far as the available literature is concerned, it does not appear that the effects of such concentrations on infants and children have even been considered.'[119]

Other doctors reported success in treating polio patients with dimercaprol, a chelating agent still used in hospitals to treat heavy metal poisoning.  In 1951 Dr. Irwin Eskwith reported he thus cured a child with most severe form of polio, bulbar paralysis.[120] I was also surprised to read that Dr. F. R. Klenner reported in the July 1949 issue of the *Journal of Southern Medicine and Surgery* that he had cured 17 acute cases of polio with large doses of another anti-toxin, ascorbic acid![121] He reported: "In the poliomyelitis epidemic in North Carolina in 1948, 60 cases of this disease came under our care. ... In 15 of these cases the diagnosis was confirmed by lumbar puncture. ... The treatment employed was vitamin C in massive doses every two to four hours. The initial dose was 1,000 to 2,000 mg, depending on age. ... Children up to four years received the injections intramuscularly  ... All patients were clinically well after 72 hours.'

But this remarkable news left the government totally unmoved. This led to angry and extremely frustrated complaints. These medical professionals could not understand why government health officers would not question the viral theory of polio despite it providing no cures. Why was their work ignored, when they had solved the enigma and provided a cure? Yet public health officials stubbornly ignored their reports as 'illogical and impossible.'

Nevertheless, Biskind in 1950 gained an invitation to present his evidence to a US Congressional Hearing.[122] By now he  was by no means alone. Dr. Ralph Scobey had found clear evidence of poisoning when analysing the blood of polio victims: '*There are two abnormal findings in cases of poliomyelitis that point strongly to poisoning as the cause of this disease. One consists in the appearance of increased amounts of porphyrin in the urine; the other is the presence of increased amounts of guanidine in the blood. It is a well-known fact that porphyria can follow poisoning by a number of chemicals. Guanidine has been found in increased amounts in the blood in arsenic, chloroform, and carbon tetrachloride poisonings.*'[123]

I had not heard of this before. However, on checking, I found his work is by no means out-dated. Today it is established in toxicology that certain kinds of poisoning can be measured by analysing the amount of the chemical porphyrin in a patient's urine.[124]

Dr. Scobey was invited to testify at Congress in 1951. That year also the US Public Health Service reported: 'DDT is a delayed-action poison. Due to the fact that it accumulates in the body tissues, especially in females, the repeated inhalation or ingestion of DDT constitutes a distinct health hazard. The deleterious effects are manifested principally in the liver, spleen, kidneys and spinal cord... DDT is excreted in the milk of cows and of nursing mothers.' For a while it even seemed just about possible that Scobey and Biskind might succeed, and that the virus theory of polio would be abandoned.

---

[119] MS Biskind; Statement on clinical intoxication from DDT and other new insecticides, presented before United States House of Representatives to investigate the use of chemicals in food products; *Journal Of Insurance Medicine;* May, 1951

[120] I.S. Eskwith; American Journal of Diseases of Children; 81: 684-686; May 1951

[121] Pages 211-212.

[122] MS Biskind; Statement on clinical intoxication from DDT and other new insecticides, presented before United States House of Representatives to investigate the use of chemicals in food products; *Journal Of Insurance Medicine*; May, 1951

[123] Dr Ralph R. Scobey The Poison Cause of Poliomyelitis Archives of Pediatrics, vol. 69, p172 (April 1952).

[124] For example: 'Previous studies from this laboratory have described metal-specific changes in the urinary porphyrin excretion pattern (porphyrin profile) associated with prolonged exposure of animals and humans to low levels of mercury, arsenic, lead, and other metals (reviewed in Woods, 1995 http://toxsci.oxfordjournals.org/cgi/content/full/61/2/234

But it seems the medical establishment was so wedded to the viral theory of polio that it was adamant that this theory could not be questioned. Instead some doctors subjected their ideas to ridicule. This made Biskind absolutely fume. He angrily reported, in a 1953 paper published in the *American Journal of Digestive Diseases*: '*It was known by 1945 that DDT is stored in the body fat of mammals and appears in [their] milk... Yet, far from admitting a causal relationship [between DDT and polio] that is so obvious, which in any other field of biology would be instantly accepted, virtually the entire apparatus of communication, lay and scientific alike, has been devoted to denying, concealing, suppressing, distorting and attempts to convert into its opposite this overwhelming evidence. Libel, slander and economic boycott have not been overlooked in this campaign.*' [125]

He had inadvertently made enemies. If he were believed, his explanation might well bring an embarrassing halt to the career of many prominent virologists and as well as to government health advisors.

Yet, I have discovered recent research that indicates Biskind and Scobey might well have been right. A recent paper has concluded: 'A very specific effect of exposure to some poisons such as the organophosphate insecticides (e.g. malathion, parathion) relates to their anticholinesterase effect.' This meant the pesticides impede nerve messages to muscle cells, causing 'weakness of muscles and paralysis including of respiration.' In other words, these pesticides cause the key symptoms of paralytic polio. [126]

I have also learnt that patients suffering today from 'post-polio syndrome' – the reoccurrence of paralytic symptoms decades later in the victims of the polio epidemics – are now being successfully treated by toxicology – again, as if their symptoms are due to toxins not a virus. An example: a group of 17 individuals suffering from post-polio syndrome were placed in a toxin-free environment and were treated with antidotes to toxins. 'Long-term follow-up of the 14 improved patients showed general return of wellbeing and renewed vigour,' and 'eight became totally pain-free'. The researchers concluded that 'post-polio syndrome' was due to an 'overload of environmental pollutants on wounded target organs.' [127]

But the toxicologists in the 1950s had failed to win their case. Their findings were not accepted as relevant by the health authorities, despite no one else finding a cure for polio. (A vaccine is a preventive, not a cure.) The germ theory advocates were just too powerful and dug in.

During the first great polio epidemic in 1916, the national polio case rate reached a high of 41.1 cases per 100,000 but then sharply dropped. Between the two World Wars it mostly stayed below 12 per 100,000. But after the Second World War, after the introduction of DDT, the polio rate tripled to reach a peak of over 37 polio cases per 100,000 in 1952. In that year 58,000 Americans got polio – and 1,400 died of it.

However, from the early 1950s the public had started to become aware of the danger of overusing pesticides. This was after the 1951 report from the US Public Health Service that warned: 'DDT is excreted in the milk of cows and of nursing mothers after exposure to DDT sprays and after consuming food contaminated with this poison. Children and infants especially are much more susceptible to poisoning than adults.'

The regulatory authorities responded. The US Congressional Delaney Committee decided to investigate chemical contamination of food and laid the foundation for the 1954 Miller Pesticide Amendment. It was, however, a cumbersome progress, with none of the urgency required.

---

[125] MS Biskind; 'Public health aspects of the new insecticides'; *American Journal of Digestive Diseases*; 20: 330; 1953

[126] http://www.agius.com/hew/resource/toxicol.htm

[127] WJ Rea et al; 'The environmental aspects of the post-polio syndrome';[ www.aehf.com/A56.htm

Jim West has reported: 'The decline of polio actually occurred after heated discussions regarding the dangers of DDT that began with in-house government/industry reviews of DDT in 1951, following Biskind and others' criticism of pesticides which began in 1949. These discussions were followed by a phase-out through industry compliance, a huge shift of sales to third-world countries, a phase-in of less-persistent pesticides, which was facilitated by legislation in 1954 and 1956, a renewed public image regarding the proper use and dangers of pesticides, the cancellation of DDT registration by 1968, and eventually the official ban of many of the persistent organochlorine pesticides by 1972 (in U.S. and developed countries).'[128]

This increasing awareness of pesticide dangers went alongside a sharp drop in polio incidence rates between 1952 and 1955. By 1954 it was down to 23.9 cases per 100,000. By the time the vaccine was introduced in 1955, the rate was down to 17 per 100,000. Thus, by the time Jonas Salk's polio vaccine was released in 1955, the level of infantile paralysis in the US was less than a half of what it had been in 1952. The figures for the UK dropped even more dramatically: by more than 82 per cent between 1950 and the first mass administration of the vaccine in the UK in 1957.

But, by 1957 the polio incidence rate in the US was down far more, to just 3.2 cases per 100,000. I thus had to ask, was this large drop due to the just released vaccine – or to the elimination of the worst of the pesticides? Was it possible there was some other answer? A lot hinged on the answers to this.

I had wondered, as I said, if the answer lay in polio having several causes, if exposure to pesticides might weaken immune systems, leaving children susceptible to polio infection? I was not then convinced the pesticide theory gave a full answer – for how could it, if we are today protected by a vaccine?

I thus left the company of the toxicologists and their challenging ideas, to look again at the work of the scientists studying the poliovirus, engaged in what they saw as the noble task of preventing it from infecting us, of stopping the epidemics and preventing them from ever returning.

We forget what it was like then, during the first half of the 20th century, when the hunt to find the poliovirus, isolate it and make a vaccine with it, consumed nearly as much time and money in the US as the campaign against HIV and AIDS has in the past 26 years. These two campaigns for a century have dominated the history of virology.

The danger presented by pesticides would not reach the forefront of public attention until 1962 when Rachel Carson published *Silent Spring* in which she graphically documented the dangers of pesticides to wildlife. Her book launch was sensationally successful. Ironically it was the danger of pesticides to wildlife, rather than to humans, that had grabbed public attention. By 1968 DDT had lost its certification and it then officially went out of use in the US – but only for a number of years.

But, despite its importance, investigating the cause of polio had been something of a distraction from the task I originally set myself. I had set out to discover just how pure and safe was our polio vaccine. It had been extremely troubling to learn it was contaminated with a dangerous monkey virus now linked to cancers. It was even more troubling to find this virus was probably still in the vaccine. I was growing more and more worried that the vaccine, and the poorly regulated procedures employed in making it, had inadvertently spread HIV.

But – had it stopped polio? I had another riddle to resolve that goes to the heart of the credibility of modern virology. Despite all the work done to regulate pesticides, DDT is still widely used in the world. So, why don't we have polio epidemics in the countries still heavily using it? Did the virologists finally somehow get the vaccine right?

---

[128] See Jim West's website 'Images of Poliomyelitis.' Unfortunately, as of April 2008, this is not on line – but there is a new edition of his work available at http://www.westonaprice.org/envtoxins/pesticides_polio.html

# Chapter 6

# A hidden epidemic

I have been told again and again by health authorities that the polio vaccine is a marvellous lifesaver – and I had accepted this on trust. As no one I knew doubted this, I had no reason to question it. I knew, however, that it is easy to invent history. If a false history is repeated often enough, the chances are that people will believe it. It is simply a matter of most of us not having time to check all the facts for ourselves.

But – now I knew of the possibility that pesticides might cause polio, I had a very clear question to answer. There were no great American polio epidemics after 1956. What stopped them: the withdrawal of the pesticides – or the introduction of the vaccine?

Most modern histories of the polio vaccine say its launch went smoothly – although many mention a brief hiccup early on called the 'Cutter Incident,' describing this as a simple error that was quickly rectified. But what I learnt from reading contemporary newspapers and medical reports was very different.

I found the triumph and relief accompanying the launch of the Salk vaccine was extremely short-lived. A medical historian of the time, Dr. M. Beddow Baily, reported: 'Only 13 days after the vaccine had been acclaimed by the whole of the US press and radio as one of the greatest medical discoveries of the century, and 2 days after the British ministry of health had announced it would go right ahead with the manufacture of the vaccine, came the first news of disaster. Children inoculated with one brand of the vaccine [the Cutter] had developed poliomyelitis. In the following days more and more cases were reported, some of them after inoculation with other brands.'

Within two weeks nearly 200 vaccinated children had gone down with polio. This produced near panic in the White House. It was not yet summer. Polio normally did not strike at this time. President Eisenhower had publicly endorsed this vaccine – and did not want any failures on his watch. US Health Secretary Oveta Hobby thus went to see the Surgeon General to sternly say the president needed to be spared further embarrassment!

Within days, on 8 May 1955, the Surgeon General suspended the entire US production of the vaccine and called for emergency meetings with Salk and the manufacturers. They then agreed that these cases were caused by polioviruses surviving the formaldehyde poisoning by being inside 'lumps in the vaccine'. The manufacturers agreed to stir their vaccine better, the public were told they had no further need to worry, and the distribution of the vaccine resumed after only a five-day break.

However, this was not the end of the trouble. It was now reported by the media that the vaccine still seemed to be causing a polio epidemic rather than preventing it.

In Boston during the next 4 months, more than 2,000 of the vaccinated went down with polio – yet in the previous year there were only 273 cases. The number of cases doubled in vaccinated New York State and Connecticut, and tripled in Vermont. There was a five-fold increase in polio in vaccinated Rhode Island and Wisconsin. Many children were paralyzed in the vaccine-injected arm.

In June 1955 the British doctors' union, the Medical Practitioners' Union reported: 'These misfortunes would be almost endurable if a whole new generation were to be rendered permanently immune to the disease. In fact, there is no evidence that any lasting immunity is achieved [by vaccination].'[129] The following month Canada suspended its distribution of Salk's vaccine. By November all European countries had suspended their distribution plans, all that is apart from Denmark

As I learnt of this, I remembered what went into this vaccine. I could not presume these cases were caused by the poliovirus in the vaccine. These children were having a host of potential toxins and viruses injected into their arms, for anything smaller than a virus could not be filtered out. Did this explain why many were paralyzed in the arm vaccinated?

The *New York Times* of May 11, 1956 reported the '*Supplement No. 15 of the Poliomyelitis Surveillance Report*' for that year revealed there was 12% more paralysis in 1956 than in 1955. By January 1957 seventeen US states had stopped distributing the polio vaccine. The *New York Times* reported that nearly half of all polio cases reported were in vaccinated children.[130]

Polio cases rose from 300 to 400% in the five states or cities that made the Salk vaccine compulsory by law. The following table gives their results.

—North Carolina: 78 cases in 1958 before compulsory shots; 313 cases afterwards in 1959.
—Connecticut: 45 cases in 1958 before compulsory shots; 123 cases afterwards in 1959.
—Tennessee: 119 cases in 1958 before compulsory shots; 386 cases afterwards in 1959.
—Ohio: 17 cases in 1958 before compulsory shots; 52 cases afterwards in 1959.
—Los Angeles: 89 cases in 1958 before compulsory shots; 190 cases afterwards in 1959.[131]

From contemporary reports there were nine times more polio cases in 1957 than in 1956, and that they were more serious than ever before. In the first 8 months of 1957 the Public Health Service reported, out of a total of 3,212 polio cases, there were 1,055 cases of paralysis, or 33.5% of the total. From January 1st to August 1958 there was a total of 1,638 cases of polio, with 801 of them paralytic, or 49% of the total. This was, as far as I can discover, a far higher proportion of serious cases than had ever been recorded.

These contemporary accounts were utterly unlike what I had expected, for today the polio vaccine is said to work extremely effectively.

It is perhaps also relevant to note that the immediate profits made from the vaccine were very considerable. Wyeth's profits went up 50% between 1955 and 1956, all on the back of the Salk vaccine. Merck's profits went up from $16 million to $20 million. Eli Lilly nearly doubled its profits from $16 million to $30 million.

But by 1964 very few cases of polio were being reported. So, what happened after 1959 to make the polio vaccine effective?

I do not know how to express convincingly what I found when I looked into this. I avoid conspiracy theory as too many chance events are thus explained – but this does not mean that some conspiracies have not happened.

I found firm evidence that the regulatory authorities had employed from 1960 another weapon from their armoury to bring down the numbers of reported polio cases. They promulgated new regulations that rewrote the rules for polio diagnosis, effectively wiping polio nearly out of existence by simply changing the rules for polio diagnosis!

In 1956, the health authorities instructed doctors that they were in future only to diagnose polio if a patient has paralytic symptoms for 60 days or more. As polio was diagnosed previously if there were just 24 hours of paralytic symptoms, and as the disease

---

[129] *Medical World Newsletter*, June 1955

[130] M Beddow Bayly; 'The story of the Salk anti-poliomyelitis vaccine'; www.whale.to/vaccine/bayly.html These press reports contradict part of the otherwise excellent information presented on the Jim West's 'Images of Poliomyelitis' website. He presented graphs that showed polio had been practically eliminated in the US by 1956.

[131] http://americandaily.com/article/15680

in milder cases frequently lasted less than 60 days, this automatically meant vastly fewer cases of polio would be reported.

Furthermore, it was now decreed that all cases of polio occurring within 30 days of vaccination were to be recorded, not as possibly caused by the vaccine, but as 'pre-existing'. This regulatory change also ensured that far fewer cases of vaccine failure would be recorded.[132]

Another regulatory change had an even greater impact. Most polio diagnoses during the epidemics had not involved paralysis but muscular weakness and widespread pain. In many cases this was produced by inflammation of the membrane that protects the brain and spinal neuron cells. The CDC described such cases as 'serious but rarely fatal'.[133] But doctors were now instructed that all such cases must no longer be diagnosed as polio but as viral or aseptic meningitis! The Los Angeles County health authority explained: 'Most cases reported prior to July 1 1958 of non-paralytic poliomyelitis are now reported as viral or aseptic meningitis' in accordance with instructions from Washington.'

As a result, the number of cases of meningitis diagnosed went from near zero to many thousands while polio came down equivalently. Between 1951 and 1960 in the United States 70,083 cases of non-paralytic polio were diagnosed - and zero cases of aseptic meningitis. But under the new diagnostic rules this was reversed. Over the next twenty years over 100,000 cases of aseptic meningitis were diagnosed and only 589 cases of 'non-paralytic polio'.

Extraordinarily, non-paralytic cases were now to be renamed as meningitis even if the poliovirus were present! In future, the reported figures for polio were officially to exclude 'cases of aseptic meningitis due to poliovirus or other enteroviruses.'[134]

These changes did not go entirely unnoticed. Dr. Bernard Greenberg, then head of the Department of Biostatistics at the University of North Carolina, testified at a 1962 Congressional hearing that infantile paralysis cases had increased after the introduction of the vaccine by 50% from 1957 to 1958, and by 80% from 1958 to 1959. He concluded that US health officials had manipulated the statistics to give entirely the opposite impression.[135]

This change was not only in the US. In Canada, the Dominion Bureau of Statistics issued in June 1959 an official bulletin entitled *Poliomyelitis Trends, 1958.* This noted; 'data shown in this report are confined to paralytic poliomyelitis only. It may be noted that the Dominion Council of Health at its 74th meeting in October 1958 recommended that for the purposes of national reporting and statistics the term non-paralytic poliomyelitis be replaced by 'meningitis, viral or aseptic,'' They also now allowed for other viruses to be found in polio cases, saying that these ' specific viruses [should be] shown where known.' When they were found, these cases also were said not to be polio.

Other cases previously diagnosed as polio would in future be classified as 'cerebral palsy', as 'Guillain-Barre syndrome' and even as 'muscular dystrophy.' Some were called 'Hand, Foot and Mouth Disease', which can also cause paralysis. (And recently the Coxsackie virus was found in cases of Chronic Fatigue Syndrome (CFS), which is also sometimes associated with polio-like symptoms of muscle damage.)

But this reclassification of polio cases seemingly did not satisfy the regulatory authorities. Apparently there were still too many cases of the worst kind of polio,

---

[132] The diagnostic guidelines also specified that the patient must have, 'No history of immunisation' if they are to be diagnosed with the illness they were vaccinated against. (*'Textbook of Infectious Diseases.'* - University of Colorado School of Medicine. 1982). In other words, if they are vaccinated against an illness, it is presumed they cannot have already had it.

[133] www.cdc.gov/ncidod/dvrd/revb/enterovirus/viral_meningitis.htm

[134] EIS Officer, Division of Immunization, Center for Disease Control, Dept of Health and Human Services, USA (personal communication to Dr Isaac Golden dated 26 August 1988).

[135] Walene James; www.vaccinetruth.org/polio_vaccines.htm

'paralytic polio' – so it was finally decided that these cases must also be removed from the polio case registry, thus eliminating nearly all the remaining cases of polio in the world – giving the heath authorities a stunning and utterly fraudulent victory.

This was achieved by instructing doctors that in future they were not to diagnose polio. This decision was to be left to the regulatory authorities. If patients came to them with the classic symptoms of paralytic polio, these were to be diagnosed as 'Acute Flaccid Paralysis' (AFP). The doctors were, and still are, told to send samples of two turds from such a patient to the official laboratories. There these turds are inspected to see if the poliovirus is in them. If signs of its presence are not found, [136] it is declared not to be polio – no matter that the children have all the classic symptoms and distress found in the worst cases of polio during the great US epidemics.[137]

This astonishingly revealed that the 'poliovirus' is rarely to be found in these paralysed children. Logically, one would think that this would force the health authorities to conclude that the virus could not be the cause of polio – but that idea seems to be unacceptable. Instead it seems they are more interested in claiming a victory.

Thus they triumphantly declare large parts of the world polio free, even where AFP is relatively common, and give the credit for this solely to the vaccine and its manufacturers, as well as to Sabin and Salk. I did not know how to characterize this except as an incredible act of medical fraud. I struggle to find any excuses for those involved. It begun in the 1950s but, I am afraid to say, it still continues.

This has had the most serious of consequences. One of these is that the power to diagnose polio has been completely taken away from ordinary doctors. Before 1958 they were taught to diagnose 'paralytic polio' as they did other diseases – by observing specific symptoms, particularly acute paralysis and great pain. But doctors are now instructed not to look for the poliovirus itself, as 'the virus is very hard to find.' Instead this task is to be left to WHO and the other governmental agencies that inspect turds. This would be comical if it were not so tragically deceptive.

Under these new rules, patients previously diagnosed with paralytic polio were re-diagnosed. When patients in Detroit, diagnosed as having paralytic polio during a 1958 epidemic, were re-tested as required by the new rule, 49% were found not to have poliovirus and were therefore told they did not have polio.

Should it find a case in which the poliovirus is present, the vaccine will be administered on a national scale. This has happened now so many times that in populous countries like India many cases of 'provocation' polio are diagnosed in the arm vaccinated. 'Unnecessary injections were associated with paralysis in the outbreak reported by Kohler et al.[138] The WHO estimates that over 12 billion injections are given every year, and most are unnecessary. Multiple injections can increase the risk of paralysis from OPV as well as wild-type viruses.'[139] These cases of paralysis are caused by many types of repeated injections and inconsistently are still called 'polio.'

This is all extraordinary. The Detroit patients, the children with AFP today, all are ill with the same symptoms and pain as found in the earlier cases of paralytic polio. Wasn't the polio vaccine devised to prevent such cases? The new rules for polio diagnosis are a perfect way to hide total vaccine failure –and have thus apparently served both the Public Health Authorities and vaccine manufacturers well. This deceit has

---

[136] /The virus is said to be present if cell damage is observed in a culture – and this damage is prevented by adding an antibody believed specific to the poliovirus. WHO 1997 Manual for the Virological Investigation of Polio.

[137] http://www.who.int/vaccines/casecount/case_count.cfm.

[138] Kohler KA, Hlady WG, Banerjee K, Sutter RW. Outbreak of poliomyelitis due to type 3 poliovirus, northern India, 1999–2000: injections a major contributing factor. Int J Epidemiol 2003;32:272–77

[139] *The International Journal of Epidemiology* Vol. 32, 2. Pp 278-9
http://ije.oxfordjournals.org/cgi/content/full/32/2/278

protected them from being sued for producing a useless vaccine. The poliovirus is scientifically classified as a human virus that naturally replicates only in the human gut, so the WHO excrement inspection is surely meaningless? Its presence in excrement is natural – and finding it there does not prove that it causes paralysis in the motor neuron cells of the human backbone.

When I went to look at the statistics provided by the World Health Organization (WHO), I found that Acute Flaccid Paralysis (AFP) remains a little mentioned epidemic in many parts of the world where pesticide use is high. Its figures for the East Asian/Pacific region reveal the number of cases of AFP between 1994 and 1998 went up by 50% in China, 400% in Malaysia, and 1,500% in the Pacific islands. In 2007 WHO inspected 156,795 excrement samples from patients with acute flaccid paralysis, finding only in 2,320 the wild poliovirus and in 5,631 the mutant poliovirus spread in the Sabin vaccine.[140]

The rest of the severely paralysed children, about 190,000 in number, despite having all the symptoms that were once diagnosed as severe polio, but without the designated poliovirus in their excrement, are now abandoned without a cure and a vaccine while WHO boasts that it has very nearly conquered polio.

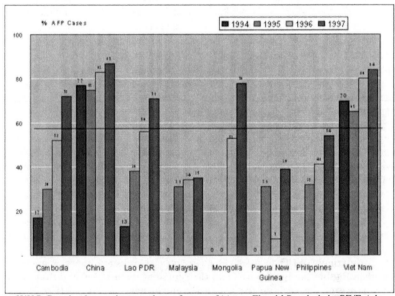

**WHO Graph.** *'Increasing numbers of cases of 'Acute Flaccid Paralysis in SE/E Asia region 1994-1997.'* This reveals, not only a growing epidemic of what was once called polio, but also that the polio vaccine is not effective against the disease it was developed to fight.

WHO makes even bolder claims for Europe and the Americas. It declares both are now free of polio and AFP. But on closer inspection, its figures prove to be extremely dubious. It declares that there is 'no data' for the number of cases of AFP in the UK and the US. It then interprets 'no data' as if it means 'zero'![141]

WHO's interpretation is contradicted by the US government's own figures. The Centers for Disease Control (CDC) today report many thousands of cases of AFP in the

[140] WHO Weekly Epidemiological Report, 5 September 2008. http://www.who.int/wer/2008/wer8336.pdf

[141] http://www.who.int/vaccines/casecount/case_count.cfm.

US every year, but it gives these every name but polio. For example, it says that Guillain-Barré disease, formerly called polio, causes 17 cases of AFP per 100,000 of the US population. That translates into around 50,000 cases annually – equal to the number affected in the worst year of the 20th century polio epidemics. The CDC also reports that every year there are some 30,000 to 50,000 cases of aseptic meningitis in the USA serious enough to require hospitalisation. These also were previously diagnosed as polio.

Thus, by the original polio definition, there are vastly more cases of what would have been diagnosed as poliomyelitis in the US today than there were at the height of the US polio epidemics. This is not too surprising if neurotoxin pesticides are partly or wholly to blame; as these pesticides are now back into very widespread use.

The level of pesticide pollution on farmland in America is now so bad that the US Environmental Protection Agency 'estimates that there are 10,000 to 20,000 cases of physician-diagnosed pesticide poisonings' every year among agricultural workers. The CDC now reports that approximately one billion pounds of pesticides are used every year in the US.

To this tally of 'Acute Flaccid Paralysis' one could add the many more cases of AFP occurring in another epidemic that has swept across the US over the past few years, one that virologists attribute to the 'West Nile' virus (WNV). The CDC states that WNV can cause a 'polio-like' paralysis. Many scientists have been less ambiguous. They say AFP caused by WNV is clinically indistinguishable from poliomyelitis.[142] A paper recently published by the British Medical Journal suggests WNV may be 'rapidly evolving to fill new ecological niches.'[143]  In 2003 in the US there were 9,389 cases of this disease, of which 2,773 had damage to the nervous system and 246 that were fatal.

Today the WHO encourages developing nations to use cheap DDT to kill malaria-spreading mosquitoes, while it organises vaccination campaigns in the same countries to fight the polio and other illnesses caused by DDT. Effectively, the pesticide companies are now partners with WHO in its war against viruses.

WHO today states on its website: 'There is no cure for polio: its effects are irreversible.' But this totally ignores the results obtained by doctors who have treated it with antitoxins. WHO has failed to find a remedy to what was once called polio because public funds are wasted on an ineffective vaccine – and because they cannot admit that toxins might be causing the illness and not a virus. This stubbornness is nothing other than tragic for the many tens of thousands of children involved.

But then, one cannot sue a virus unlike a pesticide manufacturer so this is a comfortable stand that evades litigation! But I must confess at the time I did this research, I did not see all the consequences that now seem evident to me.

Amazingly WHO today states on its official website **'there is no relationship between finding the [polio]virus and the course of the disease' and that the presence or absence of the virus in the patients' central nervous system (CNS) 'appears to have no diagnostic significance.'** But damage to the CNS is at the core of the poliomyelitis illness.  If the virus need not be present in these tissues for polio to be diagnosed, then I am afraid that it is most illogical to continue to insist that this virus causes polio.

How do I go on from this?  I am staggered by what I am discovering. Polio vaccine research has turned out to be a veritable tapestry of errors – and, I am afraid, of deceit. What then of the other vaccines?  They surely could not be as contaminated as the polio vaccines? Technology has much improved. Surely by now our other vaccines are pure and safe? So I went to look at recent official vaccine safety research.

---

[142] A Arturo Leis et al; 'West Nile poliomyelitis'; Reviewed in *The Lancet*, 1 January 2003

[143] Tom Solomon et al, West Nile encephalitis, British Medical Journal, April 19th, 2003.

# Chapter 7

# The Dangerous Impurities of Vaccines

A year after I met with the top government regulatory scientists at the NIH Emergency Workshop on SV40 in 1997, they met again in Washington for another workshop on vaccine safety. At this there were representatives of all the major US government health organisations and of the vaccine manufacturers. A third similar meeting would be held a year later in 1999.

The main issue at the November 1998 meeting was whether or not it would be safe for manufacturers to produce the viruses needed for vaccines from cancer cells. Pharmaceutical companies were seeking government approval for this, on the basis that cancerous cells, as 'immortal' and permanent, would be cheaper to use than cells they had to regularly replace by, for example, buying more monkeys.

These workshops looked at the issue broadly, by comparing the safety of the different ways available for making our vaccines. As everyone present was a scientist, the discussions were much more open and frank than they are when journalists are present.

They started with the Measles, Mumps and Rubella vaccine (MMR). One of the first speakers on this was Dr. Arifa Khan from the federal Food and Drugs Agency (FDA) and what she had to report was very disturbing. [144]

'Today I would like to present an update on the reverse transcriptase [RT] activity that is present in chicken cell derived vaccines.' My attention was immediately grabbed. I knew that the mumps and measles viruses used for the MMR vaccine are grown in fertilised chicken eggs, as are also the viruses for the Flu and Yellow Fever vaccines. (The rubella virus for MMR is produced differently - in artificially grown cells taken originally from an aborted human foetus.)

Dr. Khan was reporting the result of a just concluded two-year investigation into the safety of MMR led by the World Health Organization. She explained this was initiated in 1996 after the discovery in MMR of RT; an enzyme whose presence they believed could indicate that retroviruses had contaminated the vaccine. This had greatly alarmed them as some retroviruses are thought to cause cancers – and AIDS.

WHO had then quietly, without telling the public, without withdrawing the vaccine, organised MMR safety studies at various laboratories to see 'whether this RT activity was associated with a retroviral particle, and even more importantly, whether this retrovirus particle could infect and replicate in human cells.'

What they then discovered confirmed their worse fears. Dr. Khan continued: 'The RT activity is found to be associated with retroviral particles of two distinct avian endogenous retroviral families designated as EAV and ALV.' Now ALV stands for Avian Leukosis Virus. It is associated with a leukaemia cancer found in wild birds, so definitely was not wanted in the vaccines. EAV was less dangerous, at least for birds as it is natural for them to have it.

---

[144] http://www.fda.gov/Cber/advisory/vrbp/vrbpmain.htm
http://www.fda.gov/ohrms/dockets/ac/cber98t.htm#Vaccines%20and%20Related%20Biol ogical%20Products%20Advisory%20Committee   meeting of Vaccines and Related Biological Products Committee  19 November 1988.

Khan added that they had also found another possible danger; 'There was a theoretical possibility that the virus [ALV] could  … infect the [human] cell' thus integrating its genetic code 'into the human DNA' to cause cancer. The only reassurance she could give was that her team had watched vaccine cultures for a full '48 hours', and, in that time period, no merger of viral and human DNA had been observed. I thought this much too short a period to guarantee safety. Cancers develop over years.

Dr. Khan then warned; 'there is a possibility that there could also be potential pseudotypes (merging between) … the measles vaccine virus and the retroviral sequences' – meaning there was a risk that bird viruses might combine with the measles virus in the vaccine to create dangerous new mutant viruses, They had not seen it, but it could happen.

She acknowledged much longer term safety studies were needed than 48 hours, but said long-term studies of measles vaccine cultures were very difficult: 'because the measles vaccine virus itself lyses [kills] the culture in about three to four days.' This had prevented them from studying the longer-term consequences of this contamination of the MMR vaccine. [145]

So far, she added, they had only managed to analyse a small part of the retrovirus contamination in the vaccines. 'Our ongoing studies are directed towards doing similar analysis' of other retroviral genetic codes found in the vaccine preparations.' It was suspected that other retroviruses might also be present. She also noted that 'about 20 years ago similar RT activity was reported' in the vaccine. Apparently nothing had been done about it at that time and the public were never told.

She concluded by explaining what the World Health Organization (WHO) had decided to do about this chicken leucosis virus (ALV) contamination. It would take the risk of quietly allowing MMR to continue to be contaminated. It would permit vaccine manufacturers to continue to use retrovirus contaminated eggs, because 'you cannot get ALV free flocks in places where you are making yellow fever vaccine.'

Dr. Andrew Lewis, head of the DNA Virus Laboratory in the Division of Viral Products, then warned. 'All the egg-based vaccines are contaminated,' including 'influenza, yellow fever and smallpox vaccines, as well as the vaccine for horses against encephalomyelitis virus' for 'these fertilised chicken eggs are susceptible to a wide variety of viruses.'

This was an eye opener for me. Before I started on this investigation, if I thought about it, I would have presumed our vaccines were made of selected viruses in sterile fluid to which a small amount of preservative chemicals has been added. I think this is what most parents presume.

It was thus a shock to discover from this top-level scientific workshop that the viruses in our current vaccines are not in a sterile fluid as I had presumed, but in a soup of unknown bits and pieces; a veritable witches' brew of DNA fragments, added chemicals, proteins and, even possibly prions and oncogenes, all of which would easily pass through the filters used, to be injected into our children.

Our vaccines, I thus learnt, are not filtered clean but are suspensions from the manufacturers' 'incubation tanks' in which the viruses are produced from 'substrates' of mashed bird embryo, minced monkey kidneys or cloned human cells. These suspensions are filtered before use but only to remove particles larger than viruses. The point of the vaccine is that it contains viruses, thus these must not be filtered out. This means there

---

[145] How measles virus is isolated is described in the next chapter. The cells used 'to produce the virus' are made first cancerous, probably being exposed to radiation, then given Epson Barre Syndrome and exposed to toxins. Only after this are these cells exposed to a fluid sample from the patient who is suspected of having measles. If by now half of the cells re ill, this is oddly judged to be definitely caused by the virus. The CDC says that this cell culture should be now put in the fridge as a 'measles virus isolate!' The cells illness and deaths thus has many causes. At no point is the virus actually observed.

remains in the vaccine everything of the same size or smaller, including what the manufacturers call 'degradation products' – parts of decayed viruses or cells.

I also learnt that the only official checks made for contaminants in vaccines are for a few known pathogens, thus ignoring a vast host of unknown, unstudied, small particles and chemicals. These eminent doctors reported at these vaccine safety meetings that it is simply impossible to remove these from our common vaccines – and this would of course also apply to vaccines for pets, farm animals and birds.

I went to the published reports of the MMR manufacturers and found these confirmed what the scientists at this workshop had reported. A manufacturer stated in 2000 that it made the MMR vaccine with 'harvested virus fluids.' It stated frankly that their 'Measles vaccine bulk is an unpurified product whose potency was measured through a biological assay for the active substance rather than through evaluation of integrity of physical form. Degradation products are neither identified nor quantified.' In other words, it left the latter in the measles vaccine along with all contaminants that lay there quietly, or worked slowly. The pharmaceutical company admitted checking the measles vaccine only for obviously active contaminants. It did not measure how much the vaccine was polluted with genetic code fragments, other viruses, or with parts of bacterial, animal, bird or human cells. [146]

I looked also to see how the checks on known pathogens in vaccines are done. The main method involves PCR – and detects incredibly small DNA fragments. These cannot be identified unless they are found to be identical to a fragment that has been proved unique to a pathogen, something that is complex and difficult to do. That is why the scientists checking the avian leucosis virus contamination of the MMR vaccine had admitted that, in several years of work, they only managed to check a small part of this contamination.

In any case, PCR is utterly unable to prove a vaccine pure. A recent report stated: 'A negative PCR signal could be obtained when the total batch [of 10 litres] still contained 106 undetected viral particles.' [147]

Another common method of testing for the presence of a particular pathogen, whether a toxin, virus or bacteria, is to use an antibody test such as the HIV blood tests (ELISA and Western Blot). Such tests only work if the antibody searched for in a blood sample, cell culture, or vaccine substrate, is already proved to mark only a molecule unique to this pathogen for destruction.

But can any molecule be proved unique to a specific pathogen? Proving this is virtually impossible to carry out with complete accuracy. There is always the chance that the molecule targeted can be found in more than one thing – including many yet unidentified viruses. In other words, there is always some degree of uncertainty with these tests. As far as I can discover after a rigorous search, the accuracy of even the HIV test has never been so verified.

A major problem is that we have so far only identified a very small part of the microbial world – and therefore we just cannot verify a particular molecule is only from one type of virus. If antibodies are detected, then all that can be said with certainty is that these antibodies fit to molecules that were at some point present in the patient.

David Relman wrote in *The Atlantic:* 'Much of the microbial world is still as mysterious as an alien planet…It has been estimated that only 0.4 percent of all extant bacterial species have been identified. …. Even the germs that inhabit our bodies, the so-

---

[146] http://www.emea.eu.int/humandocs/PDFs/EPAR/mmrvaxpro/060406en6.pdf.

[147] Virus Clearance Strategies for Biopharmaceutical Safety
http://www.pall.com/applicat/bio_pharm/pdf/Bp5560.pdf.

called 'human commensal flora,' such as the swarming populations of organisms that live in the spaces between our teeth, are largely unknown.'[148]

But despite all these possible sources of error, virologists have found ways that they hope will minimise error. A way has been discovered to separate out particles found in cell cultures according to their densities – thus distinguishing particles such as retroviruses that are defined as of specific density. A sample of fluid thought to possibly contain viruses is put into a thick sugar suspension and then spun extremely fast for many hours in a centrifuge, often at 5000 to 12000g – gravity forces humans could not live under.[149] This makes the particles band according to their density. But great care needs to be taken. This is reportedly not a good way to try to find HIV – for it is said to be extremely fragile and to easily disintegrate. In general, high speed centrifuging and freeze-drying may considerably damage results prior to microscope imaging.[150]

The micrograph below is said to be of purified polioviruses, but the extraordinarily regular shapes of these particles made the molecular biologist and virologist Dr. Steven Lanka wonder they might have been shaped out of soft fragments by filtration meshes and hours of rapid centrifugation. (Contrast the micrographs of viruses later in this book.)[151] Lanka concluded: 'The "isolated" polio viruses are artificial particles, generated by suction of an indifferent mass through a very fine filter into a vacuum.'[152] (If he is right –

then where is the evidence for the isolation of the poliovirus? I clearly would have to seek this elsewhere.)

The next stage involves the use of the electron microscope. The appropriate density band for the type of virus sought is micrographed. This hopefully reveals some particles that look like viruses – but does not prove that they are. Next they must be tested in a cell culture to see if the cells exposed to these same particles will fall ill.

If they do, what are observed are cell deaths, mutations or distortions. The normal diagnostic symptoms of the disease under study are not usually seen. This is a serious difficulty as if a causal link between the particle and this disease is being sought.

We also cannot assume that these cells, living artificial lives in laboratory vessels, in conditions that often bring about mutations,[153] are producing the same viruses as those they are exposed to in the culture. The new viruses may contain variations in genetic codes. They may be entirely natural and harmless particles, as cells also produce these. It's thus very difficult to tell if the illness in the cell culture is the same

---

[148] *The Atlantic* February 1999

[149] Higher speeds of 30,000 to over 100,000g are used to separate out the internal parts of cells, for these break apart at such speeds. Presumably much damage is also done at such speeds.
http://www.beckmancoulter.com/localization/subinfo/germany/pdf/rotor_3english.pdf

[150] Pembrey R. et al  Cell Surface Analysis Techniques: What Do Cell Preparation Protocols Do to Cell Surface Properties? Applied and Environmental Microbiology, July 1999, p. 2877-2894, Vol. 65, No. 7
http://aem.asm.org/cgi/content/full/65/7/2877

[151] See Stefan Lanka in an English translation on http://www.neue-medizin.com/lanka2.htm

[152] Lanka cited above.

[153] Reported by Nobel Laureate Barbara McClintock. See chapter 20 below.

as in the original patients. But, if cells die in the lab, it is often simply assumed that the correct viruses are present. (For more on this, see chs.19-20.)

The genetic codes of viruses produced by the exposed cells are also very rarely checked to see if they are identical to the added particles – for they may share many code sequences simply because the same cells can make many types of viruses out of near identical materials – and because cells often vary the viruses they produce to some extent.

If it is finally judged that these tests have been successful in growing the right viruses, a sample of the virus-rich fluid from the cell culture is taken, and this may then be used as a 'vaccine seed' that is added to monkey or other cells in an incubator, with 'growth' chemicals, to make them produce more of the viruses wanted for vaccines.

The latest information I could find on the retroviral contamination of the MMR vaccine was in a 2001 scientific paper from the CDC. This reported that 100 MMR recipients were tested to see if they were contaminated by either of the two types of retroviruses identified by Dr. Khan and others. The conclusion was dramatic. '**The finding of RT activity in all measles vaccine lots from different manufacturers tested suggests that this occurrence is not sporadic and that vaccine recipients may be universally exposed to these [chicken] retroviral particles.**'

They then concluded: 'Despite these reassuring data, the presence of avian retroviral particles in chick embryo fibroblast-derived vaccines [like MMR] raises questions about the suitability of primary chicken cell substrates for vaccine production.' They recommended considering stopping production in fertilized eggs, and growing the vaccine viruses instead on 'RT-negative cells from different species, such as on immortalized [cancerous] or diploid [laboratory grown] mammalian cells.' I was amazed to learn this, for, to the best of my knowledge, nothing has been done since this report was made to render MMR safer. The measles vaccine is still produced from contaminated chicken embryos.

A year later, on September 7th, 1999, another Workshop was convened in Washington DC to consider these issues.[154] Representatives from all the largest public health institutions in the West were at this, including the World Health Organization whose representative co-chaired it. The UK government's vaccine safety bodies had a top-level representative in Dr. Philip Minor. Apparently no press were present– but the importance of the meeting meant that it was taped, as was the earlier conference, to ensure an accurate record.

Dr. Bill Egan, the Acting Director of the Office of Vaccines at the Center for Biologics opened the meeting with this statement:

'I think we need to remind ourselves that viruses can propagate only in live cells, and this of course holds true for whole viral vaccines... They can only be produced in cells [substrates]... We have only to think back to the finding of SV40 in poliovirus vaccines to realize the extent of the risk that any cell substrate may pose, there is still great need for concern... we have been given the task of identifying these concerns...'

The scientists present then told that our vaccines are widely contaminated by viral and DNA genetic code fragments, many viruses and proteins. They openly worried that among these could also be dangerous prions or oncogenes.

They reported that they had found monkey viruses in still more vaccines. Dr. Andrew Lewis of the FDA gravely added that 'humans were immunized with adenovirus vaccines that contained adenovirus-SV40 hybrid viruses.' In other words, a brand-new monkey-human mutant virus was created in this vaccine. Dr. Ben Berkhout exclaimed at hearing this: 'That's the one I would like to focus on today, Is [there a danger of] the

---

[154] http://www.fda.gov/cber/minutes/0907evolv.txt
http://www.fda.gov/Cber/advisory/vrbp/vrbpmain.htm

potential reversion of an attenuated vaccine strain to a virus variant that can replicate fast and can potentially cause AIDS?'

This was a startling and horrifying question. Could our most common childhood vaccines be so affected by contaminating DNA that they will give our children AIDS? Were such mutation events in vaccines rare? Apparently not. Another doctor stated. 'Recombination among a variety of viruses and cells co-infected in tissue culture is not uncommon. This is an issue that certainly will need further consideration.' In other words, vaccine incubators can create mutated viruses.

The next speaker described the 'foreign cellular DNA' they had found contaminating our childhood vaccines. Dr. Andrew Lewis of the CDER and FDA worried that this might well include 'viral oncogenes' – in other words, contaminants that might cause cancer.

Another scientist, Dr. Adimora, asked how would the public react if they knew of these dangers? 'The general public have a variety of concerns about vaccines but, to my knowledge, the cell substrates in which the vaccines are grown has not been one of their major concerns to date.' But, 'it could conceivably be different in future.'

Dr. Lewis corrected him slightly, saying the public on one occasion had worried about substrates: 'There was a tremendous concern associated with the polio vaccine developed in rhesus monkey kidney cells associated with the SV40 infection. Two years ago we were one of the sponsors of a meeting that were dealing with the follow up to those concerns.' This was the NIH meeting that had first introduced me to these issues.

Dr. Rebecca Sheets of the CBER, the US laboratory responsible for monitoring vaccine safety, worryingly noted that as government officers they had no control whatsoever over how vaccines are made! Under current legislation they could only give 'recommendations' to the manufacturers. Nevertheless, they were highly concerned for **the 'cell substrates in which the vaccine viruses are grown ... can be the source of adventitious agents, the source of tumorigenic potential, and the source of residual cellular DNA which can have both infectivity or tumorigenic potential.'**

She continued: 'If the use of cancer cells for the growth of vaccine viruses were authorised,' then they would be concerned about 'the potential for exposure to adventitious oncogenic viruses. The screening methods for these viruses are difficult or relatively insensitive, and that there may exist currently unknown or occult agents that have never before been detected despite use of current technology.' (I was later to learn that the particle identified as HIV was first grown in such a cancer culture.)

All ways of making vaccines have their dangers. Dr. Hayflick, a well-reputed scientist involved for many years with vaccines, described how the 'Primary Culture' method of taking cells from 'sacrificed animals' or bird embryos ran into problems when *'it became apparent that these cells contained many unwanted viruses, some of which were lethal to humans.'* He noted: 'Latent viruses were such a problem with primary monkey kidney cells that a worldwide moratorium on the licensing of all polio virus vaccines was called in 1967 because of death and illnesses that occurred in monkey kidney workers and vaccine manufacturing facilities'. The contaminating virus blamed was the deadly Ebola. This was most serious, but again I could find no record of the public having been informed about this suspension or the Ebola.

The top UK government expert present at this conference, Dr. Phil Minor of the National Institute of Biological Standards and Control, added that the polio vaccine had originally been so polluted that its doses contained as much monkey virus as poliovirus! I had no idea that so much monkey virus was in this vaccine given to hundreds of millions of children. Then there was another shock for me. I had been assured two years earlier at the SV40 Workshop that the polio vaccine was no longer contaminated with SV40 – and consequently I had so assured the UK public in our resulting Channel 4 television documentary. Now I learnt I had been misled and consequently had seriously misinformed the public. Scientists reported to this meeting that 'SV40 sequences' remained in the poliovirus seed used for the current polio vaccines.

As for the rubella, measles and other vaccines produced in 'Cell Line substrates', in cells taken from the wild but now grown in laboratories, these cell cultures host 'the broadest virus spectrum of any cell population known!' It was also explained that these cultures in which are produced our children's vaccines, were safety tested, controversially and alarmingly, on 'terminally ill cancer human patients' and on 'prisoners.'

Dr. Hayflick told how, when laboratory-grown cell lines were first introduced, they were erroneously thought of as immortal. He said they had now proved them mortal, overturning a dogma that had existed from the turn of the century. This was that cells living in laboratory cultures could live and replicate indefinitely. It was wrongly presumed that 'if they do die, you simply do not have the proper culture conditions.' But, we now know that healthy cells can only divide and reproduce around 50 times. It seems to be a natural limitation.

For me this shed light on why at first the early AIDS researcher, Dr. Robert Gallo, the scientist now famous for his theory on how HIV causes AIDS, was so upset when he failed to keep alive his cell lines of CD4 white blood cells. He then had guessed this must be because an AIDS related virus was killing them. But – what if these cells were dying naturally – as we now know they would have been? If so, then this is important – for their deaths were the only evidence he produced for deciding that the viruses in his cultures were deadly to white blood cells and thus the cause of AIDS, as we will see!

A year later Gallo had tried to grow HIV on white blood cells that were previously deliberately made cancerous ('transformed') by exposing to radiation or toxins, thinking this would immortalise them – and thus prevent his virus from killing them. It is a method known as the 'Continuous Cell Line' – and it was the next item on the agenda of this workshop. Dr. Hanna Golding, an expert with the CBER, explained she was really worried about being asked to approve of the use of cancer cells in making vaccines: 'The issue that we are really concerned about is the unknown. We are dealing with 13 new cell substrates that are transformed. We don't know their history. We don't know what's the aetiology.' In other words, we don't know from where they come or what they do.

The meeting was told: 'The main disadvantage of the continuous cell line is that many [cells] express [produce] endogenous viruses, and there has always been this concern over tumorigenic potential, should we say, associated with cellular DNA.' They were saying that all of these had made their way into vaccines given to children. I felt this was getting more and more horrific.

Cancer cells can be extremely aggressive, moving around laboratories, contaminating culture after culture. Dr. Hayflick told of how the eminent Dr. Maurice Hilleman, the scientist whom I had earlier interviewed about the MMR vaccine, had used what he thought was an 'intestine-based cell line' to make an adenovirus vaccine, only to discover later to his horror that his cell line had been invaded and taken over by the aggressive cervical cancer virus known as HeLa.

I also learnt that DNA fragments contaminating vaccine lots might be from dead cells but nevertheless remained extremely active and dangerous. Dr. Golding feared these contaminating DNA codes might combine together in the vaccine lots – creating a mutant viral strain that could easily get in the individual doses of vaccine.

The removal of this contaminating DNA has proved so impossible that the US government in 1986 told the vaccine manufactures that some of it could stay. It recommended a weight limit for contaminating DNA of 100 picograms per dose. But the manufacturers could not meet this safety recommendation, as was explained at this Workshop. Their failure had led the government to relax its standards, applying the 100 picograms limit solely to the product of continuous [cancer] cell lines, and allowing one hundred times as much contaminating DNA (10 nanograms) in vaccine doses produced on other types of substrate, such as the MMR vaccines. But the meeting was told that vaccine manufacturers had now admitted that they could meet even this lower standard of 'purity' –and, since these limits were only 'recommendations', the government was not able to enforce them. Thus high levels of hazardous DNA pollution remain in many vaccines. When I read this, I wondered about the cases of brain damage and autism now increasingly reported after the administration of these DNA polluted vaccines?

This failure was also a great concern to this meeting. Many of the doctors present worried that such a great amount of DNA fragments might cause viral mutations in the vaccines. 'Naked' DNA (with no protein coat) is known to be highly reactive. Dr. Phil Krause calculated; 'If there are 10 nanograms of residual DNA per dose, which is the current WHO recommendation, and if two doses were recommended per child, as is the case with MMR vaccine, and the infectivity of viral DNA in the vaccine were comparable to that of purified polyoma virus DNA, we can calculate the theoretical infectivity risk. ... For a vaccine that is universally administered to the 4 million children born in the US every year, this would represent about 500 infections per year, clearly an unacceptable rate.'

This shocked me. If he was right, and it seemed he was (none of the experts present questioned his calculations), this surely meant the current MMR vaccine is potentially very dangerous. Krause also had only added up the risk from one vaccine. What when to it is added the contaminating DNA in the many other vaccines?

I did not realise initially what it meant for the stricter safety recommendations being only applied to vaccines made on continuous cell lines. It meant that all the common vaccines might be very DNA polluted. This realisation only came after I learnt from an expert at the workshop that: **'Unpurified viral vaccines (like MMR) ...   contain residual DNA in quantities greater than 10 nanograms.'**

Dr. Krause also stated: 'Of course, in the context of DNA vaccines, we are talking about injecting even larger quantities of DNA into people.' He was speaking here about the new DNA vaccines being developed as 'safer' than our current vaccines.

Another important safety issue was raised. 'What would this contaminating DNA do when it was injected into humans in vaccines? Could it change our own DNA? Could it cause cancers – or autoimmune diseases?' 'When you consider that almost every one of these vaccines is injected right into the tissue that is the preferred site for DNA gene therapy ... I think you couldn't do much more to get the DNA expressed [to get contaminating DNA taken up by human cells] than to inject it into a muscle in the way it's being done.' Another speaker lamely admitted: 'I chaired the committee that licensed the chickenpox vaccine, and it [residual DNA] was actually an issue that we considered at that time.  We looked among recipients of the vaccine for evidence of an autoimmune response associated with the DNA included in that vaccine.' He then added: 'Actually, we didn't look, we asked the company to look and they did not find one.'

Walid Heneine of the CDC asked: 'No one has mentioned how much DNA we now have in the licensed vaccines. I mean, how much are we being exposed to? Do we have any idea how much is in the viral vaccines, like yellow fever, measles, mumps vaccines? Do the regulators have an idea from the manufacturers, how much DNA there is?'

Dr. Loewer replied: 'I have no idea. Nobody that I know has mentioned it.' Dr. Becky Sheets from CBER confirmed the suspicions of many when she responded.  'I think that the vast majority of licensed vaccines, U.S. licensed vaccines, have not been tested for residual DNA.   The few that have been tested are the ones that have been licensed in the last few years, including varicella and Hepatitis A.'

She then added: **'I wanted to respond to an earlier question regarding how purified are live viral vaccines [like MMR] – [the answer is] minimally purified.'**

These presentations made some of the experts most uneasy. Dr. Desrosiers stated: 'I don't worry so much about the agents that one can test for. I worry about the agents that you can't test for, that you don't know about.' Dr. Greenberg agreed, He said he was: 'worried also about the agents that aren't known'. He continued: **'There are still countless thousands of undiscovered viruses, proteins, and similar particles. We have only identified a very small part of the microbial world – and we can only test for those we have identified. Thus the vaccine cultures could contain many unknown particles.'** Another doctor said: 'As time goes on, of course, new viruses are discovered and new problems arise. The foamy virus has been [recently] identified as one that we should be really sure is absent from these vaccines.'

The Chairman of the Workshop then asked Dr. Maxine Linial: 'Maxine, does anybody know if vaccines have been checked for foamy virus contamination?'

She replied: 'As far as I know, no.'

'You mean nobody has looked or as far as you know?

She responded; 'I don't know. There are very few reagents. I mean, there are reagents for the so-called human or chimp foamy virus, but as far as I know, there are no good antibody reagents.' In other words, they could not tell if the vaccines contained foamy viruses. ('Reagents' are antibodies to known virus particles.)

The experts voiced other concerns. 'And I'll be honest and say that I'm surprised that primary African green monkey kidney cells continue to be used, and I'm a little bit disappointed that FDA and whoever is involved had not had a more serious effort to move away from primary African green monkey kidneys. We all know that there are a number of neurodegenerative conditions and other conditions where viral causes have been suspected for years and no viral agent identified. Maybe they're caused by viruses, but maybe they're not.'

Another doctor said: 'We need to consider again some of the issues of residual DNA. Is it oncogenic? We had a lot of experience with chicken leucosis viruses in chick embryo cells beginning back in 1960. And the thing about them is they are not easy to detect because they don't produce any pathogenic effect.'

An unnamed participant added; 'I have to express some bewilderment [at this talk of dangerous contamination], simply because, as I mentioned last night, the vero cell, which under many conditions is neoplastic [tumour-causing], has been licensed for the production of IPV and OPV [the common polio vaccines] in the United States, Thailand, Belgium and France.' The current polio vaccines thus run the risk of having oncogenes in them. Again this was news to me. I had no idea that the polio vaccine might be grown on such cells.

Dr. Rosenberg added unreassuringly: 'When one uses neoplastic cells as substrates for vaccine development, one can inadvertently get virus to virus, or virus to cellular particle, interactions that could have unknown biological consequences.'

Dr. Tom Broker said we had to be concerned about 'papilloma virus infections' in the vaccine ... 'One of the more remarkable facts of this family of diseases is that since 1980 more people have died of HPV disease than have died of AIDS.'

Dr. Phil Minor, from the UK National Institute of Biological Standards and Control, told of another disaster. 'Hepatitis B was transmitted by yellow fever vaccine back in the 1940s. The hepatitis B actually came from the stabilizers of the albumin that was actually put in there to keep it stable'

He continued: 'For many years, rabies vaccines were produced in mouse brain or sheep brain. They have quite serious consequences, but not necessarily associated with adventitial agents. You can get encephalitis as a result of immune responses to the non-invasive protein.' 'Influenza is an actuated vaccine. Again, it's not made on SPF eggs, that is, specified pathogen-free eggs. They are avian leukosis virus free, but they are not free of all the other pathogens that you would choose to exclude from the measles vaccine production system.'

Dr. Minor, the UK's top vaccine safety officer, then added: 'So even today then you have to bear in mind that a large amount of vaccine that's made is made on really quite crude materials, from an adventitious agent point of view. It's not a trivial usage. In fact, when considering what vaccines are actually made on these days, they are quite primitive in some respects.'

These warnings were coming from a senior doctor working for the UK government who would ask me at a later meeting not to pass on vaccine information that would alarm parents.

He went on to discuss SV40 and the polio vaccine. 'It's a very common polyoma virus of old world monkeys, and particularly rhesus macaques. The difficulty with this was that, when the rhesus macaque monkeys are sacrificed and a primary monkey kidney culture made from him or her, as the case may be, a silent infection is set up. So there is evidence of infection [found] just by looking at the cultures. In fact, these cultures can throw out as much SV40 as they do polio [virus].' 'The problem was that the cell cultures didn't show any sign of having defects, when they were actually infected with SV40.'

It seemed that SV40, and its accompanying proteins and genetic codes, would never have got into so many humans if they had not contaminated the vaccine – and that they were only dangerous when moved into a species for which their presence was not natural – such as into humans and into Cynomolgus monkeys.

Dr. Minor continued: 'Wild caught monkeys were being used extensively in vaccine production. Up to a half of the cultures would have been thrown away because of adventitious agent contamination, mainly foamy virus, but certainly other things as well.'

But, they could not be certain what viruses were present. They could be mistaking SV40 for other viruses. Why? He explained because antibody tests are used to test for its presence – and such tests are not all that accurate. Antibodies don't only react to a specific viral protein. They may 'cross-react' against other things. 'What you could also argue is that you are not picking up SV40 specific antibodies at all, and they could be other human polyomas [viruses] like the BK or the JC, and it's cross-reacting antibodies that we're picking up. I think that is still a thing that needs to be resolved.'

**'The point about this long story which I have just been telling you about SV40 is that SV40 was a problem between 1955 and 1962, and it's now 1999, and we still don't really know what was going on. So if you actually make a mistake, it's really quite serious. It may keep you occupied for the rest of your working life. '**

Then Dr. Minor made a still more alarming admission: 'Now the regulatory authorities in the room will be well aware of a large number of other examples of this type which don't actually get published. I think that's not so good. I think this stuff really should be out there in the public literature.

Another UK expert then took the stand. It was Dr. Robertson from NIBSC and, as he explained, 'for those of you who don't know, NIBSC is CBER's cousin from across the pond in the U.K.' In other words, it was the top UK vaccine safety monitoring body. He started off on a reassuring note: 'There is no evidence for any increase in the incidence of childhood cancers since the onset of measles, mumps vaccination.' But he then said: **'But, I think, as a scientific community, unless we do something at least for the future, we might be in a very difficult situation to defend certain issues. If I confronted some of the violent ideologically pure Greens in our country, [telling them what we have been discussing here]: I'm sure they would say: 'Shut it down because this is unsafe, totally unsafe.'**

It was thus that I learnt that our vaccines are a veritable soup, made up not just of viruses that should or should not be there, but also thousands of bits of viruses and of cells, DNA and RNA genetic codes, proteins, enzymes, chemicals and perhaps oncogenes and prions. The vaccine was monitored for the presence of only a very few of these particles and vaccine lots are thrown away only if these are found.

In other words, the vaccines we give our children are liquids filled with a host of unknown particles, most of which came from the cells of non-humans: from chickens, monkeys, or even from cancer cells. Truly we do not know what we are doing or what are the long-term consequences. All that is known for sure is that vaccines are a very cheap form of public medicine often provided by governments to assure the public that they really do care for the safety of our children.

I have not mentioned one final addition to the vaccines – the preserving and antibiotic chemicals added to the doses. The manufacturer of a MMR vaccine noted: 'The finished product contains the following excipients: sucrose, hydrolysed gelatin (porcine), sorbitol, monosodium glutamate, sodium phosphate, sodium bicarbonate, potassium phosphate and Medium 199 with Hanks' Salts, Minimum Essential Medium Eagle (MEM), neomycin, phenol red, hydrochloric acid and sodium hydroxide.' [155] What these chemicals might do was not discussed at these workshops.

On top of this I knew from government records that vaccines sometimes contain the pork-derived trypsin used to break up monkey cells and other flesh in the vaccine cultures. Also, in the latest version of the Salk vaccine there is a surprisingly large amount of formaldehyde left behind after it has done its work of 'poisoning the viruses' (despite biology teaching us that viruses are not living particles). These workshops omitted all these issues from their consideration.

Today the Salk vaccine is back in use under the brand name IPOL, supposedly in a safer format – and the Sabin is out of use in the West as it is now blamed for causing some polio cases. But IPOL officially 'contains maximum 0.02% of formaldehyde per dose.' [156] This is 200 parts a million, yet a major Harvard University study on the CDC website reports: 'Formaldehyde is a reactive chemical that has been recognized as a human carcinogen. At levels above 0.1 parts per million, the exposure causes a burning sensation in the eyes, nose and throat; nausea; coughing; chest tightness; wheezing; and skin rashes.' [157]

This utterly shocked me, coming after learning from these reports that our top government scientists know our children are vaccinated with 'primitive' cocktails of viruses mixed among DNA fragments, chemicals and cellular debris, all potentially highly dangerous – along with many unidentified particles.

Furthermore the transcript of another scientific meeting, this one held at the Institute of Medicine in June 2000, comprised of scientists from the CDC, FDA and vaccine industry, reveals it was called because a CDC scientist, Dr. Thomas Verstraeten, found a statistically significant relationship between mercury in vaccines and several neurological conditions, including possibly autism, which today is seriously affecting very many of our children. [158]

The official US Environmental Protection Agency (EPA) safety of exposure standard for mercury is 0.1 microgram per kilogram of body weight per day, or 7 micrograms for a 70-kilogram adult. Yet, 'fully vaccinated children receive as much as 237.5 micrograms of mercury from vaccines in doses of up to 25 micrograms each.' According to 2003 research, 'thimerosal [mercury] in a single vaccine greatly exceeds the EPA adult standard.' [159]

---

[155] Op. Cit.

[156] http://www.vaccineshoppe.com/US_PDF/860-10_4305_4308.pdf IPOL produced Aventis Pasteur SA

[157] http://www.efluxmedia.com/news_Formaldehyde_Exposure_Boosts_ALS_Risk_16632.htm

[158] See article at http://www.rollingstone.com/politics/story/7395411/deadly_immunity. For the research documents see http://www.autismhelpforyou.com/Simpsonwood_And_Puerto%20%20Rico.htm

[159] Davis, Eric *Health Hazards of Mercury, at* http://www.westonaprice.org_envtoxins_mercury, citing Geier MR, Geier DA 2003, Thimerosal in Childhood Vaccines, Neurodevelopment Disorders, and Heart Disease in the United States. Journal of American Physicians and Surgeons, 2003;8(1):6-11.

Mercury is now being reduced or eliminated from vaccines, and yet, undeniably most of our children seem to have survived multiple doses with these vaccines, including those containing mercury, with no evident damage. How can this be?

My horror at discovering how little is known about the contents of our vaccines, is counterbalanced by my growing admiration for our marvellous immune system. Apparently after vaccination, if we are in a good state of health, it normally is quite capable of neutralising much of this debris, removing or reducing its great danger.

But this did not explain why top scientists, who believe with every iota of their being in the great danger presented by viruses, who see these as the great enemy, have exposed our children to such dangers, without ever informing their parents of these dangers?

In 2002 further research has found major childhood vaccines contaminated with retroviruses. 'The RT-positive vaccines include measles, mumps, and yellow fever vaccines produced by several manufacturers in Europe and the United States. RT activity was detected in the vaccines despite strict manufacturing practices requiring that chick embryos and embryo fibroblasts be derived from closed, specific-pathogen-free chicken flocks. Such chickens are screened for known pathogens' [160]

The authors also stated: 'Endogenous retroviral particles are not addressed by current manufacturing guidelines because these particles had not been associated with chick cell-derived vaccines.' But this is not so. Their paper admits. 'The presence of Avian Leukosis virus (ALV) in chick-cell-derived vaccines is not a new phenomenon; many instances of ALV contamination in yellow fever and measles vaccines have been documented.' [161] As far as I am concerned, the 'current manufacturing guidelines' should have been adjusted to take account of this.

The research paper continued: 'The finding of RT activity in all measles vaccine lots from different manufacturers tested suggests that this occurrence is not sporadic and that vaccine recipients may be universally exposed to these retroviral particles.'

So far, however, they had not detected these chicken retroviruses in the children vaccinated. But their results were inconclusive, they admitted. 'Confirmation of our molecular results by EAV-specific serologic testing may however be necessary. The lack of evidence of transmission of EAV [Endogenous Avian Virus] to vaccinees is likely due to the presence of defective particles. No infectious EAVs have yet been isolated, nor has a full-length intact EAV provirus been identified. However, our understanding of the EAV family is limited.' (They were using PCR – a tool with shortcomings in identifying viruses as described earlier.)

Their final conclusion: 'Despite these reassuring data, the presence of avian retroviral particles in chick embryo fibroblast-derived vaccines raises questions about the suitability of primary chicken cell substrates for vaccine production...'

They suggest the measles and other egg-grown vaccines should be grown instead on 'immortalized or diploid mammalian cells' but added a caveat: 'Since the cell substrate is critical to the attenuation of live vaccine viruses, any change in the cell substrate could have unpredictable effects on the safety and efficacy of the vaccine and should be approached cautiously.'

It thus seems that the reason why so far little has been done to remove the chicken virus contamination from the MMR and other vaccines – is that there is no known safer way to vaccinate, despite many decades of research, despite governments spending

---

160 Research from a Harvard School of Public Health team, led by Dr Marc Weisskopf on links between ALS and 12 types of chemicals.  http://www.cdc.gov/ncidod/eid/vol7no1/hussain.htm
Lack of Evidence of Endogenous Avian Leukosis Virus and Endogenous Avian Retrovirus Transmission to Measles Mumps Rubella Vaccine Recipients   Althaf I. Hussain,* Vedapuri Shanmugam,* William M. Switzer,* Shirley X. Tsang,* Aly Fadly,† Donald Thea,‡ Rita Helfand,* William J. Bellini,* Thomas M. Folks,* and Walid Heneine*
The title of the paper is barely commensurate with its contents.

millions of dollars to try to find a safe way to make vaccines. Toxins will accumulate in the body – so what long-term cumulative damage is being caused through the great numbers of vaccines given today?

In March 1989, MMR (Urabe AM-9) was introduced in Japan. In September 1989 the first Japanese case of aseptic meningitis, post MMR vaccine, was reported to the Japanese Public Health Council. [162] When this vaccine was introduced in the UK, reports of the same illness immediately followed.[163] These should have been predicted, as similar reports had lead to the withdrawal of the vaccine in Canada.[164] As I have reported above, many cases of this disease previously were diagnosed as non-paralytic polio. If chemical pollutants caused that illness, as the evidence above seems to suggest, might contaminants in vaccines cause, or help to cause, similar neural damage?

At that time the mumps component of this MMR vaccine was blamed (with its associated contaminants included but not mentioned), and so it was eventually withdrawn from circulation in the UK. This lead to SFK, it's manufacturer, having the other two components, measles and rubella, left unsold on the shelf. It was partially to use up these that the UK organised the MR campaign whose disastrous history I recount in the first chapter of this book. It's manufacturer, Smith Klein Beecham (SKB), was also apparently given immunity from prosecution for vaccine damage. A governmental joint working party minute of May 7th 1993 reportedly stated: 'SKB continued to sell the Urabe strain vaccine without liability.' [165]

Measles, mumps and other vaccines continue to be produced on contaminated fertilized bird eggs. WHO, and the national health authorities have quietly, but officially, permitted childhood vaccines to contain 'a low level' of viral contamination – simply because they cannot remove it economically.

WHO currently approves as acceptable a level of contamination of 106 to 107 possible viral particles per millilitre for the substrates on which are grown our vaccines. They publicly say this only presents a 'theoretical safety concern' but clearly they still are very concerned, as they stated when no journalists were present in these conferences, Vaccines have become very big business since more and more doses per child are stipulated and purchased every year. The estimated revenue from childhood vaccines in the US is now over 2.4 billion dollars a year. [166] But are the contamination and additives in the vaccines damaging many of the children they are supposed to help?

---

[162] See http://www.nih.go.jp/JJID/55/101.pdf.. This is referenced in the highly recommended piece by Alan Golding available online at http://alan-golding.blogspot.com/2008/08/time-to-revisit-decisions.html

[163] Gray JA. Lancet 1989;2:98

[164] Murray MW. Lancet 1989;2:677

[165] JCVI minutes of 7 May 1993 cited by Alan Golding above. JCVI is the Joint Working Party of the British Paediatric Association and the Joint Committee on Vaccination and Immunization.

166 Pediatric Preventive Care Cost, Estimated US Average, 2005, by Patient Age, Recommendations for Preventive Pediatric Health Care (RE9939) and Recommended Childhood and Adolescent Immunization Schedule, US, 2005. Based on 4 million births a year.

# Chapter 8

# The Vaccine Plagues?

### Autistic Spectrum Disorders, Measles, MMR and Toxins.

There is a new disease complex on the block. In the early 1980s about 1 in 10,000 American children were diagnosed with an Autistic Spectrum Disorder (ASD). By 2005 one in every 250 American children were so afflicted and the CDC now says it is as high as 1 in 150. In the UK the National Autistic Society estimates that over 1 in 100 are afflicted. In 2007 it was calculated that 1 in 58 boys were affected in the UK.[167] Tens of thousands of families have had to learn how to bring up children with varying levels of highly disturbed behaviour. Soon we will have an equal number of adults that need care. It will not be long before these cases will greatly increase the numbers of our senior citizens who need total dedication from their carers. No one seems to be taking into full account the size of this disaster.

Autistic disorders are defined by the presence of impairments affecting social interaction, communication and imagination. They frequently make social life very difficult. It affects individuals in many different ways

But ASDs are not the only illnesses that may be caused by multiple vaccinations. Our top scientists worry, as we have seen, that the contaminants in vaccines may be helping to cause autoimmune diseases, brain disorders and cancers in later life. Also, environmental pollutants may accumulate in us alongside those from vaccines to cause severe damage.

There is now a real risk that the cost in illnesses caused may exceed any possible benefit from vaccination. Let me put this into context. More children are now afflicted with brain disorders than there were victims in the worse of the American polio epidemics. On top of this, our vulnerable senior citizens are similarly coming down with brain disorders that might be linked to the same factors,

What is causing these new epidemics? This time the health authorities are not blaming a virus. Many suspect it is a side effect of intensive vaccination. Others deny this and mutter that it could be genetics – but genetics have never explained a new epidemic.

I had started out on this investigation in response to a request made by parents

---

[167] http://observer.guardian.co.uk/uk_news/story/0,,2121521,00.html *New health fears over big surge in autism.* Denis Campbell, Health Correspondent Sunday July 8, 2007 The Observer
'The number of children in Britain with autism is far higher than previously thought, according to dramatic new evidence by the country's leading experts in the field.
A study, as yet unpublished, shows that as many as one in 58 children may have some form of the condition, a lifelong disability that leads to many sufferers becoming isolated because they have trouble making friends and often display obsessional behaviour.
Seven academics at Cambridge University, six of them from its renowned Autism Research Centre, undertook the research by studying children at local primary schools. Two of the academics, leaders in their field, privately believe that the surprisingly high figure may be linked to the use of the controversial MMR vaccine. That view is rejected by the rest of the team, including its leader, the renowned autism expert, Professor Simon Baron-Cohen. The team found that one in 58 children has either autism or a related autistic spectrum disorder. Nationwide, that could be as many as 210,000 children under 16.'

whose child became brain damaged days after receiving MMR and Hib meningitis vaccines together, a child who had received previously other vaccines. They asked me: 'Is the government hiding something from us?'

Was I now coming closer to an answer? No one can deny that the explosion of ASD cases started after we began to repeatedly and intensively vaccinate children. So – could this possibly be the cause?

I have reported above how top government experts say the licensed vaccines are both crude and contaminated: that they cannot be purified. They report that they contain fragments of DNA from other species that might cause human autoimmune diseases or even cancers (another relatively new epidemic).

I had interviewed Dr Andrew Wakefield earlier. He had explained to me in his office at the Royal Free Hospital in London how he had detected measles virus in the gut cells of children suffering from Crohn's Disease and Irritable Bowel Syndrome. He told how he suspected that this virus came from the measles vaccine and could be implicated in causing these illnesses. He later added that gut perforations caused by these illnesses might cause ASD by allowing toxins to escape from the gut to damage brain cells. Was this why autism sometimes began after a measles-containing MMR vaccination?

The medical establishment fiercely attacked Wakefield for his theories, and for advocating single-virus vaccines rather than MMR, saying the former was easier on the immune systems of children. This seemed logical. The attack on him seemed very unfair– but I was puzzled. He had taken time out to explain to me that it was the measles vaccine virus that was potentially dangerous. If so, then surely the single-dose measles vaccine carried the same risk?

Later I learnt that other scientists had tested autism victims with PCR and, unlike Wakefield, could not find the segment of measles virus RNA that they searched for.[168] Others claimed a protein with the molecular weight of 74,000 Daltons from the measles virus was far more common among autism sufferers than among the healthy.[169] How could such discrepancies be explained?

The controversy had been bitter. Other scientists stated they had found genetic codes unique to measles virus in autistic children. The same code also was found in the brains of victims of Multiple Sclerosis. But, I wondered, did these codes signify more than the presence of a virus? Wasn't it likely that they indicated also the presence of the many contaminates spread with the measles virus in the MMR vaccine, including proteins, enzymes, DNA from chicken cultures and many different viruses?

Wakefield came under relentless, merciless attacks from those who defended the vaccines. Some cited research that indicated many autism victims did not have major gut illnesses. Another attack cited the case of Japan where MMR had been withdrawn and new autism cases continued to occur. But I noted that the graph produced of Japanese cases showed a spike in autism some 2-3 years after MMR withdrawal and then a decline. What if the vaccine in the child took a few years to cause autism, or what if the single-virus vaccines they gave instead were also implicated?

---

[168] http://briandeer.com/wakefield/chadwick-bruce.htm

169 'Immunoblotting of measles vaccine virus revealed that the antibody was directed against a protein of approximately 74 kd molecular weight. The antibody to this antigen was found in 83% of autistic children but not in normal children or siblings of autistic children. Thus autistic children have a hyperimmune response to measles virus, which in the absence of a wild type of measles infection might be a sign of an abnormal immune reaction to the vaccine strain or virus reactivation.' Singh VK et al. Elevated levels of measles antibodies in children with autism.
Pediatr Neurol. 2003 Apr;28(4):292-4.
http://www.ncbi.nlm.nih.gov/pubmed/12849883?dopt=Abstract
http://www.taap.info/Singh.IOM%20presentation.doc

But I was left unsure. Where was the evidence for the measles virus being the sole cause of autism? Might the antibody to it mark the presence of other vaccine contaminants, ones that are injected and can pass through our protective blood-brain barrier. There seemed no need for these damaging toxins to all come from the gut.

But, even if the measles virus were not the principal agent involved, this did not mean that Wakefield was wrong in saying that repeated jabs of MMR were too much for some children to endure. What of the MMR manufacturer's admission that its vaccines contained cellular degradation products from birds? What of the top UK expert Dr Phil Minor's statement that our current vaccines are both 'crude' and 'primitive' and grossly contaminated? Could Wakefield's discovery relate to these contaminants as well?

Since many parents have reported serious illnesses in their children after MMR, we have to ask: When measles virus is injected into our children, what else might be in the needle? How sterile is the method used to make the common vaccines?

In a paper entitled '*Isolation and Identification of Measles Virus in Cell Culture*,' the US Government's leading virus research institution, the CDC, currently lays out how isolation of this virus should be done. It instructs; first obtain from a patient suspected of having measles a small sample of urine or fluid from the nose or mouth. [170]

Next prepare a culture of cells from marmoset monkeys by making these cells cancerous and giving them Epstein-Barr disease!  (They recommend this species of monkeys as they are '10,000 times' more sensitive to the measles virus than are normal human cells, meaning they are much more likely to fall gravely ill during this procedure). The monkey cells are then settled into a monolayer (one cell deep layer) in a laboratory vessel. (In order to save money, the measles and MMR vaccine manufacturers are using instead cells from mashed chicken embryos. Otherwise the procedure is much the same.)

Next, taking care to use rubber gloves and splash goggles, add a toxin called trypsin.[171] The CDC warns to now expect some of the cells to fall away as if they are poisoned.  They are.  It then instructs: add nutrients and glucose and leave the cells alone for two or three days so they can recover.

Next, add to the cell culture the sample from the patient and place the culture in a warm incubation chamber. After an hour, inspect its cells with a microscope to see if any are rounded, distorted, or floating free as they were immediately after trypsin was added. If they are, the CDC calls this proof that measles virus is present and causing this illness! Why, when toxic trypsin has been added and the cells were already ill?

But the CDC has no doubts.  It instructs; if 50% of the cells are now distorted, 'scrape the cells into the medium' and then store at -70 C as an 'isolated measles-virus stock!' This will contains many particles and toxins from these extremely sick monkey cells – yet it is said to be an 'isolate' of measles virus that might be used for a vaccine! In fact, no measles-like symptoms were looked for in the culture. The CDC does not even look to see if the measles virus is present. It is the fluid filtered off from a culture of this 'isolate' that is used as a vaccine.

When I read this paper, I was horrified by the inadequacy of the science.  The child vaccinated would have to produce many antibodies against all the contaminants – irrespective of whether they were measles virus.

This led me to wonder how this virus was first discovered and processed to make measles vaccines. I hoped it would be nothing like the faulty process used with the poliovirus. (See Ch. 3 above)  But I found that John Enders, the scientist who developed

---

[170] CDC. *Isolation and Identification of Measles Virus in Culture,* Revised November 29, 2001.

[171] http://www.sciencelab.com/xMSDS-Trypsin-9927313

the measles vaccine in 1954, said he had modelled its development on the work he had done to help make the polio vaccines. [172]

His team had obtained some fluid, 'throat washings and blood', from an 11-year-old boy with measles called David Edmonston. When this was added to 'human post-natal' cells in his lab, these cells fell ill. This he took as indicating a measles virus might be present. This fluid was then added to human cervical cancer cells (HeLa) and to 'human carcinoma cells.' The cells became still sicker. Fluids from a culture were moved to another culture and then to another. When his microscope revealed 'giant multinuclear cells' in the cultures, Enders took this as a sign that the measles virus had distorted them, not that the cancers might be getting more malignant. After he passaged the fluid a further 23 times from one culture of human kidney cells to another and then 19 times through cultures of human amnion cells, he reported the cells in the cultures were now beginning to take highly deformed shapes like 'fibroblasts,'

When his team tested the resulting cell culture fluid on Cynomolgus monkeys they found some got a 'mild' illness that in 'some aspects' resembled measles. Enders took this as evidence that this toxic mix of mutant cells was a measles virus 'isolate.' He called it the 'Edmonston isolate' after the name of the boy.

He then decided to use fertilized bird eggs rather than monkeys to save costs in making vaccines. He used the culture with highly distorted cells that he had produced after 42 passages through cell cultures. He gave it another 9 passages though amnion cells. He observed that his culture now contained cells distorted into 'fusiform and stellate' shapes.

Enders added this to fertilised eggs. 'After incubating for 9 days at 35 degrees' in 'developing chicks,' some of the chick cells took on similar deformed shapes to those he had observed earlier. He then concluded this mutated cell culture was 'the most suitable material for the preparation of vaccines' and that this method would 'greatly reduce the cost of manufacture.' Thus the 'Edmonston strain' became the basis of some of our major measles vaccines.

This is also how the measles vaccine became as contaminated as is documented in the previous chapter. It is made from and contains mutated particles from poisoned bird cells, some of which, according to the government vaccine safety experts cited earlier, might cause 'autoimmune diseases and cancers' in the vaccinated. Could vaccines contaminated with parts of mutated bird cells play a role in causing Autism Spectrum Disorders? Surely there must be a real risk that injecting this contaminated fluid into our children may sometimes overwhelm their immune systems– or do other long term damage?

It seems all our common vaccines are made similarly; with manufacturers sometimes adding to these contaminated fluids two more potential risk factors, mercury and aluminium.

### THE MERCURY ADDED TO VACCINES

Mercury is added to some vaccines as a preservative and aluminium added as an adjuvant to 'enhance the immune response,' or so I was told. Could these metals, with the other contaminants, work together to help produce the autistic epidemic? Our children are exposed to these in the earliest years of childhood, while their brains are most vulnerable and their immune responses not fully formed. They lack the detoxification system possessed by adults and their protective blood-brain barrier is not yet fully formed.

---

[172] Enders J et al. Measles Virus: A Summary of Experiments Concerned with Isolation, Properties, and Behavior Am J Public Health Nations Health. 1957 March; 47(3): 275–282. http://www.pubmedcentral.nih.gov/articlerender.fcgi?artid=1551024. Whole text.

It is not just the children who are at risk. Could the mercury in the flu vaccines that are recommended every winter to our senior citizens increase the numbers coming down with dementia? I had to look into this.

Dr. Boyd Haley, the Professor and Chair of the Department of Chemistry at the University of Kentucky, has stated: 'You couldn't even construct a study that shows Thimerosal is safe. It's just too darn toxic. If you inject Thimerosal into an animal, its brain will sicken. If you apply it to living tissue, the cells die. If you put it in a Petri dish, the culture dies. Knowing these things, it would be shocking if one could inject it into an infant without causing damage.' He also stated: 'A single vaccine given to a six-pound newborn is the equivalent of giving a 180-pound adult 30 vaccinations on the same day. Include in this the toxic effects of high levels of aluminium and formaldehyde contained in some vaccines, and the synergist toxicity could be increased to unknown levels. ... Bilary transport is the major biochemical route by which mercury is removed from the body, and infants cannot do this very well. They also do not possess the renal (kidney) capacity to remove aluminium. Additionally, mercury is a well-known inhibitor of kidney function'.[173]

A CDC report was cited by both the US and UK governments to prove that vaccines could not possibly cause autism. But the CDC has now admitted to the US Congress that they fixed its results. It had reversed its findings by unjustifiably reprocessing the statistics. Dr. Thomas Verstraeten and co-workers at the CDC were responsible for this study of the government's 'Vaccine safety databank' statistics. They examined the health records of 110,000 American children and had initially reported:

'A. Exposure to Thimerosal [mercury]-containing vaccines at one month was associated significantly with a misery and unhappiness disorder expressed by uncontrollable crying that is dose related.' That is, the higher the child's exposure to Thimerosal the higher the incidence of the disorder.

B. With 'exposure at 3 months, there was a statistically significant increased risk of neurodevelopmental disorders' including those of speech.

But then the authors reversed these results by removing a quarter of the susceptible cases and carrying out other unjustified recalculations.

This fraud was unearthed only 'in 2005, a group of Senators and Representatives headed by Sen. Joe Lieberman wrote to the NIEHS (an agency of the National Institutes of Health) saying that many parents no longer trusted the CDC to conduct independent minded studies of its own vaccine program. Lieberman et al asked NIEHS to review the CDC's work on the vaccine database and report back with critiques and suggestions.' The NIEHS had come back with a report severely critical of the CDC.

Much to my surprise I have now learnt that this reversal was due to the discovery of a secret governmental transcript similar to the ones I cited in the previous chapter on vaccine contamination.  This transcript was of a meeting of top scientists called to consider the safety of the mercury added to vaccines.

The existence of this transcript leaked when a Congressman sent a copy of a letter he had received to a Dr. Russell Blaylock who has written powerfully on this subject.[174] This letter mentioned a previously unknown transcript of a conference entitled: 'Scientific Review of Vaccine Safety Datalink Information.' This had reviewed the above study and was stamped 'Confidential.' [175]

---

[173] Letter from Haley to Congressional committee archived on web at
http://www.whale.to/m/haley.html - also http://www.whale.to/v/haley3.html
[174] I am indebted to him for drawing my attention to the mercury transcript. I recommend this article by him available online at http://www.doctorvickery.com/vcu.cfm
[175] http://www.autismhelpforyou.com/AL%20-%201.pdf  and
http://www.autismhelpforyou.com/AL%20-%201.pdf  with thanks to www autismhelpforyou.com

It recorded a secret conference held on June 7-8$^{th}$ 2000 at the Simpsonwood Retreat Center in Norcross, Georgia, USA. In attendance were 70 government scientists, plus representatives of pharmaceutical companies and of the World Health Organization. Dr. Roger Bemier, the Associate Director for Science in the National Immunization Program of the CDC, began by making this admission: 'In the United States there was a growing recognition that cumulative exposure [to mercury in vaccines] may exceed some of the [safety] guidelines.'

They cited an earlier 1999 meeting of the same NIH committee that had discussed the dangers of vaccine contamination reported in the last chapter. Their work had helped bring about 'a joint statement of the Public Health Service and the American Academy of Science in July last year (1999) which stated that as a long term goal it was desirable to remove mercury from vaccines.'

Yet today mercury still remains in several vaccines. Why was it not been removed? From what was said at these official meetings, it seems the manufacturers are unwilling to pay for making all the replacement vaccines needed, They would remove mercury from some vaccines, but not from the tetanus and flu vaccines.

Dr Johnson explained in Georgia why he was reluctant to recommend its removal from all vaccines, despite the results of Dr. Verstraeten's investigation, despite knowing that mercury was associated with brain diseases: 'We agree that it would be desirable to remove mercury from U.S. licensed vaccines, but we did not agree that this was a universal recommendation that we would make, because of the issue concerning preservatives for delivering vaccines to other countries, particularly developing countries, in the absence of hard data that implied that there was in fact a problem.' Dr Robert Chen from the CDC added: 'The issue is that it is impossible, unethical to leave kids unimmunized, so you will never, ever, resolve that issue.'

These comments were made at a time when children were receiving perhaps 20 vaccine doses of mercury and aluminium before they were three years of age. They would continue to receive some mercury in vaccines in order to allow vaccination to continue, or so it was claimed. The real reason seems to be a lack of will to fund replacements. This was despite numerous scientists at these meetings saying they desperately needed more information on the potential harm that might be done by mercury and aluminium.

However public pressure had resulted in the pharmaceutical giant Merck undertaking to remove mercury from some vaccines, as apparently also did GlaxoSmithKline, but neither had agreed to remove from the market their current stocks of millions of doses of mercury-containing vaccines. To do so, they inferred, would be far too expensive. When these stocks were exhausted, perhaps in 2004, they would only sell vaccines for infants that had 'trace elements of mercury' in them – that is, excepting their tetanus and flu vaccines in which full doses of mercury would remain. This was despite the meeting noting that older people with mercury amalgams in dental work in their teeth, or who had eaten contaminated fish, would be at increased risk from the mercury in vaccines.

The committee members reported having little data on the toxicity of the ethylmercury added to vaccines, professing ignorance of the many toxicology reports on mercury. One of the problems, they stated, was that they now had no mercury-free children to use as a safety control study! All were now contaminated with mercury.

Dr William Weiss, a paediatrician from the Committee of Environmental Health of the American Academy of Paediatrics, reminded the doctors present: 'there are just a host of neurodevelopmental data that would suggest that we've got a serious problem.'

To this Dr Weil added: 'the number of dose related relationships are linear and statistically significant. You can play with this all you want. They are linear. They are statistically relevant.' 'I have to say the number of kids getting help in special education is growing nationally and state by state at a rate not seen before.'

Dr Johnson then concluded; 'This association leads me to favour a recommendation that infants up to two years old not be immunized with Thimerosal-containing vaccines, if suitable alternative preparations are available… In the meantime I want my grandson to be given Thimerosal-free vaccines.'

But Dr Clements insisted – and would get his way: 'My mandate as I sit here in this group is to make sure at the end of the day that 100,000,000 are immunized with DTP, Hepatitis B and if possible Hib A this year, next year and for many years to come, and that will have to be with Thimerosal-containing vaccines unless a miracle occurs and an alternative is found quickly, is tried and found safe.'

On May 20th 2003 the Rep. Dan Burton presented the *Mercury in Medicine Report* in the US Congress. I advise all to read it. It's final paragraph concluded:

**'Thimerosal … in vaccines is likely related to the autism epidemic. This epidemic in all probability may have been prevented or curtailed had the FDA not been asleep at the switch regarding the lack of safety data regarding injected Thimerosal and the sharp rise of infant exposure to this known neurotoxin. Our public health agencies' failure to act is indicative of institutional malfeasance for self-protection and misplaced protectionism of the pharmaceutical industry.**" [176]

### THE ALUMINIUM ADDED TO VACCINES

They now began to discuss the aluminium salts added to vaccines as 'adjuvants'. Dr Johnson stated: ' Aluminium salts have a very wide margin of safety. Aluminium and mercury are often simultaneously administered to infants, both at the same site and at different site … However we also [have] learnt that there is absolutely no data, including animal data, about the potential for synergy, additively or antagonistic, all of which can occur in binary metal mixtures.'

Aluminium is a normal part of our environment, one of the most common elements on earth. Our bodies have evolved to dispose of it quite safely – that is when the exposure is natural. But when injected into our bodies, bypassing our natural defences, it may act as a neurotoxin and react with other metals like mercury. Also, as Dr Harn Hogenesch reported at this conference, **an aluminium adjuvant can 'induce a type 2 immune response and set up an individual for allergic reactions to vaccine components.'**

The problem was, the doctors at the conference reported, we had no data on how quickly or efficiently our immune systems remove aluminium from our bodies, particularly after vaccination. We particularly knew very little about how quickly it is removed in very young children or the elderly. If aluminium or mercury is not swiftly removed, there is a risk that they are stored in the brain and elsewhere until they reach a critical mass. In such cases there is a risk that a person might be suddenly struck down with severe brain damage. Likewise an elderly relative might slip into dementia.

Aluminium salts are added to some vaccines as antibodies are produced for longer after vaccination when aluminium is included. It is hoped this means the child is protected for longer.

But – why are antibodies produced for longer? Extraordinarily the senior scientists at these gatherings admitted that they did not know why. Antibodies are produced by our immune system to remove dangers, including toxins. Could it be that the antibody production is against long-lasting aluminium neurotoxins? The vaccine manufactures say to this day that they do not know why antibodies continue to be made for longer after 'aluminium-enhanced' vaccination! Yet, despite being so ignorant, the manufacturers have continued to use these and our health authorities have approved them as 'safe.'

I then learnt of an 11th-12th May 2000 Puerto Rico scientific meeting on 'Aluminum Adjuvants.' I obtained a transcript and it was extraordinarily interesting. I have it here

---

[176]   http://www.aapsonline.org/vaccines/mercinmed.pdf

before me and it reads like a detective story. The meeting was called in part to hear a French team of scientists report on severe disabling illnesses caused by aluminium-enhanced vaccines – and because, as Dr. Myers, the Acting Director of the National Vaccine Program Office, stated at its start" 'Those of us who deal with vaccines have really very little applicable background with metals and with toxicological research – that is the reason why this meeting is occurring today."

I know aluminium is a common element – but I had no idea what the aluminium put into our vaccines is like. I now learnt from the experts whose evidence is in this transcript that it was nothing like what I had imagined. The usual adjuvant used is an aluminium compound in the form of large numbers of tiny metallic "fibrous crystals." This alerted me, for I have previously researched asbestosis. I had learnt that asbestos did its deadly work in lungs, cutting into cells, because it too is in the form of sharp "fibrous crystals."

Dr Stan Hem told the conference that the aluminium most often used as a vaccine adjuvant is 'aluminium hydroxide," which is also known as the mineral 'bomite.' It is hard, "fibrous" and made up of sharp crystals in the form of 'millions' of 'needles.' As bomite, a naturally occurring mineral, it has been hardened into these shapes by millions of years of heat and stress. When the French scientists gave their evidence on the second day of this conference, they reported finding these aluminium needles could remain present inside macrophage cells in the arms vaccinated for at least 8 years after the injection. Asbestos fibres are also retained in macrophages. Our macrophages try to dispose of these as they do other pathogens. But they are too hard and spiky. They cut into the cells and may take years to dissolve. But in the case of asbestosis, we are dealing with lung cells, not arm cells, and vastly greater exposure. What the French now reported was a very different, much less frequent, but damaging consequence of implanting these aluminium crystals.

The French scientists diplomatically explained at this gathering that they had discovered this before the Americans by chance – because in France they had another method of doing biopsies. They use the arm muscles where vaccines are commonly injected, while in the US and elsewhere biopsies are normally performed on different muscles. Dr Gherardi stated: 'I am absolutely convinced that you have similar patients in the US but that you do not detect them because of the biopsy procedure...' [177]

They were certain other countries would find the same; for their studies showed aluminium-enhanced vaccines readily did the same damage in many animal species. The aluminium-containing muscle lesion appeared in animals 28 days after vaccination.

The French scientists had first become concerned when they noted that patients were coming to them with an entirely new disorder. They suffered from severe disabling muscle pains that commenced in both lower legs and spread upwards. Some 85% of the patients could no longer work. Many could now only do 'basic things.' In addition, some 25% also suffered from Chronic Fatigue Syndrome and some 34% had Multiple Sclerosis. They also admitted: 'We have not tested the cumulative effects' of using aluminium-enhanced vaccines.

When these patients first came to them, the French doctors suspected the cause was a new virus: 'we believed we were facing a new emerging infectious disease.' But then they discovered from biopsies that every single one of their patients had aluminium salts in the arm muscles injected, and that every case their illness had followed aluminium-enhanced vaccination. Animal studies then revealed the vaccinations and the illnesses were causally linked. 'Aluminium appears to be an adjuvant that is very slowly eliminated [from the patient's body] as compared with many others.' Within two days of exposure, all the aluminium is taken into the cells of the vaccinated. They concluded that this new

---

[177] The first US cases were found shortly after this in 2002..
http://www.springerlink.com/content/mqq7u37k410vrn27/

disease was linked to the increased use in France of particularly the aluminium-enhanced Hepatitis B vaccine.

They called this illness macrophagic myofascitas or inflammatory myopathy. Dr Gherardi stated that; 'without aluminium-enhanced vaccination [it] does not occur. 100% of the patients had been vaccinated. This is clear and there is no question about it.' However they did not know what proportion of injected patients came down with this disease. Extensive tests had not yet been carried out. Animal tests suggested the proportion might be high but so far they had only tested around 100 victims. 'These have only recently started to be found in France – and we are convinced it is a new thing.'

They further discovered traces that showed what vaccine was used. Commonly it was the Hepatitis B vaccine. In some it was Hepatitis A or Tetanus vaccine. Most patients 'had had four such injections.' The muscle pains and Fatigue Syndrome were occurring from 3 months to eight years later. 'The median delay [after vaccination] was 11 months.' Most cases that came to them were in adults; only 2% were in children. They noted that adult vaccination for Hepatitis B had started in France some years earlier.[178]

When they tested the aluminium adjuvant on rats they found it was not the aluminium alone that caused the most damage but the aluminium combined with the vaccine. 'So we have to consider the adjuvant plus the antigen' as the cause of the illness. To this I would add the many contaminants in the vaccines, the loose proteins and DNA fragments.

They had tested their theory every way they could – and it stood up. They reported a clear and certain link between the 'aluminium-enhanced vaccines' and the illnesses. The American scientists at this meeting cross-examined the French scientists but could find no fault. Finally they applauded them for a brilliant piece of medical sleuthing.

Dr. Sam Keith noted at the meeting that the aluminium is stored mostly in our bones, followed by our kidneys, brains and muscles. When it binds to the larger proteins, he said it 'can inhibit the formation of neuronal microbule,' thus possibly affecting brains. He also mentioned that aluminium in tap water seemed to increase the risk of 'dialysis dementia.'

The Americans, and perhaps the British, are more exposed to aluminium adjuvant than the French. In France it is in three types of vaccine – all the Hep B and A vaccines and in most of the Tetanus. But in the USA it is also in acellular pertussis, anthrax, Lyme, DT Absorbed and Hib, as well as some of the rabies vaccines.

It was generally agreed at this conference that they did not know enough about the toxicity of aluminium. Dr Alison Maule said it was similar to the situation with mercury. She added: 'There are huge gaps in what we know about the toxicology of aluminium … The body has efficient mechanisms for removing metals from the circulation [but] we have not done these studies in infants in terms of mercury or aluminium.' Dr. Maule then mentioned the theory that maybe this also 'has caused the explosion of asthma and allergies.'

Dr Peggy Rennels added thoughtfully: 'Regarding immediate local reactions following injections of aluminium absorbed vaccines, we know that when they are injected… some individuals will experience severe local reactions including a lot of pain.' Dr Verdier added that the necessary data was 'missing from aluminium or incomplete.'

Yet injected or inhaled metals have long been associated with severe muscle damage. Arsenic and lead severely damage arm and leg muscles causing cases previously diagnosed as polio. Now, the evidence is that aluminium-enhanced vaccines also can produce disabling muscle damage.

---

[178]  In 2001 the French team published their discovery. R. K. Gherardi, M. Coquet, P. Cherin, L. Belec, P. Moretto, P. A. Dreyfus, J.-F. Pellissier, P. Chariot and F.-J. Authier: Macrophagic myofasciitis lesions assess long-term persistence of vaccine-derived aluminium hydroxide in muscle. Brain, Vol. 124, No. 9, 1821-1831, September 2001. Available online at ttp://www.informedchoice.info/hepB.html

Having many vaccine jabs in the same arm muscle is well known to cause paralysis in that arm, a disorder known clinically as 'provocation polio'. The British Medical Journal has carried accounts of 'massive outbreaks of provocation poliomyelitis in children who received injections of the vaccine against diphtheria, tetanus, and pertussis (DTP vaccine)' in India.[179] There are many similar reports. This is particularly in such nations as India and in Africa – as many agencies there vaccinate indiscriminately without checking records on the basis that it is 'best to be sure.' These cases are clear evidence of the damage that can come from the accumulation of vaccine toxins.

There is another added chemical that concerns me. One part in fifty of a current polio vaccine, the IPOL produced by Aventis Pasteur, is formaldehyde, a known carcinogenic. This vaccine is grown in 'a continuous line of monkey kidney cells' taken from wild-caught African Green Monkeys, supplemented by newborn calf serum. This is filtered to remove large fragments then spun rapidly. The filtered off fluid is the vaccine. To this is added up to 0.02% of formaldehyde plus several antibiotics.

Vaccines are not the only source of formaldehyde. It is also found in building materials and can be produced by unvented gas stoves. Whatever the source, the toxin is accumulative.

According to a research paper, 'exposure to formaldehyde may increase the risk of developing amyotropic lateral scherosis (ALS), also known as Lou Gehrig's disease because in 1941 it killed the New York Yankees baseball player. About 5,000 people fall ill with this every year in the USA, according to the ALS Association. It is a fatal progressive neurodegenerative disease affecting the nerve cells of the brain and spinal cord leading to paralysis.

Autism occurs more in boys than in girls, and it is reported that mercury can react with the male hormones more than with the female. It is also reported that mercury can accumulate in the mitochondria, the vital energy factories of our cells, including of the nerve cells within the brain. A major cause of autism, according to some scientists, is damage to the cells' mitochondria from toxins accumulating from vaccines.[180] In one study, three-quarters of the autistic children tested were found to have damaged mitochondria.[181] This severely limits the energy available to the child's immune system.

Both mercury and aluminium can pass through the barrier that defends our brains, as can much of the debris in vaccines. All these may damage neurone as well as other cells. The above study showed the aluminium-enhanced vaccines are more dangerous than aluminium adjuvant acting alone.

Some government scientists have claimed that, as some vaccines now have most of their mercury removed, and autism cases are still occurring, this proves autism is not related to mercury. But, they have ignored the length of time that toxins persist and have effects; and have narrowly focussed on mercury as if it were the only element in vaccines that might contribute to causing autism.

In 2007 a US court, and government experts, accepted that vaccination played a significant role in making autistic the nine-year-old Hannah Poling.[182] This major test case opened the door for compensation for many affected by this fast growing autism epidemic. The US government initially tried to play down the significance of this

[179] BMJ 25 April 1998. http://www.bmj.com/cgi/content/full/316/7140/1261/f

[180] David Kirby, *The CDC has lost control of the autism argument.* Huffington Post, April 4th 2008 http://www.huffingtonpost.com/david-kirby/cdc-has-lost-control-of-t_b_95081.html. Also April 27th 2008 posting.

[181] AAN:- Oxidative Phosphorylation (OXPHOS) Defects in Children with Autistic Spectrum Disorders [IN1-1.004] John Shoffner, Lauren C. Hyams, Genevieve N. Langley, Atlanta, GA. This reported that 75% of children with Autistic Spectrum Disorders that they assessed had mitochondrial disorder (MtD) and so were always at risk of autism caused by one or more vaccines.

[182] http://www.huffingtonpost.com/david-kirby/the-vaccineautism-court-_b_88558.html

judgement by saying Hannah's disease was mostly due to a small DNA mutation in her mitochondria – but her mother has the same mutation and it has never made her ill. Hannah also did not fall ill after vaccination until June 20th 2000 when she had 9 vaccines on the same day. It was accepted by the government that the fits she later suffered were a result of these vaccinations, although it took 6 years of illness before they began. The damage done by vaccination can take years to unfold.

On February 21st 2008 the US government made another concession. It agreed that Hannah's 'autistic' brain disease was 'caused' by vaccine-induced fever and overstimulation of her immune system. She may have had slight damage to her mitochondria from environmental toxins but she had no symptoms of illness – prior to these 9 vaccines.[183]

This reminded me of what else I had read in the transcripts. Many senior doctors asked: 'What would this contaminating DNA do when it was injected into humans in vaccines? Could it change our own DNA? Could it cause cancers – or autoimmune diseases?' Dr. Rebecca Sheets of CBER, the US laboratory responsible for monitoring vaccine safety, reported that this DNA contamination could have 'both infectivity or tumorigenic potential.'

Were these DNA fragments capable of damaging the brains of children, perhaps in combination with aluminium, formaldehyde and mercury? Nothing was said in these transcripts that alleviated such worries. On the contrary, the specialists said that this DNA might cause mutations in humans.

Could environmental toxins also play a role? They accumulate alongside vaccine toxins. One of the most common brain abnormalities found in autism is a loss of some of the brain's large Purkinje neurons. Research shows these neurons are affected by acrylamide, a chemical widely put into our drinking water to help 'purify' it. [184] According to Genetics professor Joe Cummins, studies also show that heat and light can turn the polyacrylamide, used in commercial herbicides, into acrylamide – and that acrylamide is also in some fast or junk foods.[185]

But, from all that I have read, it is likely to be the cumulative effect of vaccination that finally overwhelms the children who come down with autism or similar disorders, for parents frequently report their child's illness begins within hours or days of a vaccination. From the above transcripts, vaccines are full of chemicals, toxins and biological particles from different species. These are directly injected into the child's blood and muscles, bypassing most of their immune systems. This is a hazard that children are particularly exposed to. They are injected with 30 or more vaccines in the first two years of life during a time when their brain is being formed and is thus particularly vulnerable - and both autism and attention deficit disorder are brain disorders that begin in early childhood.

Some have treated autistic children with some success by having their blood detoxified and providing regular oxygen-breathing sessions – thus removing some toxic contaminants and assisting the damaged mitochondria – but even this has not led, as far as I know, to a full recovery.[186] Then of course there are the cases of epilepsy in children following MMR and other vaccines that started me on this investigation, particularly the case of the now teen-aged loving but brain-damaged son Robert of John and Jackie Fletcher. It seems the febrile fits he suffered after vaccination on November 23rd 1992, with one fit lasting 45 minutes, starved his brain cells of oxygen, causing permanent

---

[183] David Kirby - http://www.ajc.com/opinion/content/opinion/2008/03/19/autismed_0320.html
[184] http://www.springerlink.com/content/u7h47v564m8k3283/
http://www.epa.gov/ogwdw000/contaminants/dw_contamfs/acrylami.html
[185] http://en.wikipedia.org/wiki/Acrylamide#cite_note-8

186 Report about the child Zac in MetroWest Daily News Jun 14, 2008

impairment. Such fits are a recognized vaccine risk. Remember that in Hannah Poling's legal case, her illness started with a fit that is now acknowledged to be vaccine related. Robert was only 13 months old when he received MMR and Hib meningitis vaccinations. He had been a healthy 7lbs 15ozs at birth and was at that time seen by everyone as a normal healthy boy starting to speak. He began to fall ill ten days later. Soon his speech skills vanished. Some 16 years later, Robert suffers from convulsions and much else. He has both parents as permanent carers. [187]

While ASDs have been rapidly increasing among our children, more and more of our senior citizens are coming down with severe mental disorders. The authorities say this is because we are living longer – but what if it is the accumulation of toxins from many sources, including the mercury in the flu vaccines, that is causing this tragedy? Alarmingly, aluminium is also being found in the brains of people with Alzheimer's.

All cosmetics are tested on the 'Precautionary Principle.' This mandates that a cosmetic be withdrawn if a test shows a possible serious side effect. The same should apply to our vaccines. Nevertheless, doctors responsible for public health continue to reassure us on television that our vaccines are proved totally safe and effective, while behind closed doors they say something else entirely – as shown in the above transcripts. Away from the presence of journalists, they acknowledge our current vaccines are based on primitive science, crude materials and have many worrying risk factors. But the health authorities continue to knowingly give contaminated vaccines to our children on the basis that the benefits of vaccination are worth the risk of discarding the Precautionary Principle. This is a decision they reserve to themselves. They do not trust parents with the facts. Instead they tell them there is no risk.

Even the replacement vaccines on the horizon, spun to us as safer, are not proving safe in the laboratory. Up until now, parental concerns have mostly been about the additives put in the vaccines – but the vaccine manufacturing process really needs to be at the centre of our concerns. If it cannot produce uncontaminated vaccines why are we using it? Adding aluminium, formaldehyde and mercury to its products is like pouring petrol on flames.

The fact that many children survive vaccination without evident long-term damage is a tribute to the entirely marvellous immune systems that nature normally gifts them with. These systems are capable of neutralising a thousand different toxins simultaneously – that is, when the child is healthy, is naturally exposed to these and has not been accumulating toxins. When toxins bypass our immune system, damage the mitochondria power stations in the cells, the immune systems of children will lack the energy needed to protect them. The same is of course true in adults.

Unfortunately many children have to endure vaccination while at the same time being deprived of breast milk, with its rich, living and protective content that changes as the needs of the child change, in a manner for which there is no substitute.

I still had other questions about the usefulness of vaccines. Do our children really need all these vaccines, when they have for centuries gained life-long immunity to most diseases from natural exposure coupled with what our cells need beyond all else, good nutrition, low levels of stress and clean water?

But at this point in my inquiry, before I could find answers to these questions, a major debate occurred at the eminent and ancient Royal Society in London on just how HIV had spread, a debate in which a vaccine given to hundreds of millions was implicated. This was the subject that had enticed me deeper into this investigation. I had to be present.

---

[187] The story of Robert is now told by his parents in the highly recommended book: "Silenced Witnesses: the parents' story.' This also contains accounts by parents of some of the other cases mentioned in the first chapter of this book, as well as other cases.Published by Cryshame with Slingshot Publicaitons 2008 London.

# Chapter 9

# The Royal Society Debate

# And Cover up

By 1999, three years after I began this research, any illusions I had about the purity and safety of our childhood vaccines had been shattered. It seemed they were all contaminated, that government health safety officers had long known this but opted to say nothing, – and that it is only the natural strength of our children's immune systems that have protected most of them from the pollutants in the vaccines.

We now know how easy it was for SV40, a monkey virus, to contaminate the polio vaccine. So if it could gain entry unnoticed, if our vaccines were so difficult to purify, it now seemed to me utterly feasible that HIV, reportedly a former monkey virus, could also have spread via the polio vaccine, as suggested to me by Professor John Martin at the SV40 NIH workshop.

He was by no means the first to think this. A gifted medical journalist, Tom Curtis, raised this possibility some years earlier in a major article in Rolling Stone [188] and, well before this appeared in 1992, Louis Pascal had presented the same hypothesis in a paper widely circulated among scientists and editors, but which was then so controversial that it failed to find it a publisher. In 1989 two South African scientists, Mike Lecatsas and Jennifer Alexander, published the same hypothesis as a 'Brief Communication' in a science journal. Then in 1993 it finally reached the public. B. F. Elswood and R. B. Stricker published it as a major paper entitled *Polio Vaccines and the origin of AIDS* in the journal *Medical Hypotheses*. This stated:

'We hypothesize that the AIDS pandemic may have originated with a contaminated polio vaccine that was administered to inhabitants of Equatorial Africa from 1957 to 1959. The mechanism of evolution of HIV from this vaccine remains to be determined.[189]

But their thesis still remained controversial, and was fiercely denied by scientists who came to the defence of the polio vaccine. When it was announced that HIV must have come from chimpanzees, since they carried a virus (SIVcpz) that was genetically alike to HIV,[190] I remembered how chimpanzees were used in the development of the polio vaccines.

From the 1920s hundreds of chimpanzees were killed for polio vaccine research. Elliot Dick in the 1963 *Chimpanzee Kidney Tissue Cultures for Growth and Isolation of Viruses* [191] commented: 'apart from the cost... chimp kidney tissue cultures may very well be the perfect substrate ... simply because it's the closest to us genetically.'

---

[188] Curtis T. The origin of AIDS: A startling new theory attempts to answer the question >Was it an act of God or an act of man= Rolling Stone, March 19, 1992:57.

[189] Elswood BF, Stricker RB. Polio vaccines and the origin of AIDS in Medical Hypothesis, 1994:42:347– It is available online with an update from the authors at
http://www.uow.edu.au/arts/sts/bmartin/dissent/documents/AIDS/Elswood94.html

[190] Karpas A. Origin and Spread of AIDS. Nature, 1990; 348:578.

[191] Elliot Dick: Chimpanzee Kidney Tissue Cultures for Growth and Isolation of Viruses, J Bacteriol. 1963,86, 573-576

Since polio is a disease of our central nervous system, from the beginning of poliovirus research, scientists had injected various diseased human tissues into the brains of living chimpanzees to see if these might paralyse them. After poliovirus was reportedly identified, various trial vaccines were likewise injected into the brains of hundreds of living chimpanzees as a safety test to see if these would give them polio.

We now know all apes and monkeys have retroviruses that are apparently similar to HIV in genetic code, thus named as SIV or Simian Immunodeficiency Virus, despite contradictorily not causing immunodeficiency in their hosts. But could this SIV have mutated into HIV in the vaccine or laboratory? There was then no such thing as laboratory sterility. The eminent Oxford University biologist, Professor W. D. Hamilton, acknowledged: 'contamination of tissue cultures with retroviruses is common even in the best endowed institutions.'[192]

Although all retroviruses were at first presumed to be hostile invaders, we have since learnt that healthy cells in plants, bacteria and animals normally produce them without any need for infection. So, what could make a normally harmless chimp retrovirus mutate into a form that can kill humans?

Could it be the laboratory techniques used in the development of vaccines? Sabin did much to force the poliovirus needed for his vaccine to mutate into hopefully a harmless form by transplanting it repeatedly from cell culture to cell culture; and from cells of one species to another. Of the three different types of poliovirus in his vaccine; type one was rapidly transplanted 33 times, type two 51 times and the third 34 times. These were then given to the human recipient of his vaccine. If chimpanzee viruses were inadvertently present, wouldn't the same process of transplantation also encourage them to mutate into a form that can survive in humans?

Koprowski used chimpanzees and monkeys – as well as cotton rats and mice – in the process of making his vaccine. He passaged his polio vaccine through the brains of many, before presumably, like other scientists, safety testing the vaccine by injecting it into the living brains of chimpanzees. He then tested it on handicapped American children, before testing it on the Northern Irish, on Poles and on the Congolese.

Well, if this process forced poliovirus to mutate – what did it do to monkey viruses? As far as I can judge, it seemed to me that this vaccine production process is 'tailor made' to force SIV to mutate into an HIV.

In fact that was precisely what happened to some of the SV40 contaminating this vaccine. In 1960 Sweet reported that, when growing an adenovirus vaccine; 'we found that it [SV40] hybridised [combined] with certain DNA viruses –the adenovirus had SV40 genes attached to it.' The vaccine manufacturing process had created an entirely new virus – with unpredictable results. Could this be how HIV came about?

It should also be borne in mind that the polio vaccine is not the only possibility for the spread of HIV. Dr. Deinhardt of Harvard used chimpanzee kidneys to grow virus for a hepatitis vaccine.[193] However, this was not as widely used as polio vaccine.

In 1991, an Oxford clinician, writing in the prestigious British scientific magazine Nature, suggested AIDS may have sprung from scientific experiments conducted between 1922 to 1955 in which chimpanzee and monkey blood was directly injected into human beings to try to protect them from a form of the malaria parasite that infests those primates. A total of about seventy people received primate blood or primate-tainted human blood.

In 1999 the scientist Omar Bagasra contacted me. He had just published a book entitled *HIV and Molecular Immunity: Prospects for the AIDS Vaccine,* and hoped I

---

[192] Letter to *Science* sent on 27th January 1994. He cited as evidence: C. Mulder, *Nature* 331, 562, (1988); S. Wain-Hobson and G. Myers *Nature*, 1990. 347, 18 (1990); B. Culliton Nature 351, 267 (1991)

[193] Deinhardt et al. 'Studies of Liver Function Tests in Chimpanzees after Inoculation with Human Infectious Hepatitis Virus.' *Am. J. Hy.* 1962

would review it. In this he hypothesized that AIDS probably began with the polio vaccine, saying it would take a mass experiment like this to break down our natural resistance to invasion by foreign retroviruses. He suggested that several kinds of monkey SIVs might have been combined in the vaccine to make HIV, for different simian species were used in manufacturing the original vaccine seed: 'The introduction of recombinant SIVs, developed during the culture of different SIV strains or pre-HIVs, into humans could potentially have formed HIVs.' [194]

The evidence for this thesis was growing stronger. If HIV originated in the polio vaccine, it would not have been detected, as there were then no tests for this virus.

HIV also might have evolved very quickly, Dr. Mae-Wan Ho of the Institute of Science in Society has pointed out that there are 'many genome processes that can rapidly change genomes. These include hypermutation, or mutations rates that are up to a million times faster than usual, recombination, and horizontal gene transfer.'[195]

She also pointed out: 'Another factor that would give an overestimate of divergence time is artificial genetic engineering. Artificial genetic engineering involves rampant recombination and transfer of genes across divergent species barriers.' (More about this in the next chapter.)

Retroviral mutation can occur when various retrovirus species are mixed together, as reported by Drs. D.W. Goodrich and P.H. Duesberg, the latter a member of the US National Science Academy. In a paper entitled *Retroviral Recombination during Reverse Transcription,* they reported that up to half of the related retroviruses produced after a mixed infection are recombinants.

The evidence was mounting up. Not only did the polio vaccine contain numerous simian viruses, as well as probably those of chimpanzees, the very manufacturing process of the vaccine favoured a rapid evolution of these into forms that could potentially survive in humans.

I now thought I was ready to make a television documentary on how the AIDS epidemic began, and proposed the same to Channel 4 for its *Dispatches* series. I was most disappointed when the reply came that they had no room for such a documentary that year. I instead pressed on with this book.

However, I had no idea then just how long its research and writing would take. I then thought I understood the origins of the terrible AIDS epidemic – but I could not have been more in error. What I would discover over the next few years would dramatically change my ideas and the conclusions of this book.

In 1999 a massive book of over a thousand pages, *The River,* was published, written by a medical journalist Edward Hooper.[196] It caused fierce debate within the US and UK scientific establishments. Its thesis was that HIV spread through an experimental polio vaccine developed by Koprowski and used in the Congo between 1957-59. This brought this subject from obscurity to the forefront of public attention. I had not met Hooper – but clearly he had been working along similar lines to myself. I purchased the book, wondering if he had resolved the riddle of how HIV spread so widely in Africa.

It detailed how the US-based Koprowski set up a chimpanzee research station deep in the Congo where he kept some 400 chimpanzees for use in polio vaccine research. They were used both for local vaccine safety tests – and as a source of kidneys sent to Washington and Belgium for use in vaccine experiments. Between 1957-9 Koprowski went on to test his still experimental polio vaccine by injecting it into a quarter of a million Congolese.

---

[194] Omar Bagasra, *HIV and Molecular Immunity: Prospects for the AIDS Vaccine* (BioTechniques Books, 1999); ISBN 1-881299-10-4l page 27.

[195] For example, ISIS Report - March 21 2001 E. coli 0157:H7 and Genetic Engineering

[196] Edward Hooper *The River: a Journey back to the source of HIV and AIDS.* Allen Lane, the Penguin Press 1999

I was bemused that he picked the Congo for such a trial – for surely he must have known that there was little need to vaccinate Africans, since most were already immune to the poliovirus by being exposed to it in the soil. (As I have previously mentioned, Army doctors during the Second World War observed widespread immunity to the poliovirus in Africa and the Middle East.)

But otherwise Koprowski was a surprising person to blame for spreading extremely serious viral contamination, for it was he, not Sabin or Salk, who made a public stand in 1961 against the use of monkeys for vaccine manufacturing, pointing out the great dangers of viral contamination, ably supported by his colleague Stanley Plotkin.

However, Koprowski was a late convert to such views. He had earlier used many monkeys – and chimpanzees – in developing his polio vaccine. Had he learnt his lesson through a disaster in the Congo?

I was impressed by how the geographical region in which Koprowski trialled his vaccine in Africa matched with a region in which HIV infection was reportedly found to be most intense. It suggested that Hooper might well be right.

Hooper's book caused an immense furore partly because he had as an ally one of Oxford University's finest biologists, W. D. Hamilton, who used his position in Britain's most eminent scientific institution, the Royal Society, to obtain its sponsorship of a two-day meeting that promised to be the most controversial that they had held in recent times. It was to discuss the thesis of Hooper's book *The River*. Had the polio vaccine spread HIV? I had to be present – and was fortunate to gain one of the 350 seats in its auditorium.

Hamilton's co-organisers for the meeting were Simon Wain-Hobson of the Pasteur Institute in France and Robin Weiss, Professor of Viral Oncology at University College London. When Hamilton unexpectedly died of a disease contracted in Africa prior to the meeting, Robin Weiss took over the Chair.

The meeting was held on 11-12 September 2000. It began at 2 pm with a 30-minute talk by Edward Hooper. He told how Dr. Hilary Koprowski kept chimpanzees for experimental purposes in the Congo during the 1950s and how kidneys from these were sent to the US while Koprowski was developing his polio vaccine at the Wistar Institute in Philadelphia; also to a medical laboratory in the nearby Congolese city of Butare and to labs in Belgium. Were these used to make some of his polio vaccine? Hooper also reported that some polio vaccine might have been produced in Africa itself, perhaps at the laboratory where the animals were kept.

Dr. Stanley Plotkin followed Hooper. His indignant half hour talk was called 'Untruths and Consequences.' There is, he said, 'no gun, no bullet, there is no shooter, there is no motive. There is only smoke created by Mr. Hooper.' He denied that any chimpanzee kidneys were used, and waved in the air a sheaf of some 16 affidavits, or statements, from scientists involved at the time, all fiercely denying they had used chimpanzees. He instead maintained that the only feasible theory for HIV's evolution was through chimp's blood infecting a cut on a hunter in Africa, a theory that provided little explanation of what could provoke such a rare mutation – for chimps have been eaten for millennia in Africa without AIDS appearing.

The affidavits saying they would not have dreamt of growing poliovirus on chimp kidneys, made me sit up. Given what I knew about the polio experiments of the 1950s, this just did not ring true. I knew scientists then had not hesitated to use chimpanzees. When I got the chance, I asked: ' Can you explain why they would not have used chimp kidneys for vaccine manufacturing? They then knew nothing of HIV, and surely chimpanzee tissues would then have been considered safe?'

The answer came with a smile as if I had asked a schoolgirl question. 'Why would we use chimpanzees from Africa when Rhesus monkeys were so readily available?'

I sat down but was highly unsatisfied. I knew Rhesus monkeys at that time were suspected of being contaminated with a cancer-causing agent – while chimpanzees were thought to be relatively safe. And surely rhesus had to be imported from India – from further away than Africa! When a white-haired academic got up to repeat my question, he too was fobbed off with no real answer.

Hooper replied by saying he had recorded interviews with many of the scientists involved, and some had admitted on tape to using chimpanzees, contrary to these affidavits. What I knew supported this. Chimpanzees were not then spared from laboratory 'sacrifice' – and were certainly not treated as so 'special' that they could not have various toxins injected into their brains and their organs extracted.

Another issue then surfaced. It was the length of time it might take for HIV to evolve from SIV. A paper published that year by Hahn and others and presented at the workshop argued that this might take up to 30 years. It therefore suggested the process must have started around 1930 – but admitted this estimate had a 'margin of error' of 15 years, so HIV could have started to evolve in 1945. As this pre-dated the polio vaccine, the speaker concluded that this proved it was not to blame.

But I was not impressed. This was a weak argument, as from the 1930s onwards chimpanzees were widely used in polio research laboratories, with frequent passaging of fluids through their brains, with ample opportunities for the spreading of chimpanzee viruses. There were thus plenty of opportunities for HIV to evolve from the 1930s – within the timescale suggested by Hahn.

However, Hooper seemed firmly wedded to his theory that this contamination must be linked to Congolese facilities that came into use after 1956. He seemed not to have seriously considered what was happening in the US polio research laboratories right throughout the first half of the 20th century.

This meant to defend his theory he had to resort to the possibility of rapid recombination events that might allow HIV to evolve quickly. This too seemed reasonable – for Hahn's 1930s estimate apparently did not take recombination into account.

Hooper's focus dominated the meeting as it had done his book. In order to test his theory, Professor Hamilton and Hooper had previously suggested that a sample of the vaccine used in the Congo by Koprowski and preserved at the Wistar Institute could be tested to see if it had chimpanzee material in it – and perhaps SIV.

The next event after the Plotkin talk was the announcement of the result of such a test done at the Wistar Institute on a single vaccine vial, the last of the many that once existed. It was reported free of all chimpanzee material. It was triumphantly declared that this proved Hooper's theory wrong.

At the end of the meeting there was a press conference – and the results of the tests on the Wistar vial were its prime focus. They were interpreted as meaning that HIV could not possibly have spread through the polio vaccine – and so it was reported next day in the press. I thought it a gross exaggeration  - for tests on just one vial could not prove anything except that one particular batch of vaccine was not contaminated with chimp material.

This press conference was presided over by Robin Weiss  - the same man who presided over the SV40 Washington workshop that I had attended – and it had much the same feel. The establishment position was stated as incontestably true. The vaccine was pronounced harmless.

But another theory had been put forward at this conference that could explain the spread of HIV in Africa. It had been met with approval but sadly neglected at the press conference. Dr. Preston Marx, in a talk entitled '*Serial Human Passage of SIV: the role of unsterile injecting*' had proposed that HIV was spread by the use of dirty needles in vaccinating African children. He said the serial nature of injections would allow HIV to evolve fast, saying that Simian viruses had been shown to become 1,000 times more pathogenic when 'serially passaged' through as few as three monkeys. His theory did not explain how a chimpanzee virus had contaminated these needles, but it did not blame the vaccine manufacturers or scientists. Perhaps this explained why his thesis was extraordinarily greeted with general acclaim. Robin Weiss told the New Scientist magazine: 'It has the ring of truth about it.'

Finally, Koprowski himself, now in his 80s, rose to defend his life's work. 'My achievement of developing oral polio vaccines saved millions of lives, but now I am held up before the world as the father of AIDS - a mass murderer.' He charged that Hooper 'operated with preconceptions without much attention to contradictory data.' He continued; 'Hooper's book could be blamed for undermining the global effort to eradicate polio, for it undermined public confidence in the polio vaccine.'

When I left the meeting, I chanced to meet with Dr. Phil Minor, the very senior UK government vaccine safety scientist who at the 1999 vaccine safety conference had said that 'a huge amount of vaccine is made on really quite crude material.' Out of the blue, he asked me not to publicise this polio vaccine issue as it might 'undermine public confidence in vaccination.'

I was then still of the view that the polio vaccine might have spread HIV. None of the arguments presented had convinced me otherwise. As far as I could see, the evidence was that there was ample opportunity for a chimpanzee virus to have mutated into HIV and to contaminate the vaccine. I thus found the affidavits presented at this meeting both historically inappropriate and suspect. I felt there was much more opportunity for chimp viruses to get into vaccines in polio vaccine labs than there was from dirty needles.

But I was by now aware of other issues. The African focus of this debate did not explain all the facts. The first medical report identifying what we now call AIDS concerned cases of sickness among gay white males in Los Angeles. How could an African virus infect them? They were not unusually exposed to the polio vaccine. The AIDS-related diseases they suffered were unlike those found in Africa. There were various theories that a gay airline steward or a sailor must have transported the illness from Africa to North America – but the evidence for such a relationship seemed slim.

In any case, just what did we know about HIV? How did a retrovirus come to be blamed for causing AIDS – when no other retrovirus causes a significant human illness? As I started to research this I discovered that it was not only doctors who were interested in this virus.

--------------------------------------

SOME READING

    Curtis, T. (1992a). 'The Origin of AIDS' *Rolling Stone* 626 (19 March): 54-61, 106, 108.

    Weiss, R.A. (2001). 'Polio Vaccines Exonerated.' *Nature* 410: 1035-36.

    Weiss, R.A. and S. Wain-Hobson, ed. (2001). 'Origins of HIV' *Philosophical Transactions of the Royal Society of London, Series B: Biological Sciences* 356: 777.

    Wistar Institute (2000). 'No AIDS-Related Viruses or Chimpanzee DNA' Press statement, 11 September.

# Chapter 10

# Bioweapon Research, Cancer and the AIDS Virus

I knew HIV is said to be a 'retrovirus' I knew little about these save that, when they were first discovered, they were thought to cause cancer. Well, cancer is not AIDS – but there was a link and a theory that I had not yet investigated. It was that the monkey retrovirus, SIV, mutated into HIV and started the AIDS epidemic; not in the polio vaccine as I thought, but during experiments with monkeys and retroviruses in Pentagon-funded biowarfare laboratories.

I soon learnt this was not so crazy an idea as it first sounded. America has possessed a secretive bio-warfare research program since May 1942 when President Roosevelt put in charge of such a program a Dr. George W. Merck, the founder of the giant pharmaceutical Merck Corporation. This work was centred at the highly secretive Army Chemical Warfare Service at Fort Detrick, a large military research facility located north-west of Washington DC. [197]

Its early research was partially documented in a 1977 two-volume report to the US Congress entitled *U.S. Army Activities in the U.S. Biological Warfare Program*. This told how the Pentagon funded scientists to create germ warfare weapons against crops, animals and the citizens of hostile nations, as well as protective measures against such weapons.

One of its recruits was surprisingly Dr. Bernice Eddy, the scientist who had first sounded the alarm over monkey virus contamination of the polio vaccine. Although those responsible for vaccine safety had ignored her warnings, her cancer-causing agent had gained the attention of the military. She was sent to work on military-funded experiments at the National Institutes for Health (NIH).

The NIH, in partnership with a private company, Litton Bionetics, planned to mutate SV40 for the Pentagon to make it more dangerous by infusing it with genetic codes from other species of viruses. It was hoped thus to develop entirely new species of viruses. If a virus were new, the argument went, the enemy would have no vaccines and no natural protection against it – making it a powerful weapon. However, there was a problem. It might spread to friendly troops – or even create a worldwide pandemic!

But this did not deter the researchers. If such viruses were not researched, they argued in funding applications, then no protection could be developed against them. Therefore it was imperative this work be done. Of course strict biosafety would be maintained. No such virus would be allowed to escape from laboratories – or so they assured Congress.

They then gambled by trying to mutate SV40 by inserting genetic codes into it from a cat retrovirus (FELV), then codes from avian myeloblastosis virus (AMV) and from many other suspected pathogens. In this search many chimpanzees and monkeys were

---

[197] Dr Leonard Horwitz has documented this theory from government sources in his 1996 book *Emerging Viruses: AIDS and Ebola. Nature, Accident or Intentional?*

injected with these mutants and killed, creating a real risk of mutant monkey viruses contamination, and of these in turn mutating into new and dangerous human-infecting germs.

A significant part of this Pentagon-funded research was focussed on the theories of Bernice Eddy and Sarah Stewart that had linked viruses and cancers. Cancer cells had damaged DNA. Did viruses cause this damage? If they did, this opened the welcome possibility of anti-cancer vaccines – but also the possibility of terrifying new weapons.

They used electron microscopes to search cancer tissues for any sign of particles that might be new cancer-causing viruses. The eminent virologist Dr. J. W. Beard had noted that all cells, whether infected or not, could be made to generate a heterogeneous assortment of particles. These now needed to be sorted out and studied.

Some of these viruses were found to carry tiny lengths of DNA in the form of a single or double-helix strands. Others carried strands of another kind of genetic code called RNA. Similar particles were also found to act as 'messengers' inside cells.

DNA is essentially a vast amount of information recorded in patterns of four nucleotides strung along very thin long strands of alternating sugar and phosphate molecules, five feet long in the centre of each of our cells. The four varieties of DNA nucleotides are adenine, guanine, cytosine and thymine. RNA differs by having uracil instead of thymine.

In 1965 Dr. Howard Temin created great excitement by describing a particle produced by cells that might be one of the long-sought cancer viruses. It contained double-stranded RNA and was initially called an RNA Tumour Virus, but it is now known of as a retrovirus.

The excitement this caused was due to the discovery that the RNA in this retrovirus changed into DNA when it 'infected' cells, and that this DNA was then inserted into the cells' own DNA, thus seemingly mutating them. Was this how cells became cancerous? Temin proposed this was so.

Retroviruses were thus seen as committing a major scientific heresy. Up until then it was thought that DNA ruled through a strict hierarchy. It made RNA and this made proteins. DNA was seen as the rulebook of the cell, and thus as governing RNA. But retroviruses heretically reversed this direction, by turning mere messenger RNA into DNA. How could the RNA of a retrovirus change a cell's DNA without creating genetic chaos?

Soon the enzyme was discovered that enabled retroviruses to achieve this amazing feat. It was promptly named 'Reverse Transcriptase' (RT) as it wrote genetic code from RNA to DNA, in the reverse of what had previously considered the 'normal' direction. For this discovery yet more Nobel Prizes were allotted – to Renato Dulbecco (whose excrement-based polio research is described above) and his student, David Baltimore. Retroviruses were distinguished from other viruses by saying, wrongly as we now know, that only they had this extraordinary ability.

Baltimore theorised that the polyoma viruses discovered by Eddy and Stewart might similarly put their genetic codes into the codes of their host. Seemingly this was how SV40 created cancers. The cancer-producing DNA they were thought to insert was named as an 'oncogene.'

But these theories and research failed to find an answer to cancer, despite the many Nobel Prizes allotted to the scientists in this hunt. The thousands of experiments carried out in the next few years found surprisingly that retroviruses seemed fairly harmless. Many of the cells they 'invaded' and 'mutated', much to everyone's surprise, seemed to function afterwards as if entirely healthy.

This led to the development of the theory of 'lentiviruses' (slow-viruses) that would not produce cancers, or other illnesses, until ten to thirty years after infecting their victim cells, leaving them seemingly entirely healthy in the interim. Apparently the need to wait for verification did not bother its advocates.

But, I thought there was something slightly odd about this theory. Viruses only survive a few days at most (measles virus only two hours[198]) and are thus said to cause illnesses very quickly, but this new theory involved waiting for an illness to occur until after many hundreds of thousands of healthy cellular generations had taken place since the purported infection. It was like saying a virus infected a builder of Stonehenge and was only now causing an illness in a distant descendent.

However, by 1969 most retroviruses had been exonerated. Drs. Harold Varmus and John Bishop found the putative causes of cancer, the oncogenes, were not made by retroviruses but of cellular origin, and thus deduced that cancer could occur without any help from a virus. Varmus and Bishop were later awarded a shared Nobel Prize for this discovery. [199]

The US that same year tested their new biological warfare agents during a massive fleet exercise in the Pacific Ocean. This involved many ships, stacks of caged monkeys and the release of the lethal agents into the atmosphere – all monitored by Soviet agents, as we now know.

But this exercise turned out to be a 'last hurrah' for openly carried out American biowarfare research. For years there had been demonstrations against this research. In 1968, Seymour Hersch publicized the US biowarfare weapons program in an article entitled 'America's Hidden Arsenal' – and in 1969, Senator McCarthy called for the ending of biowarfare weapons research, after documenting thousands of careless and dangerous research errors.

The public pressure brought results. On Veterans Day, November 11, 1969, President Richard Nixon asked the US Senate to complete the long-overdue ratification of the 1925 Geneva Protocol prohibiting the use of chemical and biological weapons. On November 25 he signed an executive order outlawing offensive biological research in the United States and ordering stockpiles destroyed within five years. From now on biological research at Fort Detrick would be officially 'defensive' in character, although there is evidence that offensive work quietly continued.

Lieutenant Colonel Lucien Winegar, deputy commander of Fort Detrick, said at the time that it would 'be fair to assume' that they would continue to work with dangerous organisms since any defence required knowledge of those agents. For such purposes, the facility was then consuming every year some 4,000 monkeys and nearly a million rodents.

By 1970 this research was developed in alarming directions. At the Department of Defense Appropriations Hearings of that year, the Acting Assistant Secretary of the Army for Research and Development, Charles L. Poor testified: 'within the next five to ten years, it would probably be possible to make a new infective microorganism which could differ in certain important aspects from any known disease-causing organisms.'

Poor explained what would be so new about these germs. 'Most important of these is that it might be refractory to the immunological and therapeutic processes upon which we depend to maintain our relative freedom from infectious disease.' In other words, they were trying to design it to destroy, or critically damage, the human immune system.

Was he talking about making something like HIV? His description seems to fit. His words certainly aroused the suspicion of many. When a Dr. Robert Strecker did a Freedom of Information Search, he found documentary evidence of a $10m US

---

[198] CDC Manual on Measles. Second Edition.

[199] Huebner and Todaro 1969

government grant made to develop this new immunosuppressant virus. It was estimated this development would take five years. [200]

Some of the scientists involved, Drs. Stanley Cohen and Herbert Boyer, published their initial results in 1973. However, their report did not mention a virus. Instead they reported success in splicing a gene into a common, usually harmless intestinal bacterium, *escherichia coli*, to make it immune to penicillin.[201] They had thus created a dangerous super-bug that hospitals would find hard to fight.[202]

Dr. David Baltimore has since denied that the researchers of this period deliberately created 'HIV,' saying they were incapable of such a feat. In a 2004 interview for WGBH's 'Frontline' television program he said: 'People have accused biological engineers of making HIV. No biological engineer could have made HIV because none of us had ever seen these capabilities before. We not only hadn't seen them in a virus; in many cases, they affected processes that we didn't even know were going on in cells at that time. We've learned a lot about cells by following what HIV is capable of doing, and we're still uncovering mechanisms that HIV has. This is now 20 years later.'

But what if cells subjected to the stress of these experiments had created retroviruses transformed by recombination? What if a cell mutated under this stress and produced malformed retroviruses? But I mostly wondered, when monkey viruses are put into human cells, or allowed to contaminate human cells, would they not try to change themselves into a form that can replicate in humans in order to survive – and if they did, could they not produce new epidemics? From what I had read, I then believed viruses had this ability. Are we not being constantly warned today that bird flu viruses might thus mutate to infect humans?

But at this point in my research I found more believable the polio-vaccine theory for the origin and spread of HIV. For me, military research could not explain the spread of AIDS as well as did the vaccine theory, for the polio vaccine was rapidly distributed to millions around the world. If a monkey virus might have evolved to infect humans during this military research, it would have had much more opportunity to do so during the polio vaccine research.

From what I read, and what Baltimore wrote, the science of this period was only stumbling towards an understanding of viruses. If HIV evolved out of this research, it would, I thought, have been by error rather than by deliberate means. But if it had – then AIDS would have probably started among military scientists and virologists – for which I could find absolutely no evidence.

But, the research that eventually linked a retrovirus, HIV, to AIDS did develop out of this hive of virology research. It began shortly after the National Cancer Institute expanded to include some of the biological warfare facilities. President Richard M. Nixon on October 19th, 1971, flew by helicopter to Fort Detrick to announce that the Fort would now house the 'Frederick Cancer Research Facility of the National Cancer Institute (NCI)'. One of the scientists working at the NCI was a Dr. Robert Gallo, a specialist on leukaemia, or cancers of the blood.

Nixon poured funds into the NCI. He named cancer as 'America's No. 1 enemy' and declared a 'War on Cancer' on December 23, 1971, predicting victory within 5 years!

---

[200] See dates of research in *The Smoking Gun of AIDS: a 1971 Flowchart* by Boyd E. Graves, J.D. December 6, 2000

[201] It seems that the insertion of DNA into the E Coli bacteria is through holes blasted in the side of the bacteria with powerful electric pulses. What these do to a cell that naturally uses very weak currents of electricity can be imagined. See 'Transformation of E. coli by Electroporation' UMBC University, Maryland. http://userpages.umbc.edu/~jwolf/m7.htm

[202] This research is documented in *Biological Weapons and America's Secret War: Germs* by Judith Miller, Stephen Engelberg and William Broad. Published Simon and Schuster 2001. Page 70.

Virologists had convinced him that cancer was a viral epidemic – and he thus thought a vaccine a distinct possibility.

The new facilities of NCI were immediately put to work in the 1971 authorized Special Virus Cancer Program – employing both Bernice Eddy and Maurice Hilleman, the former as specializing in 'leukaemia ecology,' the latter in 'immunology.' The main target was the retroviruses thought to carry 'oncogenes'. They had support from Robert Gallo who in 1972 became the Head of the NCI's Laboratory of Tumor Cell Biology, where he continued his search for cancer-causing retroviruses in leukaemia blood samples. He hoped to detect these through finding reverse transcriptase activity. He believed this enzyme practically unique to retroviruses.

That same year Temin and David Baltimore published a paper explaining how they thought retroviruses caused cancer. They said they highjack the cells they infect by inserting viral DNA, including the suspect oncogene, into the cell's DNA, thus forcing the cells to do the virus's bidding and at the same time making them cancerous.[203]

In 1975 a paper produced by R. Junghans, Peter Duesberg and C. Knight analysed the genetic codes of cells and chicken retroviral particles by breaking them apart with detergent, seeking the genome of this retrovirus incorporated as DNA into the cells' DNA. They stated they had then synthesized from fragments what they believed to be a complete DNA version of these retroviruses' RNA.[204]

But – this war against cancer finally failed. Viruses were not proved to be major causes of cancer. Toxins, such as asbestos, were shown to be quite capable on their own to poison cells and make them cancerous. After this virology textbooks conceded: 'Viruses alone do not cause cancers in nature.' [205] However, virologists were reluctant to give up completely on the viral hypothesis. They even labelled chicken, cat and mouse retroviruses as 'defective' for the sin of being unable to produce a cancer!

I was now starting to understand why some scientists I consulted while researching SV40 in 1997 had been reluctant to concede that any virus, including SV40, could play a major role in causing a cancer. I had been surprised by their reluctance– but that was due to my ignorance. I now knew that their opinion was formed by the defeat of the viral theory of cancer between the 1960s and 1980s.

In the 1970s virologists did not only get cancer wrong. They also lost much credibility by predicting a flu disaster that never happened. In 1976, when an army recruit at Fort Dix reportedly died of an influenza virus similar to one that infected swine, the CDC panicked. It declared this was the start of a 'respiratory epidemic' that could kill 55,000 or even many more! It could even result, the CDC terrifyingly warned, in an epidemic like that of 1918-19 that killed over half a million Americans. They thus felt compelled to take emergency measures. On 24 March 1976 President Ford announced that 'every man, woman and child' in America must be vaccinated to stop this danger – and by November some 45 million were,

But the vaccine proved more deadly than the flu. Within 3 weeks of vaccination commencing, there were 41 deaths among the vaccinated – and not one case of flu.[206] On 16 December, the vaccination program was suspended pending investigation of adverse side effects – and never restarted.

In all, 52 persons had died of reactions to the vaccine, 500-600 were impaired or hospitalised, compensation claims reached $1.7 billion, and not one case of human-to-

---

[203] Temin HM, Baltimore D: RNA-Directed DNA Synthesis and RNA Tumor Viruses. Adv. Virol. Res. 1972;17:129-186.

204 R. P. JUNGHANS, P. H. DUESBERG, C. A. KNIGHT. In vitro synthesis of full-length DNA transcripts of Rous sarcoma virus RNA by viral DNA polymerase   Proc. Nat. Acad. Sci. USA Vol. 72, No. 12, pp. 4895-4899, December 1975

[205] Dimrock and Primrose 1987 *Introduction to modern virology* p272

[206] http://reviewingaids.org/awiki/index.php/Document:Mirage_3

human swine flu infection was reported outside Fort Dix. Finally, it was discovered that the one fatality had collapsed and died, not of flu, but while on a strenuous Army training exercise.

The CDC in its panic had also overlooked vital earlier research by the Yale Professor Emeritus of Epidemiology and Public Health, Robert E. Shope (and are today still overlooking it). He discovered in 1931 that the deaths during the major 1918 'Flu' epidemic were primarily due to the victims being infected with bacteria, namely the bacillus *haemophilus influenzae suis*, and thus not primarily due to a flu virus.

I was astonished to find his research – for there is no mention of it today. Instead virologists frequently warn us that a lethal bird flu virus, the one they hold solely responsible for the dreadful epidemic of 1918, is certain to evolve again and to unleash a similar massacre of humans – just as they mistakenly warned in 1976. This too is now forgotten – and thus these virologists are today massively funded to monitor every suspicious bird death.

Professor Shope reported finding the responsible bacteria in mucus and fluid taken from the lungs of pigs infected alongside humans in 1918 and 1929. When he filtered this fluid and mucus to remove the bacteria but not the viruses (or toxins I should add), the remaining fluid only caused a mild flu – from which he deduced flu viruses were present alongside the bacteria.

He also tested human survivors of the 1918 epidemic and found they were immune to the bacteria infecting the pigs – deducing from this that they had been exposed to this bacteria during the 1918 epidemic and had thus gained immunity.[207] He published his results in a series of papers in *The Journal of Experimental Medicine*. [208]

How could such important research be so totally forgotten – or is this an absent-minded rewriting of history? There is no evidence of it ever being discredited. Forgetting it has certainly benefited the funding of virological research – for it has left our governments ready to panic and throw more funds in the direction of virologists whenever a suspicious bird death is reported.

Professor Shope was eminent in his field and confidently reported: 'Mixing the filtrate with the bacterium reproduced the severe disease'. He suspected that a filterable agent, presumed to be a swine virus, not a bird virus, might facilitate the deadly infection with the bacterium – but he did not concede any greater role to the virus. He had thoroughly researched the flu virus – and reported it could not cause severe illness by itself.

So both the flu virus and retroviruses were cleared of blame for much of the damage with which they had been associated. Up until the 1980s no retrovirus was shown to cause disease in humans. Indeed scientists had publically wondered if humans had retroviruses at all – partly because of their assumption that, if human retroviruses existed, they would be found in association with a disease. Robin Weiss reported in 1982, although 'several retroviral isolates from human material were described, closer scrutiny relegated all of them to the category of contaminants from animal sources.'

There was another experiment done around this time that did not involve the military but which some today suspect could have created and spread AIDS. Dr. Alan Cantwell has set forth the evidence for this in two books.[209] He tells how an experimental Hepatitis B vaccine was tested on a large group of homosexual males, selected for their

---

[207] Shope, R.E. 1936. *J. Exp. Med.* 63:669–684.

[208] Lewis, P.A., and R.E. Shope. 1931. J. Exp. Med. 54:361–371. Shope, R.E. 1931. J. Exp. Med. 54:373–385.

Also Journal of Experimental Medicine, Vol. 203, No. 4, April 17, 2006 803

www.jem.org/cgi/doi/10.1084/jem.2034fta – the abstracts attached to them are somewhat misleading as they omit some of his work on the bacteria

[209] Cantwell, Alan. 'AIDS and the Doctors of Death' and 'Queer Blood: The Secret AIDS Genocide Plot.'

promiscuity, in Manhattan in 1978 at the New York Blood Centre. This vaccine was highly unusual. The pharmaceutical company Merck made it from the pooled blood of 30 gay men who tested positive for Hepatitis B. The vaccine was then safety tested on chimpanzees. [210]

Given what we now know about the purification of vaccines, we can assume that it would have had many contaminants in it, including cellular debris from the sick men whose blood was used. Cantwell suggests HIV might have been introduced to Africa through some of the chimps used being released back into the wild in West Africa. He also notes that a similar experiment was made in Amsterdam between December 1980 and December 1981. He suggests that this was in effect a genocidal plot against gay men.

This theory has gained wide circulation in America – and was even quoted famously by Barack Obama's pastor in a controversial sermon. However, I see many weaknesses in it. For example, there was simply not enough time between the return of a few chimps to Africa and the discovery that many Africans tested positive. More particularly, I find unconvincing a genocidal plot against gays that relies on a relatively small vaccine trial. As I will show, other factors convincingly explain the appearance of AIDS in this gay community.

The scientists involved in the 'War on Cancer' were by 1980 so thoroughly depressed at not finding viruses that caused cancers that, half-jokingly, some renamed 'cancer tumour viruses' as 'cancer rumour viruses!' This time it seemed toxicology would defeat virology. It was soon recognized that the major cause of cancers are toxins such as asbestos, tar and tobacco smoke, or damaging radiation.

But Robert Gallo of the National Cancer Institute was not ready to give up on a hunt in which he had invested so much time. When in 1975 he detected RT activity in a blood sample from a leukaemia patient, he excitedly claimed that this definitely proved a retrovirus was present – and must cause this cancer. With no more ado he named it as 'Human Leukaemia 23 Virus', HL23V. He hoped this would guarantee his tumour lab's further funding. The next step, he predicted, would be a vaccine against leukaemia. Then, when he found he could only detect RT in a few cases of leukaemia, he theorized that this was because his retrovirus was a 'slow virus' that hid in cells for hundreds of cellular generations before causing leukaemia. It was like condemning a child for murder due to a prediction that a descendent would kill. Nevertheless he was in a hurry to justify his lab's funding by finding a cancer virus so published his speculative new theory immediately, rather than wait to see if it proved to be true. [211]

But he was deeply embarrassed when he presented this 'leukaemia virus' discovery to a science conference.  Others had tested his virus and declared it a mixture of contaminating retroviruses from woolly monkeys, gibbon apes, and baboons. He tried to save his reputation by speculating that perhaps a monkey virus caused human leukaemia. This excuse did not fly on this occasion, and he later described the event as a 'disaster' and 'painful,' 'I was depressed, dumbfounded, angry. It was the low point of my whole career. It was almost the last nail in the coffin of the field of retrovirology. The programme died.' He darkly and conspiratorially added: 'I became more cynical, tougher, less happy. I mean, what could it be but sabotage?' But I think the real problem was the similarity of the harmless retroviruses that are indigenous to humans, apes and monkeys.

---

[210] Cantwell, Alan 'HIV-AIDS was created with the use of Gay men as targets for Eugenic experiments suggests U.S. Doctor.' *The Canadian*, 21 April 2008
http://www.agoracosmopolitan.com/home/Frontpage/2008/03/29/02309.html
211 Similarly today a measles virus is said to sometimes cause SSPE some 30 years after an infection. This is often based on the presence of antibodies, but have these been proved to be only against measles? McKendall and Stroop Handbook of Neurovirology. 1994. p 544

His major problem at that time was not being able to find a retrovirus actually engaged in turning normal human cells into cancer cells. How then could he prove they caused cancer?

But in 1980 he claimed a minor success. He announced his lab had found a retrovirus that indirectly spread cancer through the lymph system. He claimed it caused a rare itchy skin cancer previously thought caused by fungi and thus called Mycosis Fungoides. Gallo named his discovery as Human T-cell Lymphoma Virus 1 (HTLV-I), and speculated, for no reason that was obvious, that it was spread by sex.[212] But the evidence for his virus was very slim. His claims were based on extremely few cases, on detecting the production of virus-like particles that might not be viruses, and on finding activity of the enzyme RT, not the virus itself – and thus it did not convince many. The British Association of Dermatologists currently reports of this disease, 'Its cause is unknown.'[213]

Gallo had to gain credibility if he were to win funds. When, at a social meeting with Japanese virologists, he heard of cases of unexplained leukaemia on a Japanese island, Kyushu, he guessed this could be just what he was looking for. The cancer involved was in T-Cells – blood-borne immune cells. But what he apparently overlooked was that the capital of this island was Nagasaki, which had not long ago been levelled by an atomic bomb.

The Japanese virologists were then not certain that the bomb could have caused these cancers as they were in children born afterwards. When they heard of Gallo's discovery of a possible link between retroviruses and leukaemia, they wondered if this might provide an alternative explanation. They thus had accepted his offer to have his laboratory look for retroviruses in blood samples from the children affected.[214] Gallo gave this work to his new recruit, Dr. Mikulas Popovic from Czechoslovakia – of whom we will hear much later.

Popovic soon reported finding the 'signs of' retroviral presence in the children's blood. Gallo claimed this was firm evidence that HTLV-1 had given these children Adult T-Cell Leukaemia (ATL). This was despite him having previously linked HTLV-1 to an entirely different illness in a Caribbean woman![215] But Gallo changed the name of the virus to suit, from Human T-Cell Lymphoma virus to Human T-Cell Leukaemia Virus.

But Gallo's HTLV-1 was a previously unknown virus – so from whence had it come? Gallo sent a bold memo to his NCI boss: 'I am speculating that it came with the slave trade' from Africa to the Americas, and indirectly, through the Portuguese having slaves, to Japan.' But if so, where had his virus hidden in the centuries that had elapsed between the slave trade and the atomic bombing of Nagasaki – and why wasn't it elsewhere in Japan? This appeared highly tenuous. As he said – it was only his speculation. (However, this was the origin of Gallo's later assertion that HIV (HTLV-3) must come from Africa as it is related to HTLV-I.)

But they had not actually seen their virus. They presumed it were present since they had detected in the children's blood the enzyme reverse transcriptase (RT). But their

---

[212] 'Detection and Isolation of Type C Retrovirus Particles from Fresh and Cultured Lymphocytes of a Patient with Cutaneous T-cell Lymphoma,' in December 1980, the first author was Bernie Poiesz, followed by Frank Ruscetti and Adi Gazdar, with Gallo bringing up the rear. Also Robert Gallo: The discovery of the first human retrovirus: HTLV-1 and HTLV-2 *Retrovirology* 2005, **2:**17

[213] http://www.bad.org.uk/patients/leaflets/mycosis.asp 2004 Website.

[214] Mitsuaki Yoshida‡ Discovery of HTLV-1, the first human retrovirus, its unique regulatory mechanisms, and insights into pathogenesis *Oncogene* (2005) **24**, 5931–5937. doi:10.1038/sj.onc.1208981
Kiyoshi Takatsuki; Discovery of adult T-cell leukemia *Retrovirology* 2005, **2:**16 doi:10.1186/1742-4690-2-16

[215] Kate Barmak‡, Edward Harhaj‡, Christian Grant‡, Timothy Alefantis‡ and Brian Wigdahl· Human T cell leukemia virus type I-induced disease: pathways to cancer and neurodegeneration: Virology Volume 308, Issue 1 , 30 March 2003, Pages 1-12

theory that this enzyme was a marker solely for HTLV-1 was very flimsily based. [216] It was known to be invalid from as soon as Dr. Harold Varmus and Professor Michael Bishop, joint Nobel laureates, learnt that the enzyme RT is in all cells; human, plant or bacterial. This enzyme is now known to be a vital constituent of healthy cellular life. Nevertheless, Gallo still claims that he really did find HTLV-1.

Today we know that radiation may damage the genetic material passed from fathers to their children. [217] This is now the most likely reason for the leukaemia among the Japanese children living near Nagasaki. But this discovery did not lead to Gallo dropping the theory linking HTLV-1 with leukaemia. The theory was instead rewritten. The virus is now said to carry proteins that disable other proteins in our blood that protect us from cancer – in particular by disabling p53, the very protein also said to be deactivated by SV40. (See chapter 2) How it can cause leukaemia when deactivated by HTLV-1 and totally different cancers when deactivated by SV40, no one has yet explained.[218]

In 1982 Gallo claimed to discover a second human retrovirus. This he named as HTLV-2, saying it caused a rare 'Hairy T-cell Leukaemia.' It was evidently very rare; found only in two to four patients. One sued unsuccessfully against the commercial exploitation of his cells[219] and another recovered when he returned to Australia and changed his diet.

## PROBLEMS WITH DETECTING RETROVIRUSES

Even when imaged with electron microscopes, retroviruses are very small. They are vastly smaller than a cell – rather like an ant next to a bulldozer. They also seem to be always mixed with other particles of similar size and shape. They are commonly described as having a density of 0.16 gm/ml, as spherical with a diameter of 100 to 120 nanometres (10,000th of a millimetre), and as covered in knobs that fall off easily if touched.

But this is a great generalization. In practice it is nothing like as simple. The Nobel Laureate Dr. Harold Varmus has co-authored a book on retroviruses that details some of the real difficulties faced by the retrovirus hunter. [220]

This book points out: 'Even the purest viral preparation showed a panoply of unidentified minor particles.' When they had tried to separate out retroviruses by centrifuging them in sucrose solution, they discovered 'vesicles from broken or intact cells have a density similar to that of the virus' and the process used is 'insensitive to size.' They noted: 'Since very few studies have compared different viruses in the same experiment, it is uncertain if size differs among the retroviral genera or if the spread in measured diameters represents other factors.'

When testing these particles to see if they could infect, and thus might be viruses, 99 out of 100 of the possible 'retroviruses' had to be rejected. (It also proved extremely difficult, perhaps impossible; to say that a particle entering a cell is identical to the one leaving it.)

---

216 Hinuma Y, Nagata K, Hanaoka M, Nakai M, Matsumoto T, Kinoshita KI, Shirakawa S, Miyoshi I. Adult T-cell leukemia: antigen in an ATL cell line and detection of antibodies to the antigen in human sera.

217 Radiation leukaemia risk 'passes from father to child.' Press Association
Tuesday September 7, 2004. This reports a Leicester University Press Release entitled 'New Evidence of radiation risk in childhood leukaemia,' It describes how a statistically significant mutation rate in the germ-line of fathers exposed by radiation was established by Dr. Dubrova Leicester University Professor of Genetics.

218 Seiki and M. Yoshida; Functional inactivation of p53 by human T-cell leukemia virus type 1 Tax protein. Oxford Journal November 23rd, 2005

219 Crewdson, John Science Fictions page 546 note b.

220 'Retroviruses' 1997 Cold Spring Harbor Laboratory Press - at the National Center for Biotechnology Information and is by John Coffin, Stephen Hughes and the eminent Harold E. Varmus. – and is at the NCBI website

When they tried to select them by shape, they found they had been distorted by the 'harsh fixation' required by electron microscopy – and perhaps also by the filters used. Even staining them could cause 'deformation.'

There were other problems too. Professor Etienne de Harven, an electron microscopy specialist, explained: 'Preparing thin sections was time-consuming and skill-demanding! Who had time for that, when research funding was getting difficult, and when major pharmaceutical corporations were starting to finance "crash programs" for speedy answers? [We were asked:] 'Why don't we try the negative staining method? It is very easy and very fast! And, after all, it gave beautiful results with unenveloped viruses like adenovirus and polyoma.'

'The results were an absolute disaster because fragile RNA tumor viruses (not yet called retroviruses.) are badly distorted by air-drying during the negative staining procedures; they appear as particles with a long tail! Unfortunately many cell debris and vesicular fragments, when air-dried for negative staining, form similar "tailed" structures. Interpreting "tailed" particles as RNA tumor viruses was therefore a bonanza for virus hunters!' He added: 'rigorous ultrastructural characterization was essential for adequate differentiation between viruses and "virus-like particles."'

De Harven also stated in 2007: 'separating retroviruses by density gradient centrifugation was always damaging to the shape of the virions,' and 'retroviruses prepared by the negative staining method were always distorted,' However, he said this was not true of 'ultrafiltration' which, according to his 1965 paper, involved spinning the suspension extremely fast (30,000g) for two hours or more. (This, he said, is a relatively easy process and should be used much more often.) When the resulting 'almost invisible' pellet was sectioned, he found it contained 'a most impressive population' of identical particles of a typical viral shape.'[221] I still have to ask – did imposing such enormous centrifugal forces for two hours on soft cellular material do anything to create this uniformity?

Varmus had initially in 1965 claimed such particles were leukaemia-causing retroviruses, saying he had proved this by animal testing; but after this, according to Paul Philpot: 'He and some other retrovirologists began to doubt that retroviruses could cause human cancer. For one thing, the retrovirus-cancer link in animals was reserved for special cases of inbred mice, chickens, and cats, and even then the link was far from perfect. Among these peculiar laboratory animals, scientists could usually isolate retroviruses from the subjects that had cancer, but sometimes they could not. And sometimes they could isolate retroviruses even in the absence of cancer. Furthermore, these retroviral isolates would not induce cancer when injected into wild mice and chickens. Nor could anybody isolate retroviruses from any wild animals, or even other laboratory animals, besides special inbred cats.' Nor could he find any retroviruses that killed cells. [222]

Varmus reported the structures of retroviruses were poorly understood. 'The structural features that underlie the different morphologies of retroviral particles and the apparently different assembly routes are not well understood.' There also seemed to be a variety of ways to assemble them.

Some particles had projections on the outside but 'the number of such projections varies greatly among different viruses and even among different strains. This variability is poorly understood and often is attributed to the propensity of the surface glycoprotein to fall off spontaneously during purification or storage. ' 'Mature viruses are so irregular

[221] Friend C & de Harven, E (1965). A new method for purifying a murine leukemia virus. Fed. Proc. 24, N° 2. And: de Harven E (1965). Viremia in Friend murine leukemia: the electron microscope approach to the problem. Pathologie-Biologie 13 (3-4):125-134. Also – 'Retroviruses, The Recollections of an Electron Microscopist Etienne de Harven in Reappraising AIDS Nov. 1998 Also Personal communication by email in October 2007.
[222] Paul Phillpot article on de Harven in Reappraising AIDS Nov./Dec. 1998

and so labile that we have been unable to apply the tools of structural analysis to good effect.' [223]

The many very different images of 'HIV' currently found on the Internet differ greatly as most, including all the colour ones, are simply products of artistic imagination. At the time of writing, the BBC website contains at least 8 totally dissimilar images of 'HIV.' One of these shows it as a purple hoop, another shows it as a sharp-spike-covered ball and another as a green wart-covered ball.

Despite the above findings of Varmus, and the similar discoveries of Professor Peter Duesberg, virology journals have mostly only reported on retroviruses as potential causes of disease – for this seems to be the only aspect of retroviruses of interest to them. Therefore little good is written of retroviruses in virology. Like other viruses, they were typed as killers before they were ever seen. Robert Gallo taught retroviruses are foreign invaders of humans – and even in 1994 maintained: 'there are no known human endogenous retroviruses.' [224] ('Endogenous' meaning originating in humans.)

But Gallo was at that time fighting a losing battle. At that time other scientists were describing retroviruses as 'the viruses in all of us' and were busy analyzing the 'biological significance of human endogenous retrovirus sequences.' [225] At the same time others were having much more success than Gallo in finding causes for leukaemia by investigating toxic environmental factors.

In fact, at that time there was little certitude about what exactly a virus was – and so even less about a retrovirus. For example, in 2005 it was reported that we still do not know the structure of the common rubella virus. Much of our description of them is based on tiny images and theoretical suppositions. Their ultimate origin was still a mystery. It is extremely hard to find any medicine that would kill them. They are inert once produced by their parent cell. This led to a debate on whether or not they were truly alive.

I wondered then if viruses might be sometimes made and shed by cells to remove the waste products of cellular illnesses? It would explain why viruses are inactive once away from the cellular 'viral factories'. Could such wastes poison other cells, and thus produce a similar reaction and expulsion? Or, to voice what to many readers might be a surprising idea: could our cells make many viruses for entirely beneficial purposes? I report on the nature of viruses in the final chapters of this book, drawing on wonderful research work that has finally utterly transformed my view of their role and importance.

But, at this point in my journey, I was not at all sure even of how HIV was proved to cause AIDS. I had started to write this book excited that I might be able to establish how the AIDS epidemic spread via the polio vaccine – and now I realised that I had simply assumed for years that the link between it and HIV was so well established that I would not need to investigate it.

Fortunately, around this time I gained access to rarely seen laboratory records and correspondence from the famed laboratory of Dr. Robert Gallo. I was thrilled to obtain these. I hoped they would greatly deepen my knowledge. They were about famed and critical experiments that are today said to be among the most cited scientific papers, the most influential papers, ever published.

But before I describe what I then found, I need to set the scene and introduce the main characters– for dramatic changes began to happen to virology from 1980.

---

223 'Retroviruses' 1997 Cold Spring Harbor Laboratory Press - at the National Center for Biotechnology Information and is by John Coffin, Stephen Hughes and the eminent Harold E. Varmus. – and is at the NCBI website

224 Gallo RC, Fauci AS. The human retroviruses in: Isselbacher KJ, Braunwald E, Wilson JD, Martin JB, Fauci AS, Kasper DL, ed. Harrison's Principles of Internal Medicine. 13 ed. New York: McGraw-Hill, 1994: 808-814.

225 Lower R, Lower J, Kurth R. The viruses in all of us: Characteristics and biological significance of human endogenous retrovirus sequences. Proc. Natl. Acad. Sci. U S A 1996; 93:5177-5184.

# Chapter 11

# A Triumph in Doubt

In 1980 the science of virology was changed for all time, for that year the US Supreme Court granted patent rights over a genetically modified oil-eating bacterium to a scientist of the University of Illinois, Ananda Chakrabarty. [226] He had invented a way of using it to clean up oil spills. The legal victory was unique, for never before had patent rights been given over a living organism.

It unleashed a stampede of patent claims for freshly analysed parts of cells, parts of viruses, even for parts of human genes, and for tests for all of them. When in 1985 the PCR procedure was discovered,[227] this made possible the isolation and patenting of thousands of fragments of natural DNA. As such a fragment was legally in 'new' state – i.e. isolated from the rest of the DNA – legally investors could 'own' it if they told the patenting office they had a vague possible use for it. All this had a vast impact on virology – changing the focus of research from whole viruses to patentable fragments of single proteins or short sequences of genetic code. These patents generated vast profits – but also impeded invaluable research – generating protests by the American Society of Genetics and the American College of Medical Genetics.[228]

These developments were initially greeted with incredulity by the more 'old-fashioned' of doctors, virologists and biologists. Their attitude was like that of Dr. Jonas Salk who, when asked if he would patent the discovery of the poliovirus, answered: 'How can one patent the sun?' In other words, they thought only invented things should be patentable, not parts of nature. They saw their work as in the public domain, done for the public good, not for private profit – and thus had not dreamt to claim ownership rights over the subjects of their research.

But the Supreme Court had decided otherwise. In future obtaining a patent over a natural part of life, or of a test or use for it, would give its holder rights for twenty years. This meant the patent-owner could license out rights to use it, to research it –and even bar others from researching it or using it in a remedy. If a patient wanted to benefit from a discovery made by scientists studying the patient's cells, they now might have to pay a very substantial fee.

Suddenly every new discovery in virology or biology became a potent source of income. Even medical scientists not interested in making such profits were forced to join in the action. If a doctor or a medical institution did not take out a patent over a new discovery, then anyone else could grab control over it. This meant its original discoverer and their medical institution could be barred from further work with it – or forced to pay substantial fees for continuing their own work.

---

[226] http://web.mit.edu/invent/iow/chakrabarty.html

[227] PCR Patent
http://patft.uspto.gov/netacgi/nphParser?Sect1=PTO1&Sect2=HITOFF&d=PALL&p=1&u=%2Fnetahtml%2FPTO%2Fsrchnum.htm&r=1&f=G&l=50&s1=4,683,202.PN.&OS=PN/4,683,202&RS=PN/4,683,202

[228] http://genetics.faseb.org/genetics/ashg/policy/pol-08.htm The protest by the American Society of Genetics against the research-hindering patenting of genetic code fragments. Also – a strongly worded protest by the American College of Medical Genetics. http://genetics.faseb.org/genetics/acmg/pol-34.htm

A colleague of Gallo, William Haseltine at Harvard, spoke to him of the fortunes that could be won – and, equally importantly, the research funds. Perhaps in future they would not be dependent on government grants, which decidedly would be a benefit as funding for research on cancer-causing retroviruses was drying up. Yet, Gallo had done well out of hunting putative cancer viruses. It had made him the Head of the largest publicly funded medical laboratory in the US, part of the National Cancer Institute within the highly prestigious National Institutes of Health in Washington DC.

To hold and market the patents he planned to acquire, Haseltine set up a biotech company, Cambridge Bioscience, and contracted with Gallo to gain marketing access to his discoveries, predicting optimistically that a quarter of all cancers would soon prove to be caused by highly profitable retroviruses. He also contracted with a virologist at Harvard, Dr. Myron 'Max' Essex – who was doing much better than Gallo out of retroviruses. He had found them in laboratory cats and was now selling a cat vaccine.

But unfortunately for their plans, retroviruses in humans failed to come up trumps. They seemed to cause only rare cancers at the very best. Thus by 1982 no commercial medical market had developed for a retrovirus test, or for a vaccine against a retrovirus

Essex, Haseltine and Gallo continued to hope – and watched for reports of any outbreak of unexplained illnesses. When, in 1981, gay young men were reported to be falling dangerously ill, they immediately wondered if an unknown retrovirus could be at work that might yet provide them with useful and profitable work.

The CDC has since stated: 'A marked increase in unusual infections and cancers characteristic of severe immune suppression was first recognized in the early 1980s in homosexual men who had been otherwise healthy and had no recognized cause for immune suppression.' This was eventually named as AIDS - Acquired Immune Deficiency Syndrome.

This is not quite accurate. The first official CDC report on what we now call AIDS was indeed issued in 1981. It focussed on five young men in Los Angeles hospitals with fungal diseases, namely fungal pneumonia (PCP) and severe Candida.  But this report expressly said their condition was unlikely to be caused by an infection as 'the patients do not know each other and had no known common contacts or knowledge of sexual partners who had similar illnesses,' and moreover they did not have 'compatible histories of sexually transmitted diseases.' One of the doctors reporting this, Michael S. Gottlieb, has since spoken of how his first case was a young gay man with his mouth full of thrush, with fever and dramatic weight loss.[229]

Moreover, 'recognized causes of immune suppression' were found in all five cases, quite contrary to what the CDC misleadingly now says. Their 1981 report had stated: 'All five reported using inhalant drugs' particularly the amyl nitrite inhalant called 'poppers'[230] These drugs were then known to be immunosuppressant as over time they restricted the supply of oxygen to the cells. The victims were in the gay partying scene that grew out of the gay liberation movement of the 1960s and 1970s. At these parties poppers were inhaled constantly, since a side effect was to relax the smooth muscles and make anal sex more pleasurable. A similar report had come in from the UK, from St Mary's Hospital in Paddington, London. Some 90% of AIDS victims were on poppers and some 60% were also taking crack cocaine. Far fewer, around 15%, were on injected drugs – it was thus these inhaled drugs that were blamed by many of the scientists who first investigated this outbreak. (More about these drugs later.)

---

229   Michael S. Gottlieb and the Identification of AIDS -- Fee and Brown 96 (6): 982 -- American Journal of Public Health

230   S. Gottlieb, H.M. Shanker, P.T. Fan, A. Saxon, J. D. Weisman and J. Pozalski. Pneumocystis Pneumonia –Los Angeles, Morbidity and Mortality Weekly Report. 30 (1981): 250-252.

Inhaled drugs obviously impact mostly the cells of the respiratory tract – and damage to this tract was a major characteristic of these early cases, resulting in Candida in the throat and mouth and a very deadly fungal pneumonia, PCP, in the lungs.

But retrovirus hunting was Gallo's skill, and so he sought to see if these initial reports might be wrong. The victims clearly had fungal infections, but this did not put him off. He thought; perhaps a retrovirus infection had made them vulnerable to fungi? It was surely possible? In this faint hope, with his colleagues Essex and Haseltine, in early 1982 he secured blood samples for analysis from AIDS patients.

Meanwhile the commercial bonding between virologists and investors grew. Around this time Haseltine applied to patent rights to more than 10,000 parts of life. In a later interview, he explained: 'During that time I was [at Harvard] essentially Chairman of two departments, both of which I founded: the Laboratory of Biochemical Pharmacology, which worked on cancer treatments; and the Division of Human Retrovirology, which conducted AIDS Research. From about 1980 on, I started creating biotechnology companies. The first was Cambridge Bioscience. I have now founded seven biotechnology companies, the most recent one being Human Genome Sciences.'

In patenting, he explained: 'you are rewarded for speculation. ... You are rewarded for intelligent and correct guesses. ... The patent office does not reward perspiration. They reward priority. They don't care if someone spent 20 years to find an invention or 20 minutes.' He soon formed a lucrative partnership with GlaxoWellcome. Others focussed on patenting the parts of plants. Thus was built a bio-industry that today is worth several thousand billion dollars.

Many AIDS victims also were coming down with a skin cancer, Kaposi Sarcoma, and Gallo already had in his portfolio a skin cancer he believed caused by a retrovirus, albeit a rare cancer found only in a few cases in the Caribbean – or in nuclear radiation-exposed Japanese. What if a similar retrovirus caused this new outbreak? What if by very good chance this turned out to be related to the two rare viruses he believed he had already found?

He immediately had remarkable luck. After testing one hundred blood samples from AIDS victims in 1982, he announced finding in their blood traces of a retrovirus that just happened to belong to the same family as his rare viruses, HTLV-1 and HTLV-2. He thus named it as HTLV-3. (It seemed all three produced reverse transcriptase – and this sufficed for him.)

There was, however, a rival laboratory engaged in the same hunt, the Institut Pasteur of Paris, and in 1983 Essex, Haseltine and Gallo listened in dismay as one of its French scientists announced at a conference that they had already found a probable cause of AIDS, a virus they called LAV, 'Lymphadenopathy Associated Virus'. From the paper they then published, they had not actually singled out and studied this virus, but had only detected RT, an enzyme found in retroviruses as well as in cells, and particles that were 'the same size as a retrovirus'. [231] The French were now testing the culture to see if these particles really were the cause of AIDS, but as a precaution, they announced they had already filed in London a UK patent application for an antibody blood test for their virus, just in case.

Gallo could not bear being beaten to such a lucrative find. He angrily declared that the French were mistaken. They had not found it first. He had sent it to them as a loan, or so he claimed. The two laboratories were in the habit of exchanging samples. He demanded the French recognize his priority and rename it immediately as HTLV-3.

The French would have none of this. When Gallo requested the courtesy of a research sample, the French politely sent him some fluid containing their virus (and much else besides, as they admitted it was not fully purified) – but only after extracting a formal

---

[231] Crewdson, John. *Science Fictions.* Pp48-49. Further on this below.

contract binding Gallo's laboratory from not using their sample commercially. The French also applied at the same time for the US patent rights for the blood test for their virus. They thought this made them commercially safe.

Fiercely competitive, in 1983 Gallo carried out test after test to try to prove that his HTLV-3 was the genuine cause of AIDS. Logically, he would have to demonstrate that HTLV-3 created vulnerability to the diseases affecting AIDS victims, particularly Candida, Fungal Pneumonia (PCP) and Kaposi Sarcoma. He could not find a direct link – but there was a possibility of a link through immune system damage. AIDS victims reportedly had low numbers of the CD4 white blood cells that are vital to the immune system. Having low numbers was not unique to AIDS, but – if his virus killed these cells, that might make patients susceptible to these and other illnesses.

So he took blood from these patients, separated out their CD4 cells and tried to grow them in a culture. But exasperatingly these cells died before he could prove anything. He did not know what was killing them. Was it the mould later reported to be in his cultures? Was it stress? Was it not nourishing them properly? Were they simply not well adjusted to living in his cultures?

Gallo would later relate how his breakthrough happened. The French suggested to him that perhaps the AIDS virus was present and killing his blood cells? This was, he later said, his Eureka moment. He had then tested the cultures for the activity of RT – the enzyme he associated with retroviruses – and found it. It was a big leap, a major assumption, but he apparently immediately concluded that it must be a retrovirus that was killing these cells.

However, his theory was still only a guess, even if inspired. He still needed to prove his suspect virus was 'cytotoxic,' a killer of cells. He would then have to demonstrate that this particularly caused an increased vulnerability to the fungal illnesses then killing most AIDS victims. If he succeeded, it would be a great and unlikely victory, for no retrovirus had yet been discovered that could kill cells or encourage fungi.

But how could he persuade the very cells he presumed his virus killed, the CD4s, not to die but continuously to produce more of his viruses so he could use these for a patentable vaccine and blood test?

He set aside the worrying problem that by 1982 many toxicologists thought they knew what caused AIDS. They had published numerous papers saying it resulted from exposure to toxic drugs, both prescribed (steroids and antibiotics) and recreational – and some doctors had even reported curing some cases of AIDS by using antitoxins. Some of these scientists worked for the federal Food and Drug Administration (FDA). (More about their research in Chapter 18.) When I learnt of this, it reminded me of the earlier debate over the causes of polio. Again a major epidemic was pitting toxicologists against virologists.

Gallo and his allies were not too worried by this, for they thought they could persuade the CDC, dominated by virologists, that as an epidemic, the cause must be a virus – and they were right. The CDC in 1982 announced the cause 'definitely' must be an unknown virus – and ordered that all the research they funded on AIDS must in future be directed to finding and combating this virus. The FDA research into AIDS-related toxins suddenly collapsed at this point, as its funds were also redirected.

The AIDS orthodoxy was now established. In 1982 the *New England Journal of Science* announced discovering how AIDS was spread. It was by viral infection through sex. It seems this was based on the observation that its gay victims commonly had oral sex many times a night, a shocking discovery for some scientists. But it was strange that they could be so sure so early. One would have thought it would be necessary to find the virus first.

But nevertheless, the evidence linking AIDS with drugs remained strong. Epidemiological surveys in numerous cities reported a 60 to 90% correlation of AIDS cases with long-term high exposure to inhaled drugs. If Gallo were to counter this evidence, and prove his theory, he knew that he had to find patients who had low numbers of white blood cells and AIDS-like illnesses, but no exposure to these inhaled drugs. He found them – among the victims of impure blood transfusions. He theorised that this meant something other than drugs must cause low numbers of CD4 blood cells. He concluded that this proved for all time that poisoning from recreational drugs was not a cause of AIDS.

But his theory was greeted with scepticism among doctors treating AIDS patients. The head of the Californian Department of Health Services, Dr. Chin, at the epicentre of the epidemic, reported: 'Even if an agent transmissible by blood [transfusions] were found to be responsible for AIDS ... a big "if", and if such an agent were found to be present ... it could not ... survive ... the chemical inactivation processes required.' Michelle Cochran, after citing this, commented in her seminal work *When AIDS Began*: 'That even the chief of the Californian Department of Health Services was sceptical that AIDS was infectious in the absence of host vulnerabilities [such as those due to heavy exposure to inhaled drugs] attests to how widespread and credible this view was in the light of the epidemiological evidence during the early years of the epidemic.' [232]

All Gallo's efforts in 1982 and 1983 to prove HTLV-3 caused AIDS ended in failure.[233] He simply could not find his putative virus in AIDS victims! It might well be thought that this would be fatal to his theory – but he then came up with an explanation. He said his virus was so good at killing CD4 cells that, by the time they examined the blood of patients it was no longer present; for it had exterminated itself by leaving itself nowhere to live. In a *Science* article of 30th May 1983 he explained: 'If infection leads to a decline in the population of infected cells, you may not find the virus by the time you get frank disease [AIDS].' He continued: 'In fact National Cancer Institute could not detect viral DNA in T-cells from blood samples taken at a later date from two patients who had earlier given positive results. The same problem might affect attempts to isolate the virus itself.'

Thus – AIDS patients would not have the AIDS virus! This explained its absence – but of course it gave his theory still more problems.

If he were right, why did AIDS persist in the absence of the virus? Also – it simply was not true that these AIDS patients had no CD4 cells. Cochrane's above-cited study of the first AIDS patients reported that some had normal numbers of CD4 cells. Many had CD4 readings of over 200 – meaning they had many thousands of these cells in their blood. Thus the virus should still be present. So, why then was it not found?

Gallo has since spoken of other theories that might explain AIDS. He wrote: 'In March of 1984, NIAID [the National Institute of Allergy and Infectious Diseases] had announced that a fungus was the cause of AIDS [Fungal Pneumonia and Candida were the principal AIDS-associated diseases]. So, there was a great reluctance to think of a retrovirus as the cause of AIDS. My friend [Dr.] Paul Black wrote a letter to the New England Journal of Medicine about why it was ridiculous to think that a retrovirus could be the cause of AIDS. After all, we know retroviruses cause cancer. Right?' [234]

But only a month later, in April 1984, Gallo claimed victory by reporting that his laboratory had succeeded in proving that a retrovirus, not fungi, was the cause of AIDS.

This meant that Gallo had triumphed over his rivals at the Institut Pasteur, or so he then thought. The French nevertheless were still ahead of him in the race to secure the US

---

[232] Cochran, Michelle. *When AIDS Began* 2003. Page 31.

[233] It was established by the later OSI and ORI governmental investigations that these 1982 and 1983 experiments were failures. More about these later.

[234] http://history.nih.gov/NIHInOwnWords/docs/page_12.html It was later discovered that fungi could test positive,, as if HIV, in the HIV test, thus compounding Gallo's difficulties.

patent rights for a test for the AIDS virus.[235] They had applied six months earlier –but he would somehow manage to gain precedence.

Gallo had thrown all his resources and contacts into this race with the French. He knew the patent would be worth a fortune in royalties (then paid to the government as his employer) and most likely a Nobel Prize for himself, as he told his friends. One of his colleagues, M.G. Samagadharen, has also related: 'Several of us had to work nights and weekends preparing [HIV test] patent applications.'

But, to obtain this patent, Gallo had to swear under oath, under penalty of criminal prosecution, that their blood test for the AIDS virus was 'the original' and the 'first'. It seems at this point in his application he conveniently 'forgot' the legal requirement to mention the earlier French application. The Patent Office seemingly also overlooked it. (Perhaps because the US government was backing Gallo in this race?)

On the 30th of March 1984 Gallo lodged four articles documenting their discovery of the AIDS virus for publication in the journal *Science* on May 4th. He then went immediately to the Department of Health to brief the Assistant Secretary of Health, Dr. Edward Brandt.

He then left for Europe to brief scientists and the BBC in advance of the publication and thus to pre-empt any possible French announcement. On April 5-6th, 1984, he lectured, first at Zurich and then, somewhat cheekily, at the Institut Pasteur in Paris, describing his laboratory's success with 'HTLV-3', saying the French virus LAV had proved a failure when tested in his lab. He recommended his audience to 'follow the literature over the next few months carefully and the story will be told in some detail.'

On April 9, 1984 Dr. Gallo gave the BBC reporter Martin Redfern an embargoed tape-recorded interview and prepublication copies of the four *Science* papers. But he had leaked the story of his success so widely by then that within a week stories about it were in the Washington Post, the Wall Street Journal, and other newspapers around the world.

This may have been a somewhat cunning ploy. Discoveries already known to the public cannot be patented. By leaking news of his potentially lucrative and high prestige research findings to journalists, Gallo had practically forced the Reagan Administration to swiftly lodge the related patent papers and thus make public his discovery well before the supporting scientific papers could be peer reviewed and published!

But the French were still in the race. Before the Administration announced Gallo's victory, they had succeeded in persuading key people at the US Centers for Disease Research (CDC) that they, not Gallo, had found the AIDS virus first – and so the New York Times were already writing up the story as a French success.

National prestige was now at stake; the Americans seemed about to lose the race. Gallo was quickly contacted – and asked to swiftly return to the USA to take part in the press conference the US Administration were rushing to organise. But the day before it was to happen, the New York Times published its article giving the victory to the French.

There was nothing for the Administration to do but to continue with the press conference and to try to drown the New York Times story in patriotic acclaim for Gallo's achievement as an American scientist. The *Science* journal rushed their peer review of the Gallo papers. They completed it by the 19th April, in less than three weeks.

Thus, on 23rd April 1984, President Ronald Reagan's Secretary of Health, Margaret Heckler, triumphantly announced at this press conference a 'miracle' produced by 'our eminent Dr. Gallo,' a glorious addition to 'the long honor role of American medicine.' It proved, she said, that their research for a cancer virus had not been a waste of time, for one of the putative cancer viruses had turned out to be the cause of AIDS. She added: 'We have applied for the [AIDS antibody test] patent today,' and President Reagan has personally authorized $54 million immediate funding for the scientists involved. She

---

[235] Ellis Ruinstein. The Untold Story of HUT78, *Science*, June 22, 1990. In this Popovic talks about the rush to complete the papers.

added: 'We hope to have a vaccine ready for testing in about two years.' She concluded with: 'Yet another terrible disease is about to yield to patience, persistence and outright genius.' [236]

This made headlines around the world. It was the greatest celebration of American medicine's achievements since President Eisenhower announced the polio vaccine in 1955. There has been nothing like it since.

At the press conference the journalists were all given preprints of the four papers to be published in *Science*, and Gallo was generous in his speech. He began by praising his senior scientist and co-author, Mikulas Popovic, for 'playing a very major role' in the discovery. In fact, earlier that year Gallo had extraordinarily left Popovic to prove the virus in their test tubes was the cause of AIDS, while he went to Europe to prophetically boast of their success as if it had already happened. Popovic was, however, not at the press conference to receive the applause, or to answer questions, for with apparent thoughtlessness Gallo had sent him off to an obscure medical conference in Florida. [237]

At the conference the press ignored as far too modest the Health Secretary's caution in saying Gallo had only found the 'probable' cause of AIDS, for Gallo had already privately briefed them. Just 3 days later, the leading science journal *Nature* had no hesitation in headlining 'Causation of AIDS Revealed' - and so too was it heralded around the world.

But the French were furious, and immediately began legal action, claiming that Gallo and Popovic had illegally used the loaned French-discovered cell virus LAV. They insisted: the Americans had proved LAV caused AIDS, not HTLV-3. They demanded the lucrative patent rights to the AIDS virus test. They also demanded that the key laboratory records be handed over to them for the purpose of their legal action. It was later reported by Nobel Laureate Harold Varmus that the images of HTLV-III that Gallo held up at the press conference were identical to images of the French virus LAV's cell culture.[238]

On December 14th 1985, the Chicago Tribune reported; 'France's Pasteur Institute, which pioneered research into AIDS, said Friday it has filed suit against the United States to establish its claim that it discovered the deadly virus before American researchers. The institute's director, Raymond Dedonder, told a news conference that 'very large sums' could be at stake in royalties from worldwide testing for AIDS.'

Gallo's claims were not helped by his subsequent behaviour. He adamantly insisted that his approval was necessary before anyone received a sample of his virus to research it. He denied samples to many scientists, and, when he did agree to share, he imposed conditions that specifically forbad the researchers from repeating or trying to verify the experiments done by Gallo's team to prove it caused AIDS! This prohibition raised very strong suspicions, as it is normal for scientific findings to be thus confirmed.

Perhaps Gallo remembered how he had been undone when scientists checked his first claim to have discovered and named a deadly virus?

The US Administration stoutly defended their scientist's claims – and its income from the patent. But it soon started to dawn on its lawyers that they were in a cleft stick. At a 'Lawyers' Meeting' on the 8th April 1986 it was explained that, to defend Gallo's claim, they had to establish that his virus was different from that of the French. But, if they did succeed in this – then this would take all value from the patent!

---

[236] http://www.avert.org/his81_86.htm

[237] Crewdson, John. *Science Fictions* p. 136.This well-reviewed book, published in 2002, is by the Chicago Tribune journalist who in 1989 revealed the evidence for Gallo having stolen the French virus. It documents this theft excellently – but totally misses the evidence for Gallo and Popovic hiding their failure to prove any virus caused AIDS.

[238] Harold Varmus Papers http://profiles.nlm.nih.gov/MV/Views/Exhibit/narrative/aids.html

If it were concluded that two different viruses caused AIDS, this 'would substantially narrow the scope of the patent to make it almost useless.' The value of the patent relied totally on a single virus being the one and only cause of AIDS. The lawyers thus concluded that the only possible way of saving the value of the patent was to admit that both the American and the French viruses were the same, perhaps by blaming inadvertent contamination at one or the other of the laboratories. The US would have to share the profits with the French, but this would be far more lucrative than having two viruses causing AIDS.

It must have been hard for him, but Gallo now found he had no choice but to agree with the decision of the government lawyers – for he was after all a government employee. It was made much easier by the decision that both he and Popovic would receive $100,000 a year as patent royalty payments – with Montagnier of the Institut Pasteur receiving the same. Around the same time members of a committee, including Montagnier but not Gallo, announced in *Nature* that the AIDS virus would be known as HIV in future.[239]

The French had to agree to this sharing of the patent rights, for they simply did not have the documentary proof they needed to establish what went on in Gallo's laboratory and whose virus was in his test tubes. The Americans had hidden from them the vital evidence; illegally as the French had the right to see it. The Federal Department of Health Chief of Staff (1983-87), C. McClain Haddow, would later explain why the French were denied these documents; 'Bob Gallo, as strong as he was on his views, couldn't support the claims he was making from a legal standpoint ... The French attorneys ... didn't know how weak our case was and they never discovered it. So we were able to craft an agreement that probably disadvantaged the French, but it was because we hid our weakness fairly effectively.' They feared going to court as this would give the French the right of 'discovery' to the Gallo laboratory documents, wherein they might learn the truth. So they engineered a quick solution in which the President could take the credit. Haddow concluded: 'We felt in a political sense that it was important for President Reagan to show that he had an interest in the AIDS problem. ...'

And that was exactly what happened. President Ronald Reagan arranged to meet at the White House with the French Prime Minister, Jacque Chirac, to seal an agreement and a cover-up to end this dispute. It was agreed that both governments would share the revenues from the patent and that the names of each side's scientists would be added to the other side's patent, under the fiction that an inadvertent error had been made in listing the inventors. Also, both would rename their virus as 'HIV.' It was finally agreed that Montagnier and Gallo would publish a joint amiable account of their discoveries.[240] (Reportedly in the hope for a shared Nobel Prize and reward. [241]) But as to who had found the virus first, this was not agreed at the White House! The agreement was all about patent revenues – although most of the press got this wrong.

It seems only *Newsweek* reported it accurately. 'The three-year tussle between United States and French medical researchers ... involves big money for both countries – at least $100 million annually, and more probably as the disease spreads. That may explain why the argument ended last week, not in the pages of a medical journal, but in the Rose Garden of the White House ... with an agreement in which both countries could

---

[239] Harold Varmus Papers http://profiles.nlm.nih.gov/MV/Views/Exhibit/narrative/aids.html

[240] A later Congressional investigation into this statement found 'Dr. Gallo was adamant concerning the necessity for an agreed-upon scientific chronology as part of the settlement agreement, apparently believing he could claim by fiat what he could not substantiate by data.' Dingell Inquiry, 1994 Staff Report.

[241241] Crewdson *Science Fictions* page 428.

share profits from the [HIV] blood test – and historians could decide who had found the virus first.' [242]

In fact this was not the end of the dispute. The compromise settlement began to unravel two years later in 1989 when a Pulitzer-winning journalist, John Crewdson of the Chicago Times, published a book-length article of 50,000 words setting out the evidence for Gallo having falsely claimed to co-discover the virus, when he had in fact purloined the French virus for the vital 1984 experiments, after failing with his own virus.

This article caused a scientific tempest. The French were furious at learning what had been hidden from them and threatened further legal action. A high-level US inquiry had to be launched. The National Institutes of Health (NIH), the employer of Gallo and Popovic, decided its Office of Scientific Integrity would conduct it and appointed a scientist, Suzanne Hadley, to take charge. She was 'one of the NIH's rising stars' with a merit award from the Inspector General.'[243]

But the NIH was well aware its investigation would now be subjected to international scrutiny, so it asked the prestigious National Academy of Science and the Institute of Medicine to jointly nominate a Panel of eminent scientists to monitor and advise its investigation. This panel would to be chaired by Frederic Richards, Yale University's Professor of Biochemistry and Molecular Biophysics.

The resulting detailed investigations lasted until the end of 1994 and involved the US House of Representatives and even the US Secret Service; the latter in order to check scientific documents for forgery. These inquiries would produce reports analyzing the fundamental groundbreaking research on AIDS for scientific misconduct and criminality.

Now, I was not interested particularly in whose virus was in Gallo's test tubes. My interest lay in how this virus was proved to cause AIDS and how it had spread. I understood that Gallo had proved whatever virus they had in their test tubes in February 1984 to be the cause of AIDS – and that he had published the evidence for this in the May 4th 1984 issue of *Science* – just as the CDC currently acknowledges: 'Four papers from Dr. Gallo's laboratory, demonstrating that HTLV-III retrovirus was the cause of AIDS, were published in *Science* in May 1984'.[244]

I needed to understand these key experiments – and thought this task would surely be made easier now I had, not only the *Science* papers, but also the related laboratory documents unearthed by the above scientific and Congressional investigations, and by John Crewdson. These included original research notebooks, drafts of key papers, laboratory correspondence, all relating to the discovery of HIV. It was a priceless resource that would surely give me all I needed.

I was astonished to discover that there had been five major investigations between 1990 and 1995 into possible fraud in Gallo's HIV research, several of these overlapping with the others. The first was the one that I have already mentioned, run by the NIH's Office of Scientific Integrity (OSI) and the Richard's Panel. Its goals, set in October 1990, were to focus 'particularly' on the integrity of the first of the four papers published in *Science* in May 1984, the one on which Popovic was the lead author, since this paper described the key experiments cited in the application for the patent on the HIV Test.

The second inquiry was under a powerful Congressional Investigative Sub-Committee headed by Rep. John Dingell. It would prevent key documents from being shredded by the NIH. The third was under the Inspector General of the Department of Health and examined criminal fraud in the 'HIV Test' patent application. The fourth was under the Office of Research Integrity of the Department of Health and Human Resources and looked for fraud, deception and 'scientific misconduct' in the Gallo *Science* papers.

---

[242] John Crewdson, *Science Fictions*, page 301.

[243] John Crewdson p.422.

[244] See AIDS Timeline, 1981-1988, on US government health website linked on www.cdc.gov

And the fifth and last was by the US Secret Service, the body normally charged with safeguarding the security of the US President. It would check the related laboratory documents in the finest forensic lab in Washington. If any were forged, it would find out.

All together, this was by far the most formidable governmental investigation into the honesty of scientific research ever undertaken. Clearly the issues at stake were considered extremely important. But Gallo was by now no little-known scientist. By 1990 he was the head of an NIH laboratory with an annual budget of around $12 million, and his annual salary was over $200,000. In a letter he sent around this time, he described himself as 'the most cited scientist in the world for the decade of the 1980s.'[245] He had in truth become enormously influential.

One of the first press reports on these inquiries was in the Chicago Tribune of February 25th, 1990. The headline was '*U.S. agency probing AIDS virus discovery.*' It said 'The inquiry is examining much of the related research conducted in recent years by Dr. Robert C. Gallo, the nation's most prominent AIDS researcher.'

But, from contemporary press reports, Gallo's laboratory was not as upright as might be expected. A newspaper report of 29th April 1990 stated: 'A 16-month congressional inquiry [by Dingell into Gallo's laboratory] has uncovered evidence suggesting that rare and valuable viruses, among them the AIDS virus, were appropriated' and sold privately. HTLV-3 [HIV] went on the black market for a price of around $1000 a milligram. The person suspected was Syed Zaki Salahuddin, 'one of Gallo's long-time assistants.' He was also the lead author of one of the four *Science* papers of May 4th, 1984.

On May 1st, 1990, this investigation further found that 'hundreds of thousands of dollars in government equipment and supplies cannot be accounted for by scientists at the National Cancer Institute' and that a million dollars had been paid to a company partly owned by Salahuddin and his wife. He was later found guilty and sentenced to pay back $12,000 and do 1,750 hours of community service. [246]

I soon learnt, from the OSI investigation records, that Gallo had confessed in 1990 that he had not found the AIDS virus in 1982, as he had prominently reported in his 1984 *Science* papers. He admitted that in 1982 he had only detected the enzyme RT and not the virus itself. [247] The investigators reported that he had lied when he claimed he did 'more than fifty' detections and produced 'ten true isolates' of the AIDS virus in 1982. They concluded that he did not find the virus before 1984.

But, in the apparent belief that people have forgotten this confession, Gallo is now astonishingly repeatedly making the same claim - that he found HIV in 1982 before anyone else. He did so in his recent book[248] and he did so, even most seriously, in sworn testimony in 2007 to an Australian court. (More on this below.) So for me, discovering his earlier confession was something of a shock.

In 1990-91, more evidence of wrongdoing in Gallo's lab surfaced in the OSI investigation into his HIV research. But at this point the new head of the NIH, Bernardine Healy, intervened. She hauled in Gallo, subjected him to a severe dressing down; laying down that in future he would not be able to absent himself from laboratory duties without permission, nor even publish a paper or give an interview without permission. Then, after hopefully silencing him, she turned her attention to the OSI.

The OSI chief, Suzanne Hadley, was then drafting the final OSI report and about to conclude that Gallo's chief investigative scientist, Mikulas Popovic, had falsified the data

---

[245]   Quoted in John Crewdson: *Science Fictions* page 439 fn. 37 ch 21.

[246]   Joan Shenton, *Positively False*, p50

[247]   Gallo stated 'we had more than 50 *detections* and more than *10 true isolates* of HIV-I.' Emphasis added;
4/26/90  OSI interview; transcript p. 58.

[248]   Robert Gallo. In his book *Virus Hunters*

in the first and most significant of the four *Science* papers,– and to recommend that, as the primary author, he be condemned for scientific misconduct.

We know this from a tape recording sent to Popovic. It by error recorded not just of his testimony, but the comments made after he left the room. Learning from this that he was about to be condemned, forced Popovic in desperation to produce the key evidence. He gave Hadley his 1984 draft of this key *Science* paper that he had felt necessary to hide overseas. Among other things, the revealed that Robert Gallo had extensively changed Popovic's version of this paper at the last moment to hide their use of the French virus.

With this it seemed the evidence was at hand to prove Gallo guilty of illegal use of the French virus and thus of scientific deceit. Hadley composed her OSI report accordingly. She concluded: 'Dr. Gallo has claimed credit for the Popovic *et al.* paper and the other 1984 papers, so must he bear responsibility for the falsehoods in the Popovic *et al.* paper. Accordingly the OSI finds that Dr Robert Gallo engaged in scientific misconduct.'

This was a damning conclusion. This OSI report now should have gone to the Richard's Panel for review – but at this point Healy intervened, removing Hadley from her duties at the OSI. The indictment of Gallo was deleted from her report.

But the watered down report that was published after her departure was still highly critical of Gallo. It accused him of 'an unhealthy disregard for accepted standards of professional and scientific ethics.' It included her findings that Dr. Gallo must share responsibility with Dr. Popovic for 'imprecise and non-meticulous science', and that Gallo's alteration of a key 1983 Institut Pasteur paper prior to publication was a 'gratuitous, self-serving, and improper act.' (Gallo had served as Peer Reviewer for a Pasteur Institute paper on the AIDS virus – and had unilaterally changed it prior to publication!) But the report then strangely concluded that none of this was 'scientific misconduct!' This conclusion seems to have been added without any consideration of what the report actually documented. On the issue of whether Gallo stole the French virus, the report now came to no conclusion.

But the accusations would not go away. The Chicago Tribune was able to report on August 11, 1991: 'Dr. Robert C. Gallo, the government's most prominent AIDS researcher ... made untrue and misleading statements in a sworn declaration defending the patent from a legal challenge by French scientists.' [249]

A still more critical report appeared in this paper on September 13th 1991. It stated: 'an 18-month investigation by the NIH into the 1984 article by Robert C. Gallo which reported the isolation of the AIDS virus concludes that this report is riddled with fabrication, falsification, misleading statements and errors.' [250] This was astonishing. The report of which it spoke is the very scientific article that is cited today as establishing for all time that HIV causes AIDS – the first of the four published by Gallo et al in *Science* in May 1984. If eminent scientific bodies found it so riddled with errors, then why is it still cited?

Possibly because, when these investigations commenced, about a billion dollars had already been invested in 'HIV infection' prevention and related research. There was thus much riding on the credibility of these foundation papers of HIV research.

A year after these investigations commenced, pressure had really started to mount on Gallo and Popovic. The NIH decision to remove Suzanne Hadley, the Head of the OSI inquiry, had proved so controversial that a new inquiry had to be set up independent of the NIH to complete the work. It was to be managed by the Office of Research Integrity (ORI) of the Department of Health in the President George Bush Administration. The ORI asked the scientists previously working with the NIH inquiry to assist them– saying, if

---

[249] John Crewdson, *Chicago Tribune*, Ill.: Aug 11, 1991. pg. 1
[250] *Lies, Errors* Cited in article by Crewdson, John. Chicago Tribune, Ill.: Sep 15, 1991. pg. 11

they found reason to present charges against Gallo or Popovic, these would be sent to a departmental legal committee for assessment and action.

The talk of an NIH cover-up to protect Gallo's AIDS research that year also reached Representative John Dingell, the Democrat head of the powerful Congressional Investigative sub-committee that had previously indicted a scientist working in Gallo's lab for theft, as I mentioned above. Dingell now immediately ordered the OSI files on Gallo and Popovic moved to his office – and asked the NIH for the services of Hadley. It could not refuse him – so she resumed her investigation but now with considerably greater Congressional investigative powers. An aide to Dingell explained: 'Everything Hadley has told us has checked out 100% against documents the committee has received from NIH. She's obviously been treated very shabbily.'

That year Gallo also got into trouble in Africa. His laboratory had developed a vaccine based on transplanting into the shell of another virus a putative part of HIV. It seems this was easier than using HIV itself as it was difficult to find. This vaccine was injected into a few Congolese in Africa and Paris and three of them died. It was then discovered that his vaccine had only been approved for use on animals! [251]  But Gallo escaped with only a mild reprimand.

In May 1991, knowing what the OSI was about to deliver its report, Gallo wrote to *Nature*, confessing that he now realised that the French virus and his own were the same. He blamed his error on inadvertent laboratory contamination. Then a similar confession appeared in the UK from a leading British virologist and colleague of Robert Gallo, Dr. Robin Weiss, the scientist I had first met when he was chairing the NIH workshop on SV40, and again when he was chairing the Royal Society debate on the polio vaccine and HIV.

Weiss now confessed that the AIDS virus he claimed to isolate in 1985, a year after Gallo, was in fact the very same one that the Institut Pasteur had sent him earlier. Like Gallo, his explanation was inadvertent laboratory contamination.[252] He also, like Gallo, had used the French virus to secure a UK patent for the HIV test.

By now Dingell was pushing for a criminal investigation into Gallo's AIDS research – and was angry at the 'waffling by the Bush Administration' that his efforts met. Charges were justified, he maintained, since 'a landmark 1984 article in which Gallo reported isolating the AIDS virus contains falsified data.' [253]

Then another damning report appeared. The Richards Panel, set up to supervise the OSI investigation, had decided not to let the matter rest after NIH produced the watered-down OSI report. They were mindful that they had been appointed by two of the most important scientific bodies in the USA – and therefore had a duty to report honestly what they had discovered.

They issued their own report in January 1992. It stated there was 'a pattern of behaviour on Dr. Gallo's part that repeatedly misrepresents, suppresses, and distorts data and their interpretation in such a way as to enhance Dr. Gallo's claim to priority.' They said his failure to acknowledge his use of the French virus represented 'intellectual recklessness of a high degree' in the 'intellectual appropriation of the French viral isolate...' [254]

In February 1992 the Chicago Tribune reported a government investigation had discovered 'a landmark 1984 article reporting Robert C. Gallo's isolation of the AIDS

---

[251]  Chicago Tribune, Apr 14, 1991 *3 Dead in AIDS Vaccine Test*

[252]  Peter Duesberg. *Inventing the AIDS virus*. Page 164.

[253]  Chicago Tribune, November 6th, 1991

[254]  Chicago Times of May 27th, 1992.

virus contains numerous falsifications of data and misrepresentations of the methods employed.' [255]

In April 1992, a *Prime Time* television investigation stated: 'It may be the greatest scientific fraud of the twentieth century.' It continued over a portrait of Gallo: 'Eight years ago this man was hailed as the genius who discovered the AIDS virus.' But now it was a story 'of how a fight for wealth and glory can interfere with the desperate attempt to conquer a deadly disease.'[256]

In July that year, another member of Gallo's laboratory was found guilty of a federal crime. This time it was Prem Sarin, the second in charge of his laboratory for more than a decade. He had embezzled $25,000 that should have been spent on AIDS research.[257]

When Dingell in late 1992 discovered he was missing some of the Gallo research documents, he sought to discover why. He wrote on 24th November 1992 to the Director of the NIH: 'we have received reliable information that documents from the Gallo/Popovic investigation were being shredded at the NIH's Office of Scientific Integrity.' He continued 'NIH's actions...show a clear pattern of obstruction and attempted deception ... particularly when juxtaposed with the curious diligence the NIH showed in its efforts to seek out and destroy the person or persons suspected of blowing the whistle on the shredding.'

A year later President Clinton gave the NIH a new director, Dr. Harold Varmus, a scientist of great repute who was not inclined to protect Gallo. In June 1993 the Chicago Tribune reported that 'the government's long-running case against its star AIDS researcher, Dr. Robert C. Gallo, has been expanded to include a broader range of misconduct surrounding his decade-old claim to have discovered the cause of AIDS.'[258]

The ORI by now had drawn up a powerful Indictment ('Offer of Proof') against Gallo and Popovic. This it presented to the Department of Health's lawyer-based 'Research Integrity Adjudication Panel'. It was broad ranging and powerful. Here are some excerpts:

§ **'Research process can proceed with confidence only if scientists can assume that the previously reported facts on which their work is based are correct. If the bricks are in fact false...then the scientific wall of truth may crumble...Such actions threaten the very integrity of the scientific process.'**

§ **'In light of the groundbreaking nature of this research and its profound public health implications, ORI believes that the careless and unacceptable keeping of research records [for proving HIV the cause of AIDS by Gallo and his team] ...reflects irresponsible laboratory management that has permanently impaired the ability to retrace the important steps taken. '**

§ **[This] 'put the public health at risk and, at the minimum, severely undermined the ability of the scientific community to reproduce and/or verify the efforts of the LTCB [Gallo's 'Laboratory for Tumor Cell Biology'] in isolating and growing the AIDS virus.'**

§ **'Gallo's failings as a Lab Chief are evidenced in the Popovic Science paper, a paper conspicuously lacking in significant primary data and fraught with false and erroneous statements.'**

§ **Gallo 'repeatedly misrepresents distorts and suppresses data in such a way as to enhance his own claim to priority and primacy in AIDS research.'**

[255] John Crewdson, *Criminal inquiry urged in AIDS lab scandal* Chicago Tribune: Nov 6, 1991

[256] Cited in John Crewdson. Page 443.

[257] Chicago Tribune, July 8, 1992

[258] Chicago Tribune June 6, 1993

§     'The [lead] Science paper contains numerous falsifications... the paper was replete with at least 22 incorrect statements concerning LTCB research, at least 11 of which were falsifications amounting to serious deviations from accepted standards for conducting and reporting evidence.' Some of the captions to micrographs, descriptions of experiments and enclosed tables were 'false and misleading'.[259]

§     'The absence of virtually any assay data for the parent cell line is simply unbelievable. [Especially since this was] used to develop and patent the HIV antibody blood test.'

§     Gallo, 'in violation of all research protocols, impeded scientists wanting to follow up on his research ... imposed on others the condition that they did not try to repeat his work.'

This is only a selection from an absolutely devastating indictment.

The Adjudication Panel, to which this indictment was submitted for action, was made up of lawyers not scientists. It decided to first consider the case of Popovic – and came to an amazing conclusion. They fully accepted that Popovic had published careless inaccurate and deceptive research, but still deemed him 'innocent' since the 'intent to deceive' had not been proved. They finished by astonishingly praising Popovic's research as published in *Science* in May 1984 as important for all time.

This utterly shocked the scientists who had helped produce the ORI report. Their indictment had been supported with the testimony of over 100 scientists, and they had been expressly directed not to try to prove 'intent' in their indictment. How could the Panel now absolve Popovic from blame on the grounds they had not tried to prove 'intent'? How could they absolve him of responsibility while accepting their conclusion that the key research he did on HIV was deeply flawed, contained false statements, and might have sent AIDS research off in the wrong direction? Furthermore, how could an Adjudication Panel made up solely of lawyers conclude by praising this research, when they as scientists had condemned it? They wondered darkly just who had advised the lawyers?

The Panel was next to consider the case of Robert Gallo – but in face of the decision on Popovic, the ORI in disgust felt it had no choice but to drop its attempt to find Gallo guilty of scientific misconduct since they had been misdirected over the need to prove 'intent'. They nevertheless declared their 'fundamental disagreement' with the Panel's understanding of 'the importance of clarity, accuracy and honesty in science.'

But Gallo was not yet clear. The Secret Service now presented the evidence they had unearthed to the Dingell Inquiry. They had been charged to examine for fraud the laboratory documents that Gallo had presented as legal evidence. They had discovered that many were 'fixed' before being presented. Documents written on different dates were changed on the same day. They found incriminating overlapping imprints of the changes on the enclosing folders.

This was the clearest evidence of criminal fraud and was immediately presented to the State Attorney General in January 1994 in the expectation that a criminal prosecution would now be ordered, but he ruled it was 'out of time'. Too long had elapsed under the five-year Statute of Limitations since the fraud was carried out. Gallo thus may have escaped prosecution on a technicality. [260]

---

[259] The Office of Research Integrity – Offers of Proof Report 1993.

[260] It was reported that 'Federal prosecutors decided earlier this year not to bring Criminal charges against Gallo, citing what the Inspector General's summary calls 'several obstacles, jurisdiction concerns and procedural rules governing criminal prosecution' including the five-year statute of limitations. Chicago Tribune 26 June 1994

But the investigators were not content to leave it there. Hadley and others went to see Varmus, the new Director of the NIH, to present the new damning evidence, including more now produced by the Inspector General's Inquiry on fraud in the Patent application for the HIV test. The Inspector General had even expressed doubts on whether the related experiments were ever done! The Patent Examiner also now acknowledged 'had she been aware of (the French AIDS test research) at the time she examined the blood test application of Gallo, she would have suspended Gallo's application.' [261]

Varmus was persuaded – and had to act. In June 1994 Gallo was given a choice: prepare to leave the NIH – or face a new investigation that might be harder to escape from unscathed. He decided to leave – in a year's time. It was then headlined on July 12th that: 'US, France settle AIDS virus dispute. The NIH will give up millions in profit from Test Patent.' The Financial Times reported: 'US climb down in feud with the French over AIDS research.' The NIH had at last acknowledged that there was justice in the French claim against them as the employer of Gallo.

However, the Dingell Investigation never reached a formal conclusion. When the Republican Party took control of the House of Representatives at the end of 1994, Dingell lost his chairmanship of the investigating sub-committee –and the Republicans promptly killed the investigation of the Reagan-endorsed Robert Gallo. However, Dingell's staff would have none of this. They did not want their years of research wasted, so they issued an unofficial final 'Staff Report' of 267 pages, detailing their findings. Their report might not have been official, but it received a highly favourable review in the top UK medical journal, the *Lancet*.

The *Chicago Tribune* summarised the Staff Report's findings in two scathing pieces, one on 1st January 1995 entitled 'In Gallo Case, Truth deemed a Casualty' and the other an editorial on 6th January entitled: 'Defending the Indefensible Dr. Gallo'. This Staff Report had reported:

§ **'The cover-up ... advanced to a more active phase in mid-March 1984, when Dr. Gallo systematically rewrote the manuscript for what would become a renowned LTCB paper (Popovic et al.; *Science*).'[262]**

§ **'The evidence is compelling that the oft-repeated [HIV] isolate claim - ... dating from 1982/early 1983, are not true and were known to be untrue at the time the claims were made.'**

§ **'Many of the samples allegedly used for the pool [the supposed HIV culture] were noted in the LTCB records to be contaminated with mould.'**

§ **'The notion that Dr. Popovic used such samples in an effort to obtain a high-titre virus-producing cell line defies credulity.'**

§ **'The [early] February 1984 experiment was so faulty and so many aspects of it so questionable, that little or no confidence can be placed in any of its claimed findings.'**

§ **'Contrary to the claims of Gallo and Popovic, including claims in their patent applications [for the HIV Blood Test], several of the putative pool samples contained no HIV, while others did not even come from AIDS or pre-AIDS patients.'**

The report then concluded:
**'The result was a costly, prolonged defence of the indefensible in which the LTCB 'science' became an integral element of the US government's public relations/advocacy efforts. The consequences for HIV research were severely**

---

[261] Chicago Tribune *U.S. INQUIRY DISCREDITS GALLO ON AIDS PATENT DIAGNOSTIC TEST. CLAIMS WERE RIDDLED BY HOLES, PROBE SAYS.* **June 19, 1994.**

[262] LTCB stood for Gallo's Laboratory of Tumor Cell Biology

**damaging, leading, in part, to a corpus of scientific papers polluted with systematic exaggerations and outright falsehoods of unprecedented proportions.'**

The report presented detailed evidence that destroyed the central claim made by Gallo in these famed *Science* papers; to have isolated HIV in dozens of AIDS patients in experiments conducted in 1982 and 1983. They said he did not have the tools needed to do this – and consequently could not have isolated or identified a single AIDS virus!

The Staff report also recorded that when Gallo was asked 'to substantiate this claim' [that he had found the AIDS virus in 1982] by his immediate boss Dr. Samuel Broder, the National Cancer Institute director, he had 'responded with a list of samples, only one of which dated from 1982.' 'When that sample was checked against records, it was found to be marked 'N.D.' meaning 'Not Done' - or 'Not Determinable.' Gallo then admitted under interrogation that he had only detected the enzyme RT, not the virus, at the time. [263] The investigators concluded; 'No evidence was supplied that any of these samples had ever been tested and found positive for HIV. In fact no such evidence existed.' [264] It then added that the US Secret Service found many Gallo laboratory records were falsified prior to being presented as evidence.[265]

On May 25th 1995 came the news that 'Dr. Robert C. Gallo, the government's best-known and most controversial AIDS researcher, is departing the National Cancer Institute after a 30-year career that included the discovery of the first human leukaemia virus and a bitter international controversy over his contribution to finding the cause of AIDS. Gallo said he plans to set up his own Institute of Human Virology in a renovated warehouse in downtown Baltimore.' [266]

But, the *Science* papers he authored, despite being found scandalously fraudulent, were never withdrawn, nor corrected, which to my mind is reprehensible given the prestige of the institutions that had condemned them and the consequence of leaving them uncorrected. Thus thousands of researchers still consult them in all innocence. Today thousands of papers on HIV and AIDS refer back to them, and all medical authorities point to them too. The US Centers for Disease Control (CDC) still state on their website that the key foundation papers in AIDS research are 'four papers from Dr Gallo's laboratory, demonstrating that HTLV-III retrovirus [HIV] was the cause of AIDS.' It does not mention that they were found to be 'polluted with systematic exaggerations and outright falsehoods of unprecedented proportions.'

The findings of all these high level investigations of the 1990s were swiftly and shockingly buried. Few AIDS scientists now know that these seminal AIDS papers were thoroughly discredited by scientists belonging to the most eminent of scientific bodies. This is an extraordinary state of affairs. It is totally amazing, almost unbelievable.

It is as if these highly prestigious top-level investigations never existed – yet they only completed their work in 1995. They are not even mentioned in the AIDS research history assembled by AVERT and referenced on the UK government's AIDS website. [267]

Despite the NIH deciding in 1994 to give the prime credit to the French, the CDC in 2008 still shares this with Gallo, reporting: 'Abundant evidence indicates that AIDS is caused by the human immunodeficiency virus (HIV), discovered in 1983 by two groups of

---

[263] He said 'we had more than 50 *detections* and more than *10 true isolates* of HIV-I.'Emphasis added; 4/26/90 OSI interview; transcript p. 58.

[264] Gallo-to-Fischinger; August 14, 1985.

[265] The fraud uncovered by the Secret Service is extensively described in *Science Fictions* by John Crewdson, published by Little Brown in 2002, pages 506-510

[266] Chicago Tribune, May 25th 1995

[267] See the Timeline published in *The Scientist* in November 2006. It states the credit was equally shared between Gallo and the French in 1987 - and totally omits any mention of this later high level controversy. http://www.the-scientist.com/article/flash/23586/1/

scientists, one headed by Dr. Robert Gallo at the NIH, and the other headed by Professor Luc Montagnier at the Institut Pasteur in France.'[268]

Gallo today is still the head of his Institute of Human Virology, IHV (a spin on HIV). After he founded this, he immediately appointed Popovic to it as a full Professor of Medicine. Although Gallo often repeats the discredited claims he made in the Science papers, Popovic has remained silent on how Gallo fraudulently changed his paper.

Today the White House, the Bill Gates Foundation and the US Defence Department generously fund Gallo's IHV to advise African governments on AIDS and to develop new HIV tests and treatments.

But – my own investigation was not over. As I said, it makes little difference to me which virus causes AIDS. I was willing to accept it was the French. I accepted that Gallo lied about his own virus. But I wanted to know more about this French virus. I needed to know how it was proved to cause AIDS and spread this dreadful epidemic.

But, despite thorough searching, I had found little about the French virus in the conclusions of the above inquiries. It seems, once they decided that HIV was not Gallo's HTLV-3 , they presumed it must be the French virus LAV. This was in accordance with their stated remit. They were set up to find out whose virus it was in the vital experiments, not to verify these experiments, but for me this was highly disappointing.

But they had so discredited Gallo and Popovic, so crushingly described their many errors, so convincingly shown how Gallo impeded any check on their research, that I now found it hard to understand how anyone can rely on the four *Science* papers he produced as proof that the French virus causes AIDS – but it is still these that are cited whenever a scientist describes when and how HIV was proved to cause AIDS. They are now perhaps the most cited scientific papers in the world.

In all fields of science, there are papers that are regarded as fundamental, as papers on which an edifice of research can reliably be erected. Scientists proceed to research the details in trust that the foundations are true. They rarely, if ever, feel a need to go back to re-do the key research, especially as this is often expensive and difficult to carry out. Indeed research grants are rarely made for such purposes. Yet these fundamental papers establish the basic concepts that guide further research. In AIDS research these papers are still said to be the four papers by Gallo and his colleagues, published in *Science* on a fateful May 4th, in 1984.

Particularly disturbing for me were the investigators' reports that Gallo had so poorly recorded his experiments that they could not be repeated and thus verified, and that he also deliberately prevented scientists from trying to verify them. It suggests that he may not have believed in his own experiments. I have to ask, if no one can verify them – why on earth are we still relying on them as a firm foundation for AIDS research? Is this why all efforts based on his research to find a cure or vaccine for AIDS have so far utterly failed, despite the spending of nearly 200 billion dollars?

I cannot express my dismay any better than did the Office of Research Integrity of the US Department of Health. **'Research process can proceed with confidence only if scientists can assume that the previously reported facts on which their work is based are correct. If the bricks are in fact false...then the scientific wall of truth may crumble. ... Such actions threaten the very integrity of the scientific process.'**

---

[268] See AIDS Timeline, 1981-1988, on US government health website linked on www.cdc.gov

# Time Line

## US Governmental Investigations into the key HIV Research.

1987   President Reagan and Prime Minister Chirac agree to share royalties on the HIV test; on the legal fiction that Gallo and the French found the AIDS virus simultaneously. It is named as HIV. The French drop their legal action against the US for stealing their virus.

1989   The Chicago Tribune publishes evidence that the French found the virus first – and that Gallo had falsely claimed priority.

1989-90   Democrat Rep. Dingell investigates Gallo's lab on other criminal matters.

1990   NIH asks National Academy and Institute of Medicine to supervise its OSI inquiry into possible fraud in the Gallo HIV research – the Richards Committee is appointed to do this.  Suzanne Hadley is put in charge of the inquiry.  The Health Department's Inspector General commences its own investigation into Gallo's HIV Test Patent application.

1991 – the NIH removes Hadley from the OSI inquiry.

1991 – Dingell goes from investigating thefts and embezzlement at Gallo's lab to put Hadley in charge of its own investigation into fraud in Gallo and Popovic's AIDS research.

1991  - Late that year, the NIH's OSI issued its report – it is severely critical but does not find 'scientific misconduct'.  No conclusion on use of the French virus.

1992  - The Richards Panel objects to NIH censoring of OSI report and issues a much more critical report. The French resume their legal action.  Dingell recovers most of the OSI documents before the NIH can shred them, although some are destroyed.

1992   The ORI investigation is set up away from the NIH's control.

1992   Dingell writes to NIH re shredding of documents

1992   ORI presents its indictment of Gallo and Popovic.

1993   November. The Appeals Board clears Popovic of having 'intent' to defraud  – and praises his paper; The ORI does not proceed against Gallo.

1994   The Secret Service finds evidence of fraud in scientific records presented by Gallo.

1994   Statute of limitations invoked. No legal action against Gallo for fraud possible.

1994   February. The case prepared against Gallo by the Dingell investigation is presented to Dr. Varmus, the new head of the NIH.

1984   June. The Inspector General recommends charges be considered against Gallo, Varmus allegedly then threatens Gallo with legal action if he does not leave the NIH.

1994   June. The French are paid further royalties for the HIV Test – their prior rights acknowledged.

1994   November. The Democrats lose control over the House of Representatives and the Republicans stop the investigation into Gallo.

1995   The Dingell Staff Report is 'leaked' by concerned academics.

1995   Gallo leaves the NIH.

# Chapter 12

# Fraudulent Papers

My hunt to discover how HIV caused the AIDS epidemic was now near its end, or so I hoped, for it had taken far longer than I ever dreamt it might. I told myself, I should have gone for the jugular earlier. But I had not realized that I would need to go back to the original experiments that proved HIV to cause AIDS. I had originally presumed that this must be self-evident.

But I was now faced by a quandary. The very papers the above investigations found to be riddled with fraud were the ones I was told to go to if I wanted to know how the French HIV was proved to cause AIDS, for the American government investigators had praised as successful the last of the experiments documented in them, those carried out after February 22$^{nd}$ and before March 30$^{th}$ 1984. These, they said, had used the French virus and had finally and successfully proved it to cause AIDS. (Yet they also said these experiments were so poorly recorded that they were unrepeatable.)

I was unused to the idea that I could trust only parts of scientific papers, but this was what I was expected to do. The prestigious investigations and institutions were all in agreement. They condemned as false Gallo's claim that he and his team had isolated this virus in 1982, in other words, before the French. Instead they scathingly concluded that, as of the 22nd February 1984, that is six weeks before these *Science* papers went for publication on March 30$^{th}$, Gallo could not have identified HIV, since up until this date 'no HIV-specific reagents [antibodies] were available to prove that a particular sample harboured the AIDS virus.' [269]

In other words, Gallo could not have identified HIV in 1982 and 1983 as he has claimed, by detecting antibodies specific to it. The investigating scientists pointed out that it was impossible to prove an antibody targeted the AIDS virus before proving what virus caused AIDS!

It was not that the French had earlier proved their virus caused AIDS. They had stated in 1983, just before sending a sample of their virus to Gallo, that: 'the role of the virus in the aetiology of AIDS remains to be determined.' [270] However, it was not just viruses they sent him. It was reported that it was a sample of a culture grown in their laboratory from the blood cells of a suspected AIDS patient, but their 1983 paper stated birth umbilical cord cells were in fact used, with no mention of the mother being infected. [271] They thought some particles in the culture might be retroviruses that caused

---

[269] Dingell Congressional Inquiry Staff Report. Around mid-February [1984] further work was done by Gallo's laboratory to try to get a rabbit antiserum that was specific to the virus, but without the virus being first truly isolated and analyzed, this was still an impossible task. There is no laboratory record of such work being done – and Popovic explicitly stated in March 1984 that this work had not been done. (In his paper as he had prepared it for publication in *Science* prior to Gallo editing it.

[270] Francoise Barre-Sinoussi et al. (including. L. Montagnier). 1983. Isolation of a T-lymphotropic retrovirus from a patient at risk for Acquired Immune Deficiency Syndrome (AIDS). Science 220: 868-871

[271] Professor Etienne De Harven has pointed out to the author that the microphotographs Montagnier produced of this virus show it as grown on birth cord lymphocytes. The 1983 paper stated: 'These were detection of: 'umbilical

AIDS – but could not be sure. Montagnier later confessed, they could not find in their serum any particles with 'the morphology typical of retroviruses.' [272]

Therefore, it was evident that, as it was not the French, it must have been Gallo and Popovic who proved the French virus to cause AIDS – and they must have done this in that final six weeks of experimenting.

I began to read the account of Gallo and Popovic's final 1984 experiments in the *Science* papers with great care and some expectation. These are recorded in the first of the four papers, the one for which Popovic is the lead author.

From the reports of the US investigations and of others involved at the time, I knew that Gallo was so confident in their coming success with the French virus that he had left his senior investigative scientist, Popovic, in charge of the vital research work with the French virus while he went to France to boast that they had already discovered the AIDS virus.

In the same total confidence, before going abroad, he also made advance arrangements for Popovic's paper, and three others based on it, to be published together in the May 4th issue of *Science*.[273] He would not return until a week before the papers were to be submitted for publication on March 30th 1984.

I found this most odd – how could Gallo have been so absolutely certain of the outcome of these vital experiments before they were carried out? Otherwise, how does one explain this irrational confidence, his putting at risk of his professional status, by going off to boast of his success before it was achieved?

I needed to know more, so I raked through the Gallo laboratory documents these investigations had unearthed, including some that John Crewdson retrieved under Freedom of Information legislation. One of these turned out to be the draft of the key Science paper, as typed up by Popovic and presented to Gallo on his return from France, a few days before the papers went to the publisher.

I was thrilled to find this. I had learnt of its existence from the reports of the investigators. They told me it had only survived because Popovic had taken extraordinary steps to protect it from the shredding machine. He had secretly sent it to his sister in Austria for safekeeping, only to be made public if needed to prove who had falsified his research.

He had retrieved it when the investigations began - but had hoped not to use it. Then after an interview with the OSI, he was sent by mistake a tape that recorded, not just his answers to questions, but also the comments made after he left the room. This revealed that he, rather than Gallo, was to be found guilty of scientific misconduct. Next morning he had a lawyer give this carefully hidden draft to the OSI.

Knowing all this made me extremely curious to read the manuscript. I was keen to see what Popovic had reported before Gallo did his editing. After all, it was he who had completed these experiments, not Gallo. The Investigators had reported: 'Dr. Popovic single-handedly carried out the most important early HIV experiments.' [274] They had also verified that the handwritten changes on the draft were by Gallo.

On his return to the States from Europe, Gallo had collected this draft, started to read it and then received a terrible shock. It was nothing like what he had anticipated. Popovic had only just left for a skiing holiday in Utah. Gallo contacted him urgently on

---

cord lymphocytes showed characteristic immature particles with dense crescent (C- type) budding at the plasma membrane...' Barre-Sinoussai et al. Isolation of T-lymphotropic retrovirus from a patient at risk for acquired immune deficiency syndrome (AIDS). Science 1983;220: 868–71.

[272] Interview with Djamel Tahi-1997. Text of video interview with Professor Luc Montagnier at the Pasteur Institute July 18th 1997. Continuum 1998; 5:30-34. The original French is given in a later footnote.

[274] Staff Report of the Subcommittee on Oversight and Investigations, Dingell Committee on Energy and Commerce United States House of Representatives

the Friday 23rd of March and ordered him back. This was only 7 days before the paper had to be sent for publication.

The government investigators report that Gallo then extensively changed the paper's typed text in his own hand at the last moment before sending it for publication. His changes are the key evidence later cited to prove that he had deliberately hidden the use of the French virus. The Congressional Staff Report stated: 'The cover-up of the LTCB's [Gallo's Laboratory] work with the IP [Institut Pasteur] virus advanced to a more active phase in mid-March 1984, when Dr. Gallo systematically rewrote the manuscript for what would become a renowned LTCB paper.' [275]

I now had in front of me what Popovic saw when he got back to the laboratory in Washington on Monday 26th March, only 5 days before this key paper had to be submitted to *Science*. It was fascinating to see that his 13 page typed manuscript had been absolutely covered in Gallo's scribbled comments, redrafted paragraphs and furious notes in the margins. There were also extra pages of Gallo's rough notes added at the end.

Gallo had changed the title of Popovic's paper. When published it would claim that they had 'isolated' the virus. But there was no mention of isolation in the title originally. I was intrigued. Isolation is said to be a key step in the study of any virus. I looked over the whole draft paper with care and found there were no experiments in it designed to isolate the virus for research purposes.

It was originally entitled:

### RESCUE AND CONTINUOUS PRODUCTION
### OF HUMAN T-CELL LYMPHOTROPIC RETROVIRUS (HTLV-III)
### FROM PATIENTS WITH AIDS

The new title read:

### Detection, Isolation, and Continuous Production of Cytopathic Retroviruses (HTLV-III) from Patients with AIDS and Pre-AIDS

But where was the justification for calling the virus 'cytopathic'! I knew that elsewhere Gallo claimed that it killed T-Cells, But extraordinarily, I could find no trace in this paper, as drafted or as published, of any evidence produced to prove this – despite this claim being made in its title.

But, wasn't this paper supposed to prove this virus to cause AIDS by killing T-Cells? That is what everyone has said of it since. As far as I could see, after the most careful of readings, the paper simply stated that proteins thought to be from a virus were found in serum samples from less than half of the AIDS patients tested. This was not just weak evidence. It established no causal relationship at all. Surely I must be missing something? I went back to reading the draft with great care.

---

[275] Popovic et al.; Science, 225, 1984, pp. 497-500.

On its first page, next to its abstract, Gallo had caustically scrawled; 'This abstract is rather trivial for a putative breakthrough paper in Science.' As I read it, I had to agree. It was indeed disappointingly 'trivial' for a paper held to document the discovery of HIV. The following is the original Popovic Abstract – with handwritten changes and comments by Gallo. (The full text of this paper with the Gallo hand written alterations is reproduced at the end of this book.)

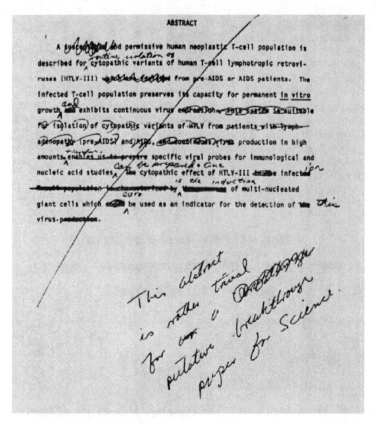

When published it would read:

Abstract. A cell system was developed for the reproducible detection of human T-lymphotropic retroviruses (HTLV family) from patients with the acquired immunodeficiency syndrome (AIDS) or with signs or symptoms that frequently precede AIDS (pre-AIDS). The cells are specific clones from a permissive human neoplastic T-cell line. Some of the clones permanently grow and continuously produce large amounts of virus after infection with cytopathic (HTLV-III) variants of these viruses. One cytopathic effect of HTLV-III in this system is the arrangement of multiple nuclei in a characteristic ring formation in giant cells of the infected T-cell population. These structures can be used as an indicator to detect HTLV-III in clinical specimens. This system opens the way to the routine detection of HTLV-III and related cytopathic variants of HTLV in patients with AIDS or pre-AIDS and in healthy carriers, and it provides large amounts of virus for detailed molecular and immunological analyses.

It mentioned that 'giant multi-nucleated cells' were produced in their cultures, and suggested that their appearance 'could be used as an indicator for the detection of the virus.' But, this suggested test was rapidly abandoned when it was soon realised that the giant cells were produced by the cancerous T-Cells selected for the cultures. They indicated the presence of a cancer, not a virus.

I shrugged aside my sceptical thoughts and started to read the body of the paper.

On its page three was the famous admission by Popovic that he had used the French virus LAV 'which is described here as HTLV-III'. Gallo deleted this and noted alongside: 'I just don't believe it. You are absolutely incredible.' It seems he must have previously instructed Popovic not to mention the French origin. The investigators commented later that these edits were 'highly instructive with respect to the nature and intent of Dr. Gallo's

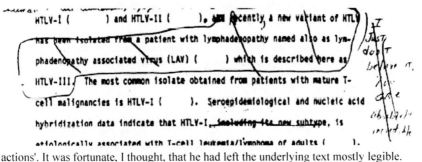

actions'. It was fortunate, I thought, that he had left the underlying text mostly legible.

From what I read, Popovic seems to have been entirely honest in reporting their renaming of the French virus, although he must have known this would make Gallo furious. This made me wonder if Popovic had wisely decided to make Gallo write the deceptive text himself. (Was this why Popovic went away to ski?) I hoped the rest of his original typed draft would be equally honest.

The rest of that page was simply a summary of Gallo's earlier work with the leukaemia-linked HTLV-I. It said: 'epidemiologic data strongly suggests AIDS is caused by an infectious agent' but presented no data to support this.

But when I turned the page, I was riveted. Gallo had deleted a statement by Popovic saying: 'Despite intensive research efforts, the causative agent of AIDS has not yet been identified.'

~~Despite intensive research efforts, the causative agent of AIDS has not yet been identified~~. Although patients with AIDS are often chronically infected with cytomegalovirus ( ), or hepatitis B virus ( ) we

This was totally unexpected. Nothing I read had led me to expect this. No one had mentioned these deleted words. Not Crewdson, not any of the investigators, no history of AIDS science. No one had reported these words, let alone their deletion by Gallo.

If Popovic had said 'prior to our research, the causative agent of AIDS had not been identified', I would not have been at all surprised. It would have been precisely what I expected. But – the sentence was unexpectedly in the present tense. Was he saying that their work with the disguised French virus had not yet succeeded? He had been brutally honest about admitting that he was using the French viruses. Was he being equally honest here?

Since then, I have repeatedly re-read the paper – and, much to my surprise, I find it contains no attempt at any point to prove that this virus causes AIDS! It is all about their efforts to grow a virus in a laboratory culture, not about research on this virus. Was Popovic admitting here that they had not yet managed to prove it causes AIDS? If so, then this would give an entirely new meaning to one of the most famous papers in virology. However, I decided that I would carefully read what else Popovic had to report before making up my mind.

Gallo clearly thought no one but Popovic would see his editing. When the paper was retyped and published a few weeks later it would be so completely changed that a government Research Integrity Adjudications Panel would report of it; 'The paper in question, it is undisputed, made a major and lasting contribution to establishing that a retrovirus was the etiological agent of AIDS.' [276]

I wondered with what Gallo had replaced these words 'despite intensive research efforts, the causative agent of AIDS has not yet been identified' in the final published document. I checked and found that they were replaced with words that said precisely the opposite. It now read 'that a retrovirus of the HTLV family might be an etiological agent of AIDS was suggested by the findings'.

I then found Popovic had upset Gallo still further in the very next sentence by calling Gallo's theory that a retrovirus caused AIDS an 'assumption'. Gallo deleted this word, replacing it with 'hypothesis', as can be seen in the clipping below, 'we

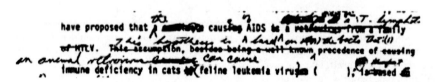

Popovic then summarized the tenuous basis of their 'assumption.' This went: as Myron Essex had found a retrovirus believed to cause in cats a T-cell leukaemia that suppresses the immune system, as Gallo had found in humans a retrovirus HTLV-I similarly said to cause a rare leukaemia, since 30 to 40% of AIDS patients had proteins in their blood similar to those from this retrovirus, and as the putative virus in their blood produced giant cancer cells ('syncytia') in the laboratory; it was assumed that the AIDS virus was a newly evolved, out-of-Africa, member of the same very small HTLV family of viruses!

But it was immediately clear that Popovic had no intention of testing and proving this theory in this paper. All he went on to report were his attempts to find a way to grow the disguised French virus in a laboratory dish.

Gallo and Popovic were well aware that their earlier efforts to prove their virus (HTLV-3) caused AIDS had ended in failure. That was why Popovic was now working with a disguised French virus. I continued to read the paper with care.

From Gallo's scribbled comments, I was surprised to learn that he clearly expected Popovic to achieve no more than to find a way of growing enough of the disguised French virus to enable them to patent a blood test for it. He never once asked for a test to be included showing it causes AIDS.

---

[276] Quoted in Crewdson, page 503. The appeal was heard by the Research Integrity Adjudications Panel

Thus in these papers there are no experiments to prove their virus killed T-cells. This was more important than one might think; given to this day no other human retrovirus is known to kill. If HIV were such an exception, if it has a unique capability, then one would expect to find here an effort to prove this.

Reading more widely, I have found scientists still do not understand how HIV can destroy T-Cells. Joseph McCune reported in *Nature* in 2001; 'We still do not know how, in vivo [in the patient], the virus destroys CD4+ T cells... Several hypotheses have been proposed to explain the loss of CD4+ T cells, some of which seem to be diametrically opposed.'[277]

But, at that time, the early 1980s, Gallo was on a rescue mission. He was trying to rescue his hypothesis that retroviruses were major causes of human diseases. He had failed to prove they were a major cause of cancer. He now wanted to prove they caused AIDS.

As I read on, I began to understand Popovic's difficulties. He explicitly stated they could not test their suspect virus or analyse its genetic code before they found a way to produce enough of it in a laboratory culture for them to experiment with it. In this paper he was thus totally concerned with achieving just this first step.

After failing to produce retroviruses in many cell cultures, Popovic had finally tested a culture that he had found abandoned in the laboratory fridge. He divided this to make a few cultures, and then tested each to see if any would grow the French virus. He was pleased to report that some of these showed signs of retroviral growth. This was the heart of his paper – his great achievement. Nothing more or less.

And how did he judge which culture was the most successful? A table in his report explained that he had worked this out by assessing 'the amount of released virus' through measuring ' RT activity in the culture.'

Now RT, meaning the enzyme Reverse Transcriptase, is naturally part of all our cells as well as of all retroviruses and of some other viruses. So, how did Popovic know the RT activity he measured was from a retrovirus? He never explained this. Yet on this depended the success of his modest experiment.

And it was not as if this 'RT activity' had appeared spontaneously. Popovic had only detected it after adding a substance to the cells that were known to provoke RT activity. (This he called the 'T-Cell Growth Factor' or TCGF). He presumed that if these provoked RT activity in the culture, then his virus must be present. He explained: 'the successful detection and isolation of HTLV was made possible by the discovery of TCGF.'

But Popovic after adding these chemicals; only detected 'transient' spikes of RT activity. This frustrated him immensely. He interpreted this as meaning his retrovirus had briefly appeared – and then vanished. He stated (before Gallo edited this): 'HTLV variants ... can only be detected transiently...'

I had to ask; what if these spikes of RT activity are part of defensive reactions by cells to this chemical? Why should they be solely linked to a particular retrovirus?

But – I then had another thought. What if the 'AIDS virus' was in fact a human retrovirus created by our cells to defend them against toxins? In recent times, evidence has been found for retroviruses sometimes being able to repair damaged DNA. (More about this in a later chapter.) Could the 'HIV' virus be in fact a particle sent out to repair damage caused by drug-based toxins – or damage caused by the diseases common in AIDS cases? This was but a thought, but Popovic had produced no evidence that proved any retrovirus to be doing damage.

Popovic wrote in his paper that, when he examined his cultures with an electron microscope, he saw particles that might be retroviruses. He had centrifuged culture

---

[277]    'The Dynamics of CD4+ T-cell Depletion in HIV Disease' by Joseph McCune in *Nature*, April 19, 2001

samples, and found RT activity in the band with the right density for retroviruses. So – retroviruses might be present – but which ones? In any case, this did not prove they caused AIDS.

He had also tested for the presence of antibodies that targeted proteins that might come from their putative AIDS virus – but without first proving this virus the cause of AIDS, the presence of such proteins could not be described as from an AIDS virus.

All cells, and all the retroviruses they make, possess the enzyme RT. Today any school child studying biology knows this. 'RT is certainly not unique to HIV,' the 17-year-old Loren Smith, the daughter of a friend, has just emphatically informed me. But was this well known at that time when Popovic did these experiments?

I put this question in August 2006 to the Emeritus Professor of Pathology at Toronto University, Etienne de Harven, one of the first to micrograph a retrovirus. He replied: 'In 1984 it was well known and published that reverse transcriptase (RT) is an ubiquitous enzyme, present in all living cells and therefore also in all cell debris.' The RT activity detected by Popovic was 'most likely the result of the presence of contaminating cell debris...and was not acceptable evidence for the presence of any retrovirus'. He has since told me that this was well known back in the 1970s.

Gallo and Popovic must have known that RT was in all retroviruses and cells. Some of their colleagues won a Nobel Prize in 1975 for discovering this. Barbara McClintock won a Nobel in 1983 for discovering a natural process in our cells that can cut and splice our DNA – and we now know that RT is involved in making RNA available for the same purpose .[278] So – why did they claim to have 'isolated' the AIDS virus by detecting RT?

If, as Popovic said, all the HTLV viruses from I to III were thus 'discovered', then, in my view, all the science about these Gallo-discovered 'viruses' is highly questionable.

The only other test documented by Popovic in this paper involved the use of rabbit antiserum, but he put little weight on this. He mentioned it only on a single line of his manuscript, where he said serum from AIDS patients was tested 'against hyperimmune rabbit serum raised against disrupted HTLV-III.' But I was excited to find this. It was the experiment I had searched for, the one that governmental investigators had credited as successful – and thus extremely important. It was the one the Staff Report of the Dingell Congressional Sub-Committee claimed to have proved the French virus the cause of AIDS. However, I was surprised by their confidence on this latter point, for they also noted that 'no primary data' were supplied to substantiate this use of the rabbit antiserum! [279]

Despite this, their report had concluded: 'In late-December 1983, MOV [one of their names for the cell-culture containing the French virus LAV] was used to inject a rabbit, with the objective of producing the first HIV-specific reagent. The experiment succeeded, and by late-February, the resulting hyperimmune rabbit antiserum was available for use to test LTCB samples for the presence of the suspected AIDS virus.'

If this was the vital experiment, the one that proved the virus to cause AIDS, then surely Popovic would have given this far more emphasis, much greater more prominence?

But on closer inspection, to my surprise I found this experiment was not designed to prove a virus causes AIDS. It was nothing more than an attempt to detect proteins thought to be the former parts of a virus. If these proteins were correctly identified, success with this test could prove no more than that the virus might have been present in these patients; not that it caused AIDS.

---

[278] Gallo thought RT a weapon used by an invading retrovirus to attack our DNA. Instead it has turned out that, although it might sometimes malfunction, RT is a vital natural enzyme that has shaped our DNA over hundreds of millions of years of evolution.

[279] The Congressional Inquiry also reported that: 'In September 1990, when he [Gallo] was asked to document LTCB [his] laboratory's isolates obtained prior to April 1984 that were tested against HIV-specific reagents, Dr Gallo listed only 9 samples that he said were tested against the rabbit antiserum; no primary data accompanied this response.'

Rabbit antiserum is often used in virology research and made by injecting a rabbit with fluid containing proteins said to be definitely from the virus in question. The rabbit will then produce antibodies against these proteins (and anything else in the fluid). A few days later blood serum that contains these antibodies is taken from the rabbit. This is the 'antiserum'. It is then used to test for the presence of the same proteins in other blood samples

But to what proteins did Popovic expose the rabbit? He said to proteins from 'disrupted HTLV,' meaning from the renamed French virus – but this virus was not yet proven to cause AIDS. Also, the word 'disrupted' in this context means the virus has been isolated and broken up, with its constituent proteins then separated out and studied to see if any are usefully unique to that virus – but nowhere had Popovic described such an experiment.

So – he could not justifiably claim to have made an antiserum to the virus that causes AIDS, or even that this antiserum identified its presence. The Investigators had previously condemned Gallo for claiming in 1982 and 1983 that he knew an antibody was specific to the AIDS virus before this virus was identified. Wasn't Popovic now making the same error?

We now know that finding an antiserum that identifies with surety the presence of a virus is difficult to accomplish. For one thing, since it is estimated less than 0.4% of all viruses have so far been identified, it is near impossible to absolutely prove any protein unique to a particular virus.

Also, proteins are tiny. Like antibodies they are just molecules. To isolate and identify these from the body of a virus is a very difficult and expensive experiment. It was very unlikely that Popovic would omit a description of such an experiment if he had attempted it.

I searched related scientific literature to see if Gallo or Popovic had described elsewhere such an experiment – and discovered that Gallo had indeed later described in *Nature* how this rabbit antiserum was made. He surprisingly said it was 'raised against p24' – a protein molecule with the molecular weight of 24,000 Daltons that he thought to come from the core of HIV. He presented no proof that it did. In fact, elsewhere in these same *Science* papers he said p24 also came from the leukaemia virus HTLV-1!

The full story seems to be that in late February 1984 Popovic injected a rabbit with a vial of fluid taken from a French LAV sample that had previously tested positive for p24 molecules. When these antibodies were found to varyingly reacted to blood serum from AIDS patients 'with a range of from 10% to over 80%', he inferred p24 was present in them and with it the French virus.

But we now know that p24 is in all human cells. It is involved in the making of the tiny transports, 'vesicles', in all cells.[280] Whenever a cell dies, its p24 molecules are released into the blood. As AIDS patients typically suffer from 'body wasting', they will have large numbers of such cellular fragments in their blood. Thus Popovic, and the French, could sometimes find much p24 in the blood serum from such patients – without any need for their virus to be present.

Gallo made the same erroneous assumptions as Popovic – as these same *Science* papers bear witness. He said that so much p24 (and p41) was in cultures made of cells from AIDS patients, that these proteins 'may therefore be considered viral structural proteins.' He summarized his quite incredible assumption thus:

---

[280] See chapters 19 and 20 below.

> HTLV-III (Fig. 2B). Extensive accumu-
> lation of p24 and p41 [see (20)] occurred
> in the virus preparation (Fig. 2B, panels I
> and II). Protein stains showed that these
> molecules are the major components of
> the virus preparation (19). P24 and p41
> may therefore be considered viral struc-
> tural proteins. Furthermore, an antigen

This was not the clear convincing experiment I was searching for that would prove that the French virus caused AIDS but the very reverse. I was totally amazed that the eminent government investigators would report this as successful – for they had been far more rigorous in assessing Gallo's tests for his own virus. I can only assume they were so focused on whether Gallo found an AIDS virus before the French, that, once they had proved he did not find it first, they simply assumed the AIDS virus must be the French.

The investigators' focus was very evident. All they had deemed worthy of note from the many deletions and changes in this Popovic draft was that: 'Dr. Gallo, chastising Dr. Popovic, extensively revised the paper, removing all references to Dr. Popovic's use of the IP [Institut Pasteur] virus and making it appear Dr. Popovic's seminal experiments had been performed with an authentic LTCB [Gallo's laboratory] isolate.'

I returned to the draft. I had now reached its concluding paragraphs. Popovic began his conclusion with these words: 'We report here the establishment and characterization of an immortalized T-Cell population which is susceptible to and permissive for HTLV cytopathic variants.'

To my great surprise, this from start to end was all of consequence that Popovic had to report in this 'key' paper – and he seemingly had got even this wrong by equating RT enzyme activity with the presence of their virus. After noting 'RT activity' in their cultures, he had felt he had no need to prove anything else before concluding: 'Thus, the data clearly indicate continuous HTLVIII production by permanently growing T-Cell population in a long term culture.'

But, the very last paragraph of his conclusion was even more revealing. (Please excuse its technical jargon. I will explain.)

*'The transient expression of cytopathic variants of HTLV in cells from AIDS patients and the lack of a proliferate cell system which would be susceptible and permissive for the virus represented major obstacle in detection, isolation and elucidation of the agent of this disease. The establishment of a T-Cell population, which, after virus infection, can continuously grow and produce the virus, provides the possibility for detailed biological, immunological and nucleic acid studies of this agent. '*

This is the sum total of his claims. Despite the enormous spin that Gallo later put on this paper; Popovic did not claim in it to prove any virus the cause of AIDS! He explained that all he had tried to do was to develop a culture of T-cells that would grow ('was permissive for') their suspect virus – as the lack of such a culture was 'a major obstacle' both to finding and studying such a virus. 'Transient expression' meant no more than that RT activity was intermittent in his culture. His last sentence states that finding such a culture provides 'the possibility' for the necessary research to be carried out.

That is it. These were the very last words of his paper - before Gallo rewrote them. They make it crystal clear that all that Popovic claimed to achieve was to have made the vital detailed tests a future 'possibility'. Without such future studies it would be impossible to identify a virus as causing AIDS, as Popovic well knew. This at last made sense of his earlier statement that the cause of AIDS remained to be discovered. It explained why Popovic's paper contained no experiments designed to prove a virus the cause of AIDS. It explained Gallo's urgent rewriting of the text. If he had not rewritten this paper and made it near impossible to verify, his gamble of announcing a major discovery before he had made it would have been revealed and, without any doubt, would have ended his career. But, before it was published Gallo would rewrite this conclusion, making subtle changes, adding the words 'previous', 'routine' and 'precise' to suggest all the obstacles listed by Popovic had been overcome. When published it would read (the text in bold being the more consequential of the changes and additions).

'The transient expression of cytopathic variants of HTLV in the cells from AIDS patients and the **previous** lack of a cell system that could maintain growth and still be susceptible and permissive for the virus represented a major obstacle in detection, isolation and elucidation of the **precise** causative agent of AIDS. The establishment of T-cell populations that continuously grow and produce virus after infection opens the way to the **routine detection of cytopathic variants of HTLV in AIDS patients** and provides the **first opportunity** for detailed biological immunological and molecular analyses of these viruses.'

The final paragraph – typing by Popovic, handwriting by Gallo:

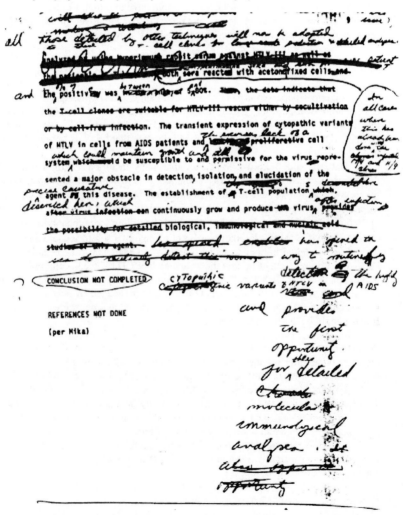

Thus, in the paper widely credited with proving HIV to cause AIDS, there is nothing of the sort. There is no mention of any experiment carried out to prove this, or even to establish that any virus present was in any way 'cytotoxic'.

If Gallo did fix and spin these papers, this might explain why, against all scientific norms, he afterwards refused samples of his culture and virus to scientists whom he suspected might want to verify his conclusions and imposed on others an outrageous agreement that they would not use them to attempt to repeat these experiments. It may also explain why Gallo documented their experiments so badly, according to the ORI ten years later, that it had proved impossible to repeat them, leaving scientists, and all of us, having to rely on trust that he got things right.

As for AIDS being spread by the sexual transmission of HIV, no evidence at all to support this was presented in the four *Science* papers. Yet, immediately after these papers appeared, the press described AIDS as caused by a sexually transmitted virus. Was this also the result of spin by Robert Gallo? I would have to search for the evidence. But first, I needed to look at the other documents unearthed by the governmental investigations to see if these might contain evidence that proved HIV dangerous.

### THE EVIDENCE THAT HIV KILLS T-CELLS

Popovic's paper calls HTLV-3 a 'cytopathic' retrovirus; that is, one that causes degeneration or disease in cells. But when I searched for evidence in his paper to support this, I could only find the observation that AIDS patients typically have low numbers of 'Helper' (DC4) T-Cells – with the implied inference that this was because the AIDS virus had killed them.

But it is widely known in science that many factors can diminish the numbers of these cells – such as chronic drug addiction, severe malnutrition and Chronic Fatigue Syndrome. Sometimes even healthy people have low numbers. As I have noted, in 2001 *Nature* reported that it still was not known how HIV could kill T-cells.[281] In 2006 a paper by Benigno Rodriquez reported that HIV can't be killing more than 4% to 6% of the CD4 cells lost in AIDS cases – in other words not enough by itself to cause AIDS. [282]

Popovic noted in his paper that there was a CD4-CD8 'reverse ratio', before Gallo deleted it. Popovic meant by this that when Helper CD4 T-Cells cells fall in number, the population of Killer CD8 T-cells goes up commensurately, and vice versa. We now know our immune system can change CD4s into CD8s as needed. It needs only a very small surface change to them. This too might explain why sometimes there are fewer CD4 cells. It may simply be that we need more CD8s.

In some frustration I have since searched for earlier papers in which Gallo or Popovic might have proved LAV, renamed as HTLV-3, able to kill or as cytopathic – but there are none, utterly none. The Institut Pasteur likewise seems not to have proved this. Neither had Popovic or Gallo proved their own virus, HTLV3, able to kill T-Cells.

All I could discover of any possible relevance is that, whenever Gallo tried to grow T-cell cultures before 1983, the T-cells died. Many factors could have caused this, such as the wrong nutrients, bacterial contamination, or mould - the latter found by the investigators to be contaminating some of his cultures.

Gallo did mention later that cells in the culture sometimes seemed to be enlarged and clumped – but that was a consequence of them being 'immortalised' by being made cancerous, not of them dying.

---

[281] 'The Dynamics of CD4+ T-cell Depletion in HIV Disease' by Joseph McCune in *Nature*, April 19, 2001

[282] Benigno Rodriguez et al., published 27th September 2006 in the *Journal of the American Medical Association*

So, did the *Science* papers contain any firm evidence for HIV killing blood cells? I had to conclude, after a thorough search, that no evidence at all of this was presented in these papers, despite Gallo adding the word 'cytopathic' to this Popovic paper's title. But, this omission is surely something anyone can confirm – so why are so few asking these vital questions?

## 'HIV IS NOT IN GALLO'S PICTURES OF HIV.'

A letter I found preserved in the inquiry records contained further disturbing evidence. It was from Dr. Matthew Gonda, the Head of the Electron Microscopy Laboratory at the National Cancer Institute, replying to a letter from Gallo of March 1984 that had asked him to prepare for publication EM micrographs of the 'enclosed samples' that 'contain HTLV' [HIV].

Gonda's reply is dated March 26th, just four days before these images were needed for publication. Gonda told him: **'I would like to point out that the 'particles' ... are in debris of a degenerated cell' and 'at least 50 per cent smaller' than they should be if they were retroviruses.** He concluded: **'I do not believe any of the particles photographed are HTLV I, II or III.'** He devastatingly added that: **'No other extracellular 'virus-like' particles were observed.'** [283] Gonda copied this letter to Popovic.

Discovering this was an enormous surprise because the *Science* articles, as sent for publication four days later, there was included in the second paper for which Gallo is the lead author, four micrographs 'of HTLV-III' credited to Gonda. In the accompanying text, Gallo declared all these particles to be of the right shape and correct size for HTLV-III - although close examination reveals most are of different shapes and sizes. (See the images below – HTLV-III is said to be the roundish dots bordering the vastly bigger cell.)

There were also images of HTLV in the third of the *Science* papers for which Gonda was named a co-author. Gallo would latter claim in *Science* that some of these images were 'inadvertently' photos of the French virus provided by the Institut Pasteur[284] but this seems also to have been part of his cover-up.

If these are the same images as referred to in Gonda's letter – then, for Gallo to initially say these are definitely of HTLV-III and later to say they were of LAV is highly puzzling since he had received Gonda's expert advice to the contrary.

Gallo was most misleading when interviewed by the New York Times for an article that appeared on 12th March 1986. In this Gallo said one of the four images published looked like LAV because 'Mathew A. Gonda had been ill and a technician pulled the wrong photograph from the file.' But Gonda did not say he was ill in this letter.

Gonda told Crewdson he had selected the images himself. But Gonda's letter of the 26th March says far more. It says he had looked at the images and found no suspect AIDS virus. Crewdson had this important letter – but, as far as I can see, he mysteriously does not refer to it in his account of what happened prior to the papers going to the *Science* journal. He also had the Popovic draft paper at the time he wrote his book *Science Fictions* about these events, but at no point does he mention the deletions from the Popovic paper that hid their failure to prove the French virus the cause of AIDS. As far as I can discover, no one that saw these papers, whether in the governmental investigations or the press, made any mention of these deletions, despite many of them citing the deletions in the same paper that hid Gallo's use of the French virus.

---

[283] Letter from Matthew Gonda, Head Electron Microscopy Laboratory; to Mika Papovic (stet), 26th March 1984

[284] Crewdson op cit. page 347

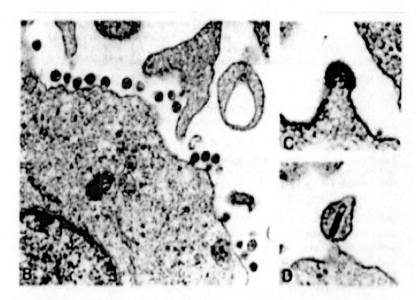

**Electron Microscope images of 'HTLV-III' as published with the *Science* articles of May 4th 1984 and attributed to Gonda. The large object on the left of the larger micrograph is part of a blood cell. The dots around it are surmised to be HTLV-III. The two smaller micrographs are said to be of the virus 'budding' out of the cell – something all retroviruses do as well as other viruses such as measles,**

The Congressional Inquiry's Staff Report spoke of an earlier incident: 'As evidence for his claim, Dr. Gallo produced an EM (Electron Microscope image) of a sample labelled 'Betsy's cells'. Dr. Gallo said this sample was sent to Dr. Gonda on March 13, 1984; according to Gallo, the sample was EM+ for HIV. But no written report was ever produced showing that Dr. Gonda had found Betsy's cells to be EM+, and Elizabeth Read-Connole told OSI that neither she nor Dr. Popovic had ever seen such a report.' I do not know if the above images are of Betsy's cells. The letter I cite from Gonda seems to have also escaped the attention of the authors of the Staff Report.

It should be noted that Gallo's micrographs of his putative 'AIDS virus' show particles quite unlike the images the Pasteur Institute produced of 'LAV'. Gallo's seem to have rod-like cores while those published by the French in 1983 show LAV to have semi-circular cores.[285] (See below) Gonda of course had gone further. He said the particles looked like cellular rubbish.

Please also note the large particles below are of 'cord' lymphocytes – thus cells from a newborn baby. Montagnier claimed to have infected these cells with retroviruses produced by the cells of an adult patient with 'pre-AIDS.' But cord tissues naturally produce harmless retroviruses. He had no way of telling one retrovirus from another. Also this 'pre-AIDS' condition had little relationship to AIDS. It was in fact said to be 'Cervical Lymphadenopathy,' in other words, ''swollen lymph glands', a condition that occurs naturally when the body is defending itself against pathogens – at a time when our cells might be making many defensive endogenous retroviruses.

---

[285] Isolation of a T-lymphotropic retrovirus from a patient at risk for acquired immune deficiency syndrome (AIDS). Barré-Sinoussi F, Chermann JC, Rey F, Nugeyre MT, Chamaret S, Gruest J, Dauguet C, Axler-Blin C, Vézinet-Brun F, Rouzioux C, Rozenbaum W, Montagnier. Science. 1983 May 20;220(4599):868-71.

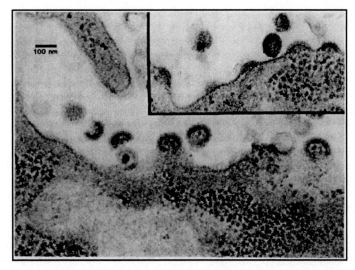

**Image produced by the Institut Pasteur. Original Caption:** "Electron microscopy of thin sections of virus-producing cord lymphocytes. The inset shows various stages of particle budding at the cell surface."

### 'HIV IS NOT IN YOUR CULTURES'

In the records I also discovered a report from Dr. Tom White of Roche. He had been asked by the OSI to do a PCR check on the cultures in which Gallo and Popovic claimed to have grown HTLV-III in the hope that this check would show if the French LAV had been substituted for HTLV-III (or HTLV-IIIb as the virus was also named). For the purposes of comparison, the OSI provided him with samples of LAV from the Institut Pasteur.

But what he reported was: **'None of the ten pool [culture] samples contained a virus that looked remotely like HTLV-3B or LAV'.**[286] In his opinion, this meant that it was 'essentially impossible' for either virus to have come out of these cultures.[287]

Popovic had reported these same cultures showed RT activity when he dosed them with his growth factor substance. White's report was surely conclusive evidence, if any were needed, that Popovic's LAV did not produce this RT activity.

Among the laboratory correspondence I found a letter from Gallo to a scientist who had written to say he could not confirm Gallo's claims, since he could not find HTLV-III (HIV) in AIDS patients. The reply was dated the 29th March 1984, just one day before the *Science* papers were sent for publication. In this Gallo confirmed; **'It is extremely rare to find fresh cells expressing the virus'.** He went on to say it was far easier to find the virus in the laboratory 'probably due to removal of inhibiting factors present in the patient.'[288] (See appendix for a copy of the letter)

---

[286] The ten viral cultures examined are detailed on pages 602-603 of John Crewdson's 2002 book *Science Fictions* Also see his page 413. Crewdson however is not entirely consistent. After quoting the OSI expert as saying that none contained HTLV-1B or LAV, he says some lines further down that 4 out of the 10 cultures contained 'no AIDS virus.' This later observation seems to be based on other tests, which looked for RT, not the virus.

[287] John Crewdson Science Fictions page 413.

[288] Gallo to Jun Minowada, 29th March 1984

Gallo has since admitted, at a 1994 meeting sponsored by the US National Institute of Drug Abuse; **'We have never found HIV DNA in T-cells'**.[289] This was a most extraordinary admission. It meant his team had not provably found a single HIV-infected T-cell. All retroviruses integrate their genetic codes as DNA into their hosts. If HIV genetic codes are not in T-Cells – HIV has not infected them.

The implications of what I was discovering by now seemed colossal to me. I was horrified by what I had learnt. On the foundation of this research has been erected the entire HIV/AIDS research edifice. Today it is almost universally held that the French HIV (LAV) was proven in these papers to be the one and only cause of AIDS.

As for the other three *Science* papers, Gallo took the lead credit for the second. It focused on his claim to have 'isolated' his virus in 48 AIDS victims in 1982 - which the investigators proved scientifically impossible and which he later confessed was erroneous. The third of the papers referred to his claim to have identified HIV antigens in 1983 in experiments also dismissed as utterly incompetent by the investigators, and the fourth included claims about antibodies against HIV on which the HIV Tests would be based – despite it being impossible to identify such antibodies if the cause of AIDS had not yet been identified, as Popovic had said.

The vital papers to my dismay had turned out to be an absolute quagmire of, dare I say it, illogical science.

I feel these errors are evidence that Gallo had decided in advance to go for broke. He had failed with his own virus. He strongly suspected that the French would beat him to the post. He felt there remained only one chance for success. He would presume the French had found the AIDS virus - and beat them by patenting a test for their virus renamed as his own! He believed they would never discover what he had done. With any luck, he would also win a Nobel Prize.

Most extraordinarily, the evidence strongly suggests that he never attempted to prove the French virus caused AIDS before going for his patent. (See also the chapter on the HIV test.)

But Gallo did not get away with everything.  On January 8th, 1993, *Science* headlined the news that the Federal Department of Health (HHS) had found Gallo guilty of trying to scientifically mislead. The headline read:

---

# HHS: Gallo Guilty of Misconduct

The verdict is that by concealing the fact that his lab put the French virus into a permanent cell line, Robert Gallo intended to mislead the scientific community

---

But, Gallo, as far as I can judge, got away with a far greater act of deception, perhaps the greatest scientific fraud of the 20th century, affecting the lives of countless millions. On the basis of his claims, all other theories about the causes of AIDS lost their funding as he boasted.[290] Even worse, so did promising ways of medically treating AIDS cases. The doctors using anti-toxins with some success were abandoned. It became practically heretical to question if HIV causes AIDS. The 1990-1995 investigations were effectively buried – as were all the papers they unearthed.

Much the same fate has met scientists who disagreed with Gallo's claims, saying that the evidence strongly suggested that AIDS had other causes. Yet, some of them have

---

[289]   Lauritsen JL (1995). NIDA meeting calls for research into the poppers-Kaposi's sarcoma connection. In: Duesberg PH, eds. AIDS: Virus- or Drug Induced. London: Kluwer Academic Publishers, pp. 325-330.

[290]   As Gallo acknowledged with pride; 'In a 2007 Court Hearing, the Parenzee Trial, he spoke of how funding to research other theories was cut off immediately. See chapter below entitled; 'Gallo fights back.'

maintained their position since 1984, with their apparent obstinacy and lack of conformity denying them much research funding.

Among these 'dissidents' are major scientists, including a Nobel Laureate and eminent professors at Ivy League Universities. They have among their number the first to describe the genetic code of retroviruses and the first to micrograph such a virus. They all have maintained, at grave risk to their careers, that Gallo's research findings cannot be confirmed and that HIV cannot cause AIDS. Their work has nonetheless attracted scant coverage in the media – so their names and positions are listed at the end of this book.

Yet, it is apparent from their papers that they came to their costly 'dissident' conclusions while not knowing of Popovic's real conclusion, and not knowing just how extensive was Gallo's last-minute rewriting of this key research, so effective has been the cover-up.

As for the far greater numbers of scientists who would not think to question the HIV theory, I have found none who have attempted to repeat what they believe Gallo did earlier. New frontiers evidently beckon them – such as being the first to develop a vaccine or a new antiretroviral drug. Today most HIV specialists focus on tiny 'HIV' genetic code fragments, in the confident belief that these were proven to come from HIV in earlier experiments.

But my own investigation could not end here. Gallo and Popovic may have got it wrong – but I had to consider if other scientists might have proved their thesis right later? I had to look at more modern research if I were to come to any kind of useful conclusion.

# Chapter 13

# Is HIV linked to sex?

As Gallo briefed the media in the days following the April 1984 press conference, a panic began among the public. Most heterosexuals had not dreamt the 'gay' epidemic could affect them, but now they learnt it was among them all, straights and gays alike.

Yet, as I have mentioned, none of Gallo's four Science papers had attempted to prove AIDS sexually transmitted, or explicitly that it would infect heterosexuals. They had not even tried to address these issues.[291] So why then this panic?

Gallo had earlier speculated that a cancer virus he had discovered, HTLV-I, was spread through sex. This was never verified, and indeed is today severely questioned, but he now surmised that HTLV-III was likewise spread as he thought it part of the same viral family. But his guesses were readily accepted for quite another reason – because of the observed promiscuity among partying gays who first fell ill with AIDS.

From the 1960s, Gay Liberation had expressed itself through sexual revolution. It was thus to be expected that the moral establishment would say that sex had made Gays ill. Nor was it too surprising that the heterosexual sexual freedom of the Flower Power generation was the very next target for suspicion. I, for one, was affected by this. I thought it a cruel fate that HIV had come along to rob me of my freedom.

But, when I looked at the figures, I had to ask: why in the first years of the epidemic did AIDS affect vastly more homosexuals than heterosexuals – and why so very few women? They were less than 5% of the reported victims. There seemed no explanation. It is a doctrine in virology that all viral infections will strike gays and heterosexuals, young adults and old, men and women alike. So they confidently predicted, as HIV is a virus it must be an 'equal opportunity infector.' Wait a year or so. It has started among the most promiscuous– it will get to the rest soon.

The first case of AIDS put down to heterosexual transmission was recorded a few months before the May 1984 papers were issued – in other words some years after the disease first appeared. The person affected denied he was gay – and thus heterosexual sex was entered on the record. It soon became routine to presume that Afro-American cases likewise were heterosexual, on the basis, it seems, of social stereotypes.

The root cause of AIDS was initially surmised to be 'promiscuity' for another reason too. The virus was so difficult to find intact in its suspected victims that it was guessed that it must be delicate. Thus the virus was surmised to be too fragile to be spread except by intimate contact. It was also said to fall to pieces if touched or washed with water.

As far as I can judge from the medical literature of that time, the sexual transmission of AIDS was simply promulgated by press releases and media interviews as self-evident – 'just look at the promiscuity of the people most affected – look at the partying gay scene.' It was not long after this that it was also predicted that Africans would be terribly devastated by AIDS because of their 'well-known' promiscuity. Dr. Robin Weiss, a leading UK virologist and colleague of Robert Gallo, declared: "Promiscuity is the common factor between U.S. homosexuals and Central African

---

[291] Padian's paper of 1997 in the *American Journal of Epidemiology*[291] that showed that, in a 10 year follow-up prospective study of heterosexual couples of whom only one partner of either sex was positive, 'no seroconversions occurred among exposed partners', suggesting no transmission of HIV via the vaginal route.

heterosexuals. Many of the young men in some African cities seem to have as many female partners as some (male) homosexuals in New York and San Francisco have male partners.' [292]

Weiss also confidently predicted that Africans would be suffering an AIDS epidemic more severe than the USA's – despite at that time 'more than 15 African countries having not reported a single case of AIDS.' [293] Africa simply had to have AIDS argued Gallo – as he had declared his HTLV-I was from there so HTLV-III must be too. His case against the French finding the virus first was based on there being a relationship between his HTLV-I and HTLV-III.

That same year, 1985, the CDC astonished and horrified America by estimating that over 1.5 million American heterosexuals 'must' be already infected. It was predicted terrifyingly that they would die within two years. In 1987 the CDC increased this to 1.8 million. The *Journal of the American Medical Association* calculated: 'With a mortality rate that, two years from diagnosis, exceeds 80%, this illness now ranks as one of the most serious epidemics confronting man in modern times.' [294]

From newspaper reports, few private physicians in Chicago would administer the Gallo-invented AIDS blood test, as they had utterly no remedy for those found positive. 'I don't want to be the first doctor to have his patient jump off the Sears Tower when he gets his results,' Dr. David Coynik told the *Chicago Tribune*, adding he discouraged patients from taking the test. There were also doubts about its accuracy. When a large number of blood donations were retested after having tested positive, they were found to be negative, which did not say much for the accuracy of the test. [295]

Nevertheless Dr. Merle Sande, the head of a Californian AIDS research task force, confidently stated: 'We are clearly in the midst of a major medical catastrophe ... the eventual magnitude ... could be absolutely enormous.' [296] In 1987 Oprah Winfrey predicted; 'By 1990, one in five heterosexuals will be dead from AIDS.' [297] It was as if she had announced the Apocalypse. These reports also brought fear of death into love making, linking it to deep phobias.

But then it turned out that the US Government's Centers for Disease Control (CDC) had based its frightful predictions solely on extrapolations from the proportion of gay men falling ill at the 1981 peak of the San Francisco epidemic. It had applied this percentage to the entire American population – without any clinical evidence of illness in the rest of the population.

They also predicted that women were far more likely than men to get AIDS, as vaginas could hold infected spermal fluid for longer. [298] This was despite clinical reports that far fewer American women were getting AIDS.

Many members of the gay community had greeted with enormous relief the declaration that a virus caused AIDS. Toxicologists had earlier told them that their lifestyle caused their illnesses, but the discovery of this virus now surely had lifted the blame from their drug taking and partying lifestyle?

It soon became politically correct to grimly warn 'AIDS will affect all' – no matter that it was still practically confined to the gay community. After all, if it were caused by a virus and transmitted by sex, it must affect women and straight men equally. Before I

---

292 Chicago Tribune (CT) - Sunday, December 22, 1985, Page: 11

293 Chicago Tribune December 22, 1985.

294 Chicago Tribune January 27, 1985 This statement was by Dr Thomas C. Quinn .

295 Chicago Tribune December 15, 1985.

296 Chicago Tribune January 27, 1985.

297 *The Myth of Heterosexual AIDS*, 1990.

298 CDC Contraception Technol Update. 1985 Dec;6(12):161-3. PMID: 12280299. This particularly quoted Mary E. Guinan, Assoc. director of the CDC's Sexually Transmitted Diseases division.

looked into its history, I had long believed the same. I presumed HIV to be relatively easy to pass on sexually. My private life was governed by this supposition.

But when I now sought confirming scientific evidence, I discovered to my surprise that in 1986 Gallo reported: 'Data from this and previous studies have shown that receptive rectal intercourse, for example, is an important risk factor for HTLV-III [HIV] infection. We found no evidence that other forms of sexual activity contributed to the risk.'[299] This shocked me. I had thought the evidence was otherwise. Surely if a virus were responsible, it would infect both partners equally?

I then found that in 1987 the major 'Multicenter AIDS Cohort Study' had similarly reported 'in gay men the only significant sexual act related to becoming HIV antibody positive and progressing to AIDS is receptive anal intercourse.'[300] This on-going massive study was founded on the presumption that HIV to be spread only by sex.[301]

Spermal fluid is itself immune-suppressant. It contains chemicals that protect the sperm from a woman's natural defensive system. Could the above findings be explained by spermal fluid weakening the immune system of a receptive partner by getting into their blood through skin tears during anal sex?[302] I was not sure.

But still no scientific evidence emerged that supported the idea that heterosexuals were equally in danger. This led in late 1987 to the Reagan Administration asking the CDC; 'How did you know that 1.8 million Americans are HIV infected?' the official who compiled AIDS case reports, E. Thomas Starcher, replied to their astonishment; 'It's just a guess.' Another CDC researcher reported: 'I was at the meeting; we were a subcommittee, and supposed to make these predictions. It was really just off the tops of our heads... The main problem we had is that there are no good data. The data do not exist.'[303]

The Education Secretary, Bill Bennett, in some surprise then asked James Mason, the director of the CDC, 'You mean this thing is not exploding into the heterosexual community?' Mason replied, 'No, it's not.' Bennett angrily responded: 'Well, why have you been telling everybody that it is?' The Chicago Times thus reported on November 15. 1987: 'Among heterosexuals, the AIDS epidemic has never really begun.'

Wiley at Berkeley also reported: 'The chances of acquiring the AIDS infection are much less than for syphilis or gonorrhoea, even herpes; less than almost any other venereal disease you can name, on the order of 1 to 1,000 contacts' A chart was produced showing in 1987 there was a 91.7% correlation between homosexuals using recreational drugs and getting AIDS – but only a 4.3% correlation with heterosexual sex.[304]

However, the CDC, backed by lurid headlines in the media, continued to warn that most of those infected would come to a terrible death, not right away but in five to ten years. The panic spread. Gays were blamed for infecting heterosexuals, evicted from their apartments and even refused medical help.

Nearly a decade later, in 1996, *The Wall Street Journal* would find the focus of the Federal AIDS education campaign was still on warning heterosexuals, rather than homosexuals, about their risk for AIDS. It also discovered that there was no scientific justification for this, since homosexuals remained at far greater risk. It reported that the CDC, in consultation with the advertising agency Ogilvy and Mather, had decided to stress the danger to heterosexuals to make it easier for politicians to fund the war on AIDS

---

[299] Stevens CE, Taylor PE, Zang EA, et al. Human T-cell lymphotropic virus type III infection in a cohort of homosexual men in New York City. JAMA 1986;255:2167-2172

[300] Kingsley et al., 1987.

[301] http://www.statepi.jhsph.edu/macs/dossier/MACS Also see report in the Chicago Times of June 1 1987.

[302] Research by the Perth Group and others has indicated that spermal fluid can itself be toxic if it gets into the blood – as it might do on the less well-protected anal route. www.perthgroup.com

[303] Chicago Tribune (CT) - Sunday May 31, 1987

[304] Chicago Tribune (CT) - Sunday November 15, 1987

and to protect gays from discrimination. A high-up 'source' told *The Wall Street Journal*; If most people in the U.S. feel they are at very low risk, there will be little support for AIDS-prevention effort.' 'There is a real concern that funding … will be cut.' [305]

The resulting investigative article was entitled '*AIDS fight is skewed by federal campaign exaggerating risk*s.' It commenced: 'In the summer of 1987, federal health officials made the fateful decision to bombard the public with a terrifying message: 'Anyone could get AIDS'.' But; 'While the message was technically true, it was also highly misleading. Everyone certainly faced some danger, but for most heterosexuals, the risk from a single act of sex was smaller than the risk of ever getting hit by lightning.'

Behind this terrible fiasco with the most horrific of consequences, lay a fundamental scientific dilemma. The reality was that in the West it was still mostly men, and gay men at that, who were going down with AIDS. This was not reconcilable with a 'virus-only' theory of AIDS causation. Many scientists knew this – but they feared to seem to question this theory. It had apparently become almost a religious doctrine.

So, despite the lack of evidence, legal measures were promoted to prevent heterosexual infection. Illinois made an AIDS test mandatory before marriage. Colorado debated making the transmission of HIV punishable with 4 years in prison. West Virginia considered making it first-degree murder. [306] Today, around the world, in many countries and states, it is a grave criminal offence to have sex after being found HIV positive without warning the partner.

But at that time, the panic created was fought by other voices that started to appeal for some sanity, pointing out that AIDS was already declining among gay men and that accidental falls in the home killed more people than did AIDS in the USA.[307]

Meanwhile the CDC struggled to get a grip on other difficulties facing the 'HIV virus' theory. As Gallo had noted, it was extremely difficult to find HIV in AIDS victims – but this was explained now by saying it mutated fast – so fast that it was hard to identify. No routine methods against viruses seemed to work against it. No anti-virus measure cured it. It was like attacking an invisible enemy.

But – what about heterosexual transmission of HIV? Surely this was later proved beyond a shadow of a doubt? I then discovered that the largest controlled scientific study ever carried out on the risk of HIV infection through heterosexual sex was by Dr. Nancy Padian in 1997. It was well designed. She identified 175 heterosexual couples with one partner HIV-positive. She then monitored them for up to 6 years to see how long it would take for the HIV infection to spread from one partner to the other.

The couples, as one would expect, were initially counselled on their need to take precautions – but were then left to make their own decisions. Afterwards it was discovered that one quarter of the couples did not consistently use condoms.

But the results of this study were totally unexpected – and apparently embarrassing for the scientists involved. They reported: 'no seroconversions occurred among exposed partners,' In other words, not one case of HIV transmission! The following is scanned from Padian's paper.

---

[305] Amanda Bennett and Anita Sharpe, *AIDS fight is skewed by Federal bodies exaggerating risks*, Wall St. Journal, 1st May 1996

[306] Chicago Tribune (CT) - May 31, 1987

[307] Papadopulos-Eleopulos, E., 1988, *Reappraisal of AIDS: is the oxidation induced by the risk factors the primary cause?* Med. Hypo 25:151

> We followed 175 HIV-discordant couples over time, for a total of approximately 282 couple-years of follow-up (table 3). Because of deaths as well as the break-up of couples, attrition was severe; only 175 couples are represented in table 3. The longest duration of follow-up was 12 visits (6 years). We observed no seroconversions after entry into the study. Table 3
> summarizes behavior change over time, comparing

('Seroconversions' here means a person becoming HIV positive. 'HIV-discordant' means one partner only was HIV positive at the start of the study.)

This study remains of high repute. As far as I know, no one has questioned its methodology. The authors noted in its conclusion: 'Neither condom use, total number of sexual partners since 1976, nor lifetime number of sexually transmitted diseases was associated with infection'." [308]

The lead author, Professor Nancy Padian, still plays a major role in AIDS research. In 2007 she is a member of the prestigious Institute of Medicine. [309] In 1991 she cast doubts also on the accuracy of earlier studies that tried to measure the risk of infection from heterosexual acts. She reported that these 'studies may not have adequately controlled for other confounding nonsexual routes of transmission such as risks associated with intravenous drug use. At first blush, cases that appear attributed to heterosexual transmission may, after in-depth interviewing, actually be linked to other sources of risk ... Furthermore, it is often difficult to establish the source of infection in such couples.' [310]

But, I am most surprised to find that Professor Padian has recently attempted to backtrack from her findings without withdrawing the paper in which they are found. She stated, on a website set up in 2006 to defend the HIV theory of AIDS: 'Individuals who cite the 1997 Padian et al. publication or data from other studies by our research group in an attempt to substantiate the myth that HIV is not transmitted sexually are ill informed, at best. Their misuse of these results is misleading, irresponsible, and potentially injurious to the public.'[311]

She then explained how she has been so seriously misinterpreted: 'A common practice is to quote out of context a sentence from the Abstract of the 1997 paper: "Infectivity for HIV through heterosexual transmission is low".' But misleadingly she had failed to quote her words immediately preceding these. They were that they observed 'no new infections' by HIV in the years in which they were monitoring heterosexuals That is not 'low transmission' but zero. I am citing the main body of her paper, not its abstract.

Padian also claimed that people have failed to understand her research correctly by not noting 'couples were strongly counselled to use condoms and practice safe sex.' She concludes: 'That we witnessed no HIV transmissions after the intervention documents the success of the interventions in preventing the sexual transmission.' [312] However, she distorts her own research. Her paper had reported that a quarter of the couples studied did not use condoms consistently. The following is also scanned from her original paper:

---

[308] Padian NS, Shiboski SC, Glass SO, Vittinghoff E. Heterosexual transmission of human immunodeficiency virus (HIV) in northern California: results from a ten-year study. Am. J. Epidemiol. 1997;146:350-7

[309] Nancy Padian is a Professor of Obstetrics, Gynecology and Reproductive Sciences at the University of California and she has worked on the heterosexual transmission of HIV since 1984. She is a frequent participant in annual NIH Office of AIDS Research planning workshops and has chaired the workshop on international research for the last four years. She is an elected member to the Institute of Medicine

[310] Padian NS, Padian NS, Shiboski SC, Jewell NP. Female-to-male transmission of human immunodeficiency virus. JAMA 1991;266:1664-7.

[311] http://www.aidstruth.org/nancy-padian.php

[312] http://www.aidstruth.org/nancy-padian.php

> the first follow-up visit. At last follow-up, couples were much more likely to be abstinent or to use condoms consistently, and were much less likely to practice anal intercourse ($p < 0.0005$ for all). Nevertheless, only 75 percent reported consistent condom use in the 6 months prior to their final follow-up visit. Forty-seven couples who remained in follow-up for 3 months to 6 years used condoms intermittently, and no seroconversions occurred among exposed partners.

She also stated in that paper:

> To our knowledge, our study is the largest and longest study of the heterosexual transmission of HIV in the United States. The consistency of results over the 10-year duration argues for the validity of our results. For example, the practice of anal sex and lack

I believe that her recent attempt to deny her own research conclusions is clear evidence of the pressure scientists are now under to protect their careers by conforming to beliefs promulgated by the AIDS establishment.

In her original paper, despite not observing any such cases, she presumes that the couples she had excluded from her study as inappropriate because both were already HIV positive at the start of her project, must have previously infected each other through sex.

Having made this assumption without having any proof of it, she then produced from this an 'estimated' risk of HIV infection 'through male to female contact' of '0.0009', with the female to male risk factor being 'eight times' less than male to female - in other words, an HIV positive heterosexual man would pass on HIV once in a thousand acts of unprotected intercourse, and an HIV-positive women would infect a man once in 8,000 unprotected acts! (It is a surprising, but exactly the same figure of 0.0009% was reported to be the Ugandan male to female risk factor for HIV infection, in a study by other authors published in *Lancet* in 2001.)

It scarcely needs to be said, but these risk levels are so low that they are scarcely detectable, are totally insufficient to maintain an epidemic – and utterly unprovable. And as I noted, she actually observed no cases of transmission at all.

This makes it very hard for me to accept as accurate the World Health Organization 1992 estimate that 30% of all pregnant women in Uganda were HIV infected through sex. These women would have had to be incredibly sexually active to achieve this. [313]

There is other evidence supporting near zero transmission through heterosexual sex. The *Journal of Infectious Diseases* reported; 'The probability of transmission of HIV-1 from male to female during an episode of intercourse has been examined in seven studies. Analysis of data from North American and European studies of heterosexual couples provide estimates of per-sex-act HIV-1 transmission of approximately 1 in 1000 (0.001, ranging from 0.0008 to 0.002).' [314] Again, these figures are based solely on 'estimates.'

---

[313] Kamali A, Quigley M, Nakiyingi J, et al. Syndromic management of sexually-transmitted infections and behaviour change interventions on transmission of HIV-1 in rural Uganda: a community randomised trial. *Lancet* 2003;361:645-52.
Gray RH, Wawer MJ, Brookmeyer R, et al. Probability of HIV-1 transmission per coital act in monogamous heterosexual, HIV-1 discordant couples in Rakai, Uganda. *Lancet* 2001;357:1149-1153.
[314] J Infect Dis 1990,161:833-877

Peterman found 'eleven wives remained uninfected after more than 200 sexual contacts with their infected spouse.' [315]   Also, in one of the largest ever studies on 'HIV positive' haemophiliacs and their wives', no wives became 'HIV positive' during the study. This was despite each couple having vaginal intercourse a large number of times. The authors 'calculated that in 11 couples unprotected vaginal intercourse occurred a maximum of 2,250 times (minimum 1,563) without transmission of HIV.' [316]

Then, in the largest of all European studies, spanning six countries, it was concluded 'the only sexual practice that clearly increased the risk of male-to-female transmission was anal intercourse...[and that] no other sexual practice has been associated with the risk of transmission'. [317]

All this is highly surprising, for the heterosexual transmission of AIDS in Africa is now the gospel accepted by nearly all media and health workers – apparently totally on the basis of not reading the relevant science papers, and trusting in a very uncritical medical establishment and the sexual stereotyping of Africans.

The official 2003 *Annual Report on HIV/AIDS in San Francisco*, the supposed centre of the American AIDS epidemic, reported that from 1999 to 2003 there was no increase in HIV infection in San Francisco – despite there being at the same time an enormous increase among homosexuals in such STD infections as rectal gonorrhoea and syphilis.

This report went on to say: 'HIV remains relatively rare among heterosexuals, blood transfusion recipients and children.' It gave figures. Out of all the US AIDS cases since the start of the epidemic, 95% were male in San Francisco, 92% male in California and 82% male in the US. Most of the victims in San Francisco were also white (72%) – with only 12% being African-Americans. Some 76% of all HIV infections were in males having sex with males. Critically, only 4% of AIDS victims in San Francisco were female and only 1% of all AIDS victims were thought infected through heterosexual sex.

As for male haemophiliacs, while they frequently have immune system problems, their wives remained HIV uninfected 'despite a high prevalence of asymptomatic clinical and immunologic abnormalities in the haemophiliacs, we found their wives, on average, to be normal with respect to T-cell subsets and other surrogate laboratory markers.' [318]

Similar figures are reported for the UK. According to government statistics, only 64 women born in the UK were found newly HIV infected in 2004. This contrasted to several thousand men. In 2007, after having made HIV testing a routine part of antenatal care, the UK's Health Agency reported that, of the 178,493 UK-born women tested in 2005, only 75 were found HIV positive – a fall to nearly half of the low incidence reported one year earlier (0.04% as against 0.07% of those tested in 2004).   The same report stated: 'The 2356 new diagnoses of HIV infection among men who have sex with men reported in 2005 was the highest ever.'  Similar statistics have now been produced for twenty years – and yet women are still being warned in the press that they are equally at risk.

The main players are simply ignoring the inconvenient official statistics.   Dr. Robert Gallo in 2007 told a trusting journalist: 'It is true that the virus is more easily transmitted from men to women. Women are at the greater risk.'   [319]

---

[315]   Peterman T A; Drotman D P; Curran J W  Epidemiologic reviews, (1985) Vol. 7, pp. 1-21.

[316]   Van der Ende ME, Rothbarth P, Stibbe J. Heterosexual transmission of HIV by haemophiliacs. British Medical Journal 1988; 297(6656): 1102-3.

[317]   European Study Group. Risk factors for male to female transmission of HIV. British Medical Journal 1989; 298: 411-414

[318]   Kreiss JK et al. Antibody to human T-lymphotropic virus type III in wives of hemophiliacs. Ann Intern Med. 1985 May;102(5):623-6.

[319]   http://aras.ab.ca/articles/scientific/200703-GalloInterview-Lambros.pdf Also see the final footnote to this chapter.  WHO and UNAIDS in 2008 reported they now accept that there has been no AIDS epidemic among heterosexual people outside of Africa and that it is unlikely to happen.

African women migrants to the UK are reported far more HIV infected than are UK-born women - but the UK Health Authorities say these African women are 'presumed infected in Africa.' So – how come that AIDS infects many more women in Africa than in the West? Why is heterosexual sex apparently much more dangerous in Africa? It has been long said that this was because Africans are much more promiscuous than Westerners, but where is the evidence for this?

Professor P.A.K. Addy, Head of Clinical Microbiology at the University of Science and Technology in Kumasi, Ghana, stated: 'Europeans and Americans came to Africa with prejudiced minds, so they are seeing what they wanted to see...I've known for a long time that Aids is not a crisis in Africa as the world is being made to understand. But in Africa it is very difficult to stick your neck out and say certain things. The West came out with those frightening statistics on Aids in Africa because it was unaware of certain social and clinical conditions.'[320]

Major studies were published in 2002 and 2003 in the *International Journal of STD and AIDS* on HIV transmission by sex in Africa. Among many papers they reviewed the following was typical. 'A recent study of HIV incidence in serodiscordant [only one partner HIV positive] couples in Africa estimated a rate of transmission per coital act of only 0.001123, comparable to rates of 0.0003± 0.0015 from similar studies in the US and Europe.' Among these couples only 1.2% reported 'consistent condom use.' These 'estimated' figures mean there is not enough HIV transmission by sex in Africa to cause or sustain a sexually transmitted epidemic.[321]

Furthermore, if WHO statistics are to be believed, African women around childbirth become HIV positive without having sex! [322] 'Many studies report HIV infections in African adults with no sexual exposure to HIV and in children with HIV-negative mothers. Unexplained high rates of HIV incidence have been observed in African women during antenatal and postpartum periods [when they were unlikely to have had sex].' (But when their bodies were naturally producing many other retroviruses to protect their embryos – as we now know.)

HIV was also reported in Romania as transmitted to children without sex and without having HIV positive parents. 'The unexpected discovery of HIV in a 12-year-old Romanian girl in a Bucharest hospital in June 1989 ... led to extensive testing and by 1990 some 1,086 Romanian children less than four years old had been found to be HIV-positive – despite not having any obvious way to acquire this infection.' [323] Likewise, in the former Soviet Union, about 250 children were similarly reportedly HIV positive in 1988-89 [324] and 'more recently, nearly 400 children attending a single hospital in Libya apparently contracted HIV', again without any sexual exposure. [325]

---

[320] Hodgkinson, N. 1994. Research disputes epidemic of Aids. Sunday Times. London, May 22nd, p24

[321] Rothernberg, Potterat and Drucker 'HIV infections in Sub-Saharan Africa not explained by sexual or vertical transmission.' *International Journal of STD & AIDS* 2002; **13**: 657± 666

[322] Taha TE, Dallabetta GA, Hoover DR, *et al.* Trends of HIV-1 and sexually transmitted diseases among pregnant and postpartum women in urban Malawi *AIDS* 1998;**12**:197± 203

Olayinka BA, Obi CL. Symptomatic HIV-infection in infantsm according to serostatus of mothers during pregnancy. *East Afr Med J* 1999;**76**:566± 70

UNAIDS. Zimbabwe. *Epidemiological Fact Sheet [2000 update]*. Geneva: WHO, 2000

Qolohle DC, Hoosen AA, Moodley J, Smith AN, KP Mlisana. Serological screening for sexually transmitted infections in pregnancy; is there any value in re-screening 664 International Journal of STD & AIDS

[323] Patrascu Dumitrescu O. The epidemic of human immunodeficiency virus infection in Romanian children. *AIDS Res Hum Retrovir* 1993;**9**:99± 104 - Hersh BS, Popovici F, Apetrei RC, *et al.* Acquired immune deficiency syndrome in Romania. *Lancet* 1991;**338**:645± 9

[324] Dehne KL, Podrovshiy V, Kobyshcha Y, Schwartlander B. Update on the epidemics of HIV and other sexually transmitted infections in the newly independent states ofthe former Soviet Union. *AIDS* 2000;**14**(suppl 3):S75± 84

[325] Quadri R, Yerli S, Posfay-Barbe K, *et al.* Outbreak of bloodborne viral infections in children attending a single hospital [abstract]. *Hepatology* 2000;**32**:281A

In 2003 Gisselquist et al reported: 'A series of sexual behaviour surveys in 12 African countries during 1989-93 shows no apparent correlation between the percentage of adults in a country reporting non-regular sexual partners in the last year and HIV prevalence.' [326] 'Moreover, a Zambian study ... reported at least 13% of sequences in newly infected person were not related to their partner's HIV.'[327]

The latter paper was bluntly entitled: *'Let it be sexual: how health care transmission of AIDS in Africa was ignored.'* [328] It went on to argue that AIDS had been spread in Africa by the repeated use of dirty needles for vaccinations. It concluded: 'Evidence permits the interpretation that health care exposures caused more HIV than sexual transmission.'

At this point in my reading I realized this was the theory that I first heard explained at the Royal Society debate in London. It seems this theory is still alive and strong – but perhaps only because sexual transmission studies have utterly failed to explain the spread of HIV in Sub-Saharan Africa.

After reviewing the scientific literature, this 2003 paper concludes that the 'post-1988 consensus that sexual transmission is responsible for 90% of adult HIV infections in Africa emerged despite, rather than from, the available evidence. ... Unfortunately, many experts have accepted the consensus as fact, and have not seen any need for further research to test its estimates. The result has been that the consensus has suppressed inquiry and dissent. Hence, from 1988 the consensus has been self-reinforcing, as researchers in Africa—and in Asia and the Caribbean—have often assumed sexual transmission without testing partners, without asking about health care exposures, and, when conflicting evidence nevertheless emerges—such as infected adults who deny sexual exposures to HIV—routinely rejecting it.'

'The consensus reflected poor management of research programmes and projects, since key questions suitable for empirical resolution ... were settled with assumptions "unencumbered by data" ... Now as then, experts may ignore evidence they do not want to see.'

I had, however, some problems with their theory. As far as I can see, they have not allowed for false positive HIV results in Africa from fungi and mycobacteria (See chapter below on the HIV test.) The mothers also would not have needed a dirty needle to order to test positive for the HIV test manufacturers list 'multiple pregnancy' as a risk factor for a false result. Also, I was not convinced by the way the authors, despite acknowledging that studies show the risk of HIV infection among health professionals from a needle stick injury are virtually zero, maintain their theory by saying these injuries were far less penetrating than a vaccination jab.

But what they had very valuably proved by their extensive review of the scientific literature was that there is now much scientific evidence that totally contradicts the consensus view that HIV and AIDS are spread by sexual transmission. [329]

[326] International Journal of STD & AIDS 2002; **13**: 657± 666

[327] Fideli US, Allen SA, Musoda R, *et al.* Virologic and immunologic determinants of heterosexual transmission of human immunode® ciency virus type 1 in Africa. *AIDS Res Hum Retrovir* 2001

[328] Let it be sexual: how health care transmission of AIDS in Africa was ignored, by David Gisselquist, John J Potterat , Stuart Brody and Francois Vachon International Journal of STD & AIDS 2003; 14: 148 ^161

329 POSTSCRIPT. In June 2008 a joint WHO-UNAIDS report stunningly admitted that they now believed there would not be a generalised epidemic of AIDS among heterosexual people 'outside of Africa!' Dr Kevin de Cock, the Head of WHO's department of HIV/AIDS, stated: 'It is very unlikely that there will be a heterosexual epidemic in other countries.' Asked to explain why were heterosexual Africans affected, he replied to say this was not fully understood. Reported in *The Independent*, London June 8th, 2008. There is a ready answer to explain the different situation in Africa and it is disingenuous of him not to give it. WHO has officially given AIDS in Africa a unique clinical definition under which symptoms common to men and women are defined as AIDS. See next chapter.

# Chapter 14

# AIDS - The Redefined Epidemic

I had always imagined that illnesses are defined according to their clinical symptoms – and that their diagnosis was strictly a scientific matter. I would think that the vast majority of people would think likewise. I had been thus shocked when I discovered polio was given new rules for diagnosis to cover-up the failure of the poliovirus vaccine. I had not thought that politics could interfere with such matters.

But I now have to report that much the same has happened with AIDS  – again, it seems, to hide the failure of a medical theory.  I have discovered that there have been several changes to the official definition of AIDS since the illness was first described – with Africa being given its own extraordinary and unique diagnostic rules. The result is that, in the USA, Africa and Europe today, it is not necessary to be HIV positive to be diagnosed with AIDS. Indeed, in the USA and Europe it is not even necessary to feel ill or to have any evident clinical symptoms of illness.

## 1982 CDC: *AIDS clinically diagnosed by symptoms of illness*

At first AIDS was diagnosed clinically like most other diseases – by the evident symptoms of illness.  In 1981-2 it was described as a condition in which two illnesses, fungal pneumonia (PCP) and severe Thrush, appeared together, often accompanied by a skin cancer, Kaposi Sarcoma. These 3 illnesses became known as the 'AIDS Indicating'. The principal cause of death was PCP, caused by a fungus that is normally harmlessly and present in nearly all of us, but which had suddenly become a killer. Once diagnosed, death was usually less than eleven months away.  A few hundred such cases were diagnosed in the UK and USA in the early 1980s. The patients were all in the urban partying gay scene in which a great deal of anal sex was fuelled by intensive and multiple drug taking.  Their illnesses were at the time varyingly said by scientists to be caused by inhaled recreational drugs, by medical immune-suppressant drugs heavily prescribed for STDs, by a new mutant form of syphilis or by a new virus spread by promiscuous sex,

## 1984 CDC: *HIV antibodies are now the key diagnostic symptom.*

AIDS was redefined in 1984 after HIV was declared its cause.  The presence of the virus became the major AIDS defining condition – as detected by finding an antibody with the HIV test.  If antibodies against an HIV protein were found, then it was predicted confidently that within 10 years one of the above AIDS-defining and death-producing illnesses would follow. If a patient already had these illnesses, but the virus were absent, then it was said that the virus had killed all the cells it could live in. As many were now found to be 'HIV [antibody] positive' despite looking healthy, a panic rapidly spread. It was soon predicted that 1.5 million Americans were already infected and well on the way to dying of AIDS.

## 1987   CDC: *HIV no longer necessary for an AIDS diagnosis.* [330]

As reported in the last chapter, the CDC in 1987 ran into trouble when it lobbied the White House for greatly increased funding for AIDS research on the basis that AIDS was a major epidemic among heterosexuals. When the White House demanded the evidence, the CDC was forced to slash its estimate of the number of Americans infected from 1.76 million to 600,000 (a cut some have since mistakenly attributed to the just-introduced antiretrovirals). [331]

The Chicago Times reported on May 31, 1987 that 'the nation has become transfixed by a fear of deadly disease not seen since the polio epidemics of the 1940s and 1950s' but this fear, it said, was ill-founded for 'AIDS still ranks as one of the rarest of diseases.' 'Deaths from AIDS are far less frequent than the various forms of heart disease that kill more than a million Americans every year, rarer even than deaths from alcohol-related liver disease, diabetes, atherosclerosis, influenza and pneumonia, motor-vehicle accidents, homicide, suicide or accidental falls in the home.'

At the same time, statistics from San Francisco indicated the AIDS epidemic might be ending. Professor Andrew Moss, an epidemiologist at the University of California, reported in 1987: 'the serioconversion rate [numbers testing HIV antibody positive} in gay men crashed quite a few years ago. San Francisco's doing new estimates and they're a lot lower than any previous estimates'[332] – in fact down from 21% in 1982 to just 1% in 1983 and continuing downwards for the next four years.[333]

Remarkably, some who previously tested positive were now testing negative, as was reported by John Hopkins Hospital in Baltimore. Professor Susanna Cunningham-Rundles of Cornell said: 'I believe there are people who have encountered the virus and successfully fought it off.'[334]

But within months the CDC regained the epidemic it was beginning to lose by the most extraordinary of tactics. It issued new diagnostic rules for AIDS that would allow it to continue to grimly warn that America was in grip of a vast AIDS epidemic. It did so by quietly instructing doctors that they should now diagnose AIDS even in the HIV negative if they suffer from any one of a very extended long list of 'AIDS-indicating illnesses.'

It thus reversed the ruling it had made only three years earlier when it made a positive HIV test a requirement for an AIDS diagnosis. It still states on the websites of both the CDC and the UK health authority that a positive HIV test is not a precondition for AIDS diagnosis.[335] This is despite these authorities maintaining that HIV is the cause of AIDS!

I am sure this is equally astonishing for many of my readers – so I invite you to go to the CDC website and check for yourselves. [336] In case you are not on the web, here is a scan of the text.

---

[330] The 1987 redefinition is on the CDC website at http://www.cdc.gov/mmwr/pdf/other/mmsu3601.pdf

[331] Chicago Tribune, November 15, 1987

[332] As above.

[333] Chicago Tribune, December 11, 1987

[334] Chicago Tribune, December 20, 1987

[335] The CDC definition of AIDS, and lists of AIDS defining diseases, are also available on http://www.righto.com/theories/aidsdef.html The 1993 redefinition was published in *MMWR* 41 (RR-17)

[336] http://www.cdc.gov/mmwr/pdf/other/mmsu3601.pdf.

## 1987 REVISION OF CASE DEFINITION FOR AIDS FOR SURVEILLANCE PURPOSES

For national reporting, a case of AIDS is defined as an illness characterized by one or more of the following "indicator" diseases, depending on the status of laboratory evidence of HIV infection, as shown below.

### I. Without Laboratory Evidence Regarding HIV Infection

If laboratory tests for HIV were not performed or gave inconclusive results (See Appendix I) and the patient had no other cause of immunodeficiency listed in Section I.A below, then any disease listed in Section I.B indicates AIDS if it was diagnosed by a definitive method (See Appendix II).

The CDC then produced a list of some 17 illnesses that it says should be diagnosed as AIDS without laboratory evidence of HIV infection. It stated that **'with laboratory evidence against HIV infection', (that is, with a negative HIV test) 'any of the provided list of diseases could be diagnosed as AIDS,'** (This is called the 'Section 1.B' list) Remarkably this list includes the three original AIDS diseases, PCP fungal pneumonia, severe Candida (Thrush) of the throat or lungs, and Kaposi Sarcoma. These were in future to be called AIDS even after a negative HIV test. Since these original AIDS diseases were diagnosed in some 63% of all AIDS cases in the UK in 2006, a positive HIV test was thus made almost redundant for an AIDS diagnosis.

### III. With Laboratory Evidence Against HIV Infection

With laboratory test results negative for HIV infection (See Appendix I), a diagnosis of AIDS for surveillance purposes is ruled out *unless*:

A. all the other causes of immunodeficiency listed above in Section I.A are excluded; **AND**

B. the patient has had either:
   1. *Pneumocystis carinii* pneumonia diagnosed by a definitive method (See Appendix II); **OR**
   2. a. any of the other diseases indicative of AIDS listed above in Section I.B diagnosed by a definitive method (See Appendix II); **AND**
      b. a T-helper/inducer (CD4) lymphocyte count <400/mm$^3$.

I am sure that if questioned, the CDC will explain that results of the test can be 'inconclusive' or even 'negative' because HIV hides very efficiently in its victims. But, I wonder if this is a case of the 'Emperor's Clothes' – the story of a naked monarch who believed he was dressed because he trusted what he was told? Likewise we are expected to trust that the virus is causing the illness despite its absence.

Onto this list, as not requiring a positive HIV test for an AIDS diagnosis but a CD4 count below 400, in 1987, went a further 14 new 'AIDS indicating illnesses,' including bronchitis 'of any duration' and a herpes ulcer suffered for more than a month. [337] This is despite these illnesses having existed for centuries before AIDS arrived and having their own bacteria, viruses or fungi, that have to be present for the illness to be diagnosed. Not for the latter the privilege of being absent on duty!

This redefinition also allowed that, after a positive HIV test, a person could be diagnosed with AIDS if he or she was diagnosed with just one of a different and longer list of illnesses provided by the CDC, including septicaemia, pneumonia, meningitis, bone or joint infection, an abscess in an internal organ caused by streptococcus or other

[337] Yet there is reportedly no mention of AIDS in three major overview studies of cervical cancer published in April 1999 in the *New England Journal of Medicine* (accessible via www.nejm.org ).

bacteria. Why such illnesses need HIV was not explained. For children, 'multiple bacterial infections' would henceforth be sufficient for an AIDS diagnosis! Thus despite the apparent absence of HIV, a child might be put for life on powerful antiviral drugs.

Finally, and even more surprisingly, the CDC ruled that people who 'have either a negative HIV antibody test' or 'an opportunistic disease not listed in the definition as an indicator of AIDS', may be diagnosed with AIDS 'on consideration of ... a history of exposure to HIV.'[338] This totally astonished me. Under this, even a person with flu could be diagnosed as having AIDS despite a negative HIV test, if a friend had a positive HIV test.

> information that would lead to a more accurate diagnosis. For example, patients who are not reportable under the definition because they have either a negative HIV-antibody test or, in the presence of HIV antibody, an opportunistic disease not listed in the definition as an indicator of AIDS nonetheless may be diagnosed as having serious HIV disease on consideration of other clinical or laboratory characteristics of HIV infection or a history of exposure to HIV.

By redefinition, AIDS thus became an illness that can have an incredible range of symptoms. No wonder this redefinition caused an immediate panic![339] In Italy the new definition immediately put up the AIDS figures by 188%. In the US it went up by 280%! AIDS became by definition a collective name for a legion of old diseases, without even the need for HIV to be present. But critically this also meant that any specialist working on just one of these disorders would now be able to tap into the growing AIDS budget.

Also most importantly, with this redefinition came a great watering down of the risk factor attached to an AIDS diagnosis. With so many people now diagnosed with AIDS in the absence of the original deadly 'AIDS Indicating diseases', the average life expectancy after diagnosis went up greatly without any need for medication.

## 1993 CDC: *Feeling ill no longer a necessity for an AIDS diagnosis.* [340]

In 1993 the last major formal redefinition of AIDS took place, one that would again greatly swell the size of the AIDS epidemic. This time the CDC did not replace the 1987 definition but added to it that AIDS could now be diagnosed in people who had none of the 'AIDS Indicating' illnesses – and even if they did not feel ill! The CDC predicted that this redefinition would more than double the number of official AIDS cases.

The new provision added to the definition was that a person without evident symptoms of illness could be diagnosed with AIDS if they had less than 200 CD4 white blood cells in a micro-litre ($\mu$L) of blood – half the level mentioned in the previous redefinition. The CDC estimated that there were at that time 120,000 to 190,000' Americans who did not know they had AIDS since they were not ill, had no AIDS symptoms but who did have a CD4 Count of below 200.

---

[338] MMWR Supplement, CDC, August 14 1987

[339] Quoted in *What if everything you thought you knew about AIDS was wrong?* by Christine Maggiore. page 14.

[340] This revised definition is available at http://www.cdc.gov/mmwr/preview/mmwrhtml/00018871.html

The CDC explained, ' the population of HIV-infected persons with CD4+ T-lymphocyte counts of less than 200/uL is substantially larger than the population of persons with AIDS-defining clinical conditions' i.e. the redefinition would more than double the numbers diagnosed with AIDS!

This time the effect of the redefinition was not just to put up the numbers in the epidemic, but also to vastly increase the numbers of people immediately prescribed the expensive chemotherapy drugs known as 'antiretrovirals'. The CDC said all American citizens with a CD4 cell count below 200 per μL now must be told that they already had AIDS – and instructed to start immediately on these drugs, even if they did not feel ill and were otherwise quite robust. However, putting such people on these drugs meant in practice that many were better able to withstand their severe side effects.

On top of this, the CDC made a further major change. They directed there was no need to wait to take the drugs until one had a below-200 CD4 count! In future, antiretroviral drugs could be prescribed if the CD4 count was below 500, in the hope to prevent AIDS starting by preventing infection.

If these people were not ill beforehand, they were likely soon to be, as they now faced a lifetime on powerful chemotherapy. (Some of the antiretroviral drugs are also marketed as chemotherapy against cancer – but for that purpose, only for a limited period because of their side effects.)

The very fact they were diagnosed with AIDS was enough to make many start to feel ill. Such a diagnosis was a major source of stress all on its own.

This time the UK only partly followed suit. It said without any symptoms of illness, a person should only be diagnosed with AIDS if they had a CD4 Count below 300 and were also HIV positive. But in the UK, as in the US, in future it would be irrelevant to ask if they felt unwell before diagnosing them with AIDS.

The new definition also added 3 diseases to the list of 23 'AIDS-indicating' illnesses. Onto the list came TB, bacterial pneumonia and invasive cervical cancer. The addition of TB greatly swelled the numbers of the poor diagnosed with AIDS – especially as TB under these rules could be, and was, diagnosed as AIDS in the absence of HIV.

Cervical cancer was added as a result of lobbying by lesbian women who were acting in solidarity with their gay brothers. Until then very few women were diagnosed with AIDS, but this could not last, or so thought Maxine Wolfe in 1993. She logically explained that, as a virus caused AIDS, it must be an illusion that women were not getting AIDS. 'We don't know if women were really asymptomatic. They simply did not have male-defined symptoms.' Cervical cancer was thus added. The result was; 'In the half-year following, over 9,000 cases in women were reported. The number of women said to have AIDS in the US went up by 300%.'

How this is reconcilable with the vaccine announced in 2007 against a different virus said to cause cervical cancer I just cannot guess. It is another mystery of government diagnostic rules.

By 1997 according to the CDC, 61% of all new AIDS patients in the US were, at the time of their diagnosis, not suffering from any of the AIDS defining illness– and yet put on antiretrovirals for the rest of their lives. They were told that without the drugs they were certain to die just as fast as did AIDS patients during the first years of the epidemic.

But they were badly misinformed. Most of the early patients were only diagnosed with AIDS after coming down with deadly Fungal Pneumonia. If patients today were similarly diagnosed with AIDS, far fewer would be diagnosed – and their life expectancy after diagnosis would be far shorter.

But, a major new killer in AIDS cases has now emerged – liver failure, a known side effect of antiretroviral drugs. It is now a major killer in AIDS cases in the West – yet is still not listed as an 'AIDS indicating' illness. Other known side effects of these drugs are cancers and heart disease – and again these are now listed as major killers in AIDS cases. But AIDS patients in the West are still surviving longer than they did in 1984 – for the redefinitions have cleverly ensured this by including those without evident symptoms at the time of diagnosis.

Yet, despite all the redefinitions, it is still mostly multi-drug-using partying gays who die of AIDS in the West. Yet our public health authorities instead emphasise the percentage rise in heterosexual cases among Westerners – without saying how many fewer these are than cases among gay men.

For example, in 2004 the UK government headlined: 'Recent increases in new HIV diagnoses have been largely driven by infections acquired through heterosexual intercourse'. And yet the small print of the same report stated; 'Men-having-sex-with-men (MSM) remain the group at greatest risk of acquiring HIV infection within the UK, accounting for an estimated 84% of infections diagnosed in 2003 that were likely to have been acquired in the UK' – and, out of 6,606 new cases of 'HIV infection in 2003, only 43 cases were among heterosexual or lesbian women born in the UK, and only 57 cases among UK born heterosexual men!

The numbers of deaths listed in AIDS statistics are also not what they seem. They are not 'deaths from AIDS', as one might be forgiven for presuming. The small print reveals these are 'deaths among the HIV-infected,' leaving open the actual cause of death. This makes these figures not only highly misleading, but meaningless. Likewise in 1997 the CDC acknowledged that: 'Reported deaths [on CDC AIDS statistics tables] are not necessarily caused by HIV-related diseases!' [341]

So how do the UK health authorities justify saying that heterosexual and female cases of AIDS are greatly increasing? Solely by adding African immigrants 'presumed infected in Africa.' It is among them that are found nearly all the heterosexual and female cases of 'AIDS'. But why? How can a virus prefer Africans to Whites? This is a question I left hanging in the last chapter. It is about time I dealt with it.

## THE AFRICAN AIDS DEFINITION

### *AIDS is to be diagnosed with different symptoms in Africa*

It is common knowledge that AIDS in Africa is rampant, that it affects men and women alike, and is destroying the population and economic prospects of Sub-Saharan Africa. Everyone also thinks, as I have for most of my life, that AIDS in the West and Africa has the same diagnostic definition and symptoms; that they are clinically the same. This is only surely sensible – the same virus must cause the same illness?

But, when I investigated, I found the truth was utterly otherwise. AIDS is diagnosed entirely differently in Africa. Officially in Africa a person only has to have a few symptoms common to many diseases that ultimately are caused by great poverty, poor water supplies and lack of sanitation. Again there is no requirement to test positive for HIV for an AIDS diagnosis. This was strangely easy to discover. I only needed to go to the official WHO website and look it up. This tells me that our media has not been doing its homework when reporting AIDS in Africa.

The unique African clinical definition of AIDS found on the WHO website and in African government manuals, was created in the early days of AIDS research. In 1983 Robert Gallo had speculated the AIDS virus was from Africa, saying that this was because he had detected a trace of one of his suspect cancer retroviruses, HTLV-I (not HIV), in a black patient on Haiti. [342] When in 1985 Gallo tested blood sera from children in Uganda

---

[341] Professor Robert S. Root-Bernstein.' The Evolving Definition of AIDS.'
[342] Gallo to Director of NCI, 4th August 1983. [342]

and discovered 67% had 'HIV' antibodies, he deduced from this that these children had no chance of survival, and that Uganda would come to a quick and disastrous end. [343]

Although this was horrific, the discovery that males and females tested HIV positive equally in Africa must also have been something of a relief for him. It was essential to his virus theory that both genders be equally infected.

But this relief did not last long. It was soon discovered that Africans testing positive were rarely falling ill with the AIDS indicating diseases of the West, with PCP, Thrush and Kaposi Sarcoma. This surely meant that they were not getting AIDS! This seriously threatened his HIV theory. If this virus caused these illnesses in the West, why wasn't it doing so in Africa?

But in 1984-5 a close colleague of Gallo's, Professor Myron Essex of Harvard, recommended that the HIV test not be relied on in Africa. He had just discovered that mycobacteria test falsely positive in the HIV test. It seemed an antibody detected with the HIV test was also against mycobacteria. He concluded that, since mycobacteria are very common in Africa, the test was unreliable in that continent.[344] (This also could explain why so many Ugandans tested positive.)

Essex stated: 'our observations ... suggest that HIV-1 Elisa and Western Blot results be interpreted with caution ... [they] may not be sufficient for HIV diagnosis in AIDS-epidemic areas of Central Africa where the prevalence of mycobacterial infections is quite high.' [345] His finding has since been confirmed by a host of other studies.[346] This is a major reason why WHO has since often not relied on HIV tests in Africa.[347]

In late 1985 a solution to this embarrassing enigma was worked out at a meeting of international health experts and representatives of Central African governments held in the West African city of Bangui between October 22nd- 25th 1985, under the auspices of the World Health Organization.

At this there were protests from African government representatives who held that the West was grossly exaggerating the AIDS problem in Africa since few Africans were falling ill with the classic AIDS symptoms.[348] But the international agencies ran roughshod over these objections and it was agreed that in future black Africa should have its own unique definition of AIDS, one that did not rely on the HIV test, nor on the presence of the main AIDS-indicating illnesses as then defined – and one that would definitely ensure that in future Africa had a gigantic AIDS epidemic.

The new rules laid down that Africans in future should be diagnosed with AIDS if they scored a total of 12 points from a new list of general symptoms of illness. These official African AIDS diagnostic rules are still current, and are called the 'Bangui Clinical Definition of AIDS.' They are also used for AIDS surveillance. This is from the WHO website:

---

[343] Saxinger WC, Levine PH, Dean AG, et al. Evidence for exposure to HTLV-III in Uganda before 1973. Science 1985;227:1036-1038.

[344] His views are in a paper he and colleagues published in 1985.

[345] Myron 'Max' Essex, Head of Harvard AIDS Institute. In a 1994 study he warned that 'existing antibody tests 'may not be sufficient for HIV diagnosis' in settings where TB and related diseases are commonplace.'

[346] Another such study found 'ELISA and WB may not be sufficient for HIV diagnosis in AIDS-endemic areas of Central Africa where the prevalence of mycobacterial diseases is quite high' Kashala, O. Marlink, R. Ilunga, M. Diese, M. Gormus, B. Xu, K. Mukeba, P. Kasongo, K. & Essex, M. 1994 Infection with human immunodeficiency virus type 1 (HIV-1) and human T cell lymphotropic viruses among leprosy patients and contacts: correlation between HIV-1 cross-reactivity and antibodies to lipoarabinomannan. Journal of Infectious Diseases 169, 296-304.

[347] In 2008 WHO reposted that 1.7 million people worldwide have TB of whom 0.2 million are positive for HIV. It did not mention that TB bacteria can themselves falsely test positive as HIV.

[348] ChicagoTribune November 24, 1985

## BANGUI CLINICAL DIAGNOSIS OF AIDS

**Exclusion criteria** (If these are present then it is not AIDS)
1. Pronounced malnutrition
2. Cancer (excluding Kaposi Sarcoma)
3. Immunosuppressive treatment

### Inclusion criteria with the corresponding scores
### Important signs
| | |
|---|---|
| Weight loss exceeding 10% of body weight | 4 points |
| Protracted asthenia (defined as 'weakness or debility' [349]) | 4 points |

### Very frequent signs
| | |
|---|---|
| Continuous or repeated attacks of fever for more than a month | 3 points |
| Diarrhoea lasting for more than a month | 3 points |

### Other signs
| | |
|---|---|
| Cough | 2 points |
| Pneumopathy (Any disease of the lungs) | 4 points |
| Oropharyngeal candidiasis (Thrush in mouth or throat) | 4 points |
| Chronic or relapsing cutaneous herpes (severe rash,) | 4 points |
| Generalized pruritic dermatosis (severe itching) | 4 points |
| Herpes zoster (relapsing) (a painful infectious skin rash) | 4 points |
| Generalized adenopathy (enlargement of lymph modes.) | 2 points |
| Neurological signs (signs pertaining to nervous system) | 2 points |
| Generalized Kaposi's sarcoma (a skin cancer) | 12 points |

### It finally stated that THE DIAGNOSIS OF AIDS IS ESTABLISHED WHEN THE SCORE IS 12 OR MORE.'

In 1994 this was modified slightly. The WHO 'Expanded Case Definition' of that year ignores Essex's 1985 advice and recommends that the HIV test be done as well – but also says, if this were not available, then the original Bangui Definition should be adhered to unchanged. Thus African states have practically identical AIDS reporting forms, with the Bangui definition on them.

Thus, most astonishingly, for an African to be told they are cursed with AIDS, it more than suffices for them to have an intermittent fever, protracted weakness, diarrhoea and 10% weight loss – all symptoms that can result from living in unsanitary conditions. With these symptoms, the African AIDS epidemic could be sharply diminished by funding sewage works, clean water supplies, and better nourishment. These are the very same measures that ended the epidemics that ravaged the British poor in the 19th century.

But by adopting this definition and calling this AIDS, the international experts had done the contrary. They had created by fiat a massive African AIDS epidemic that they claimed was caused by promiscuous sex, with death only delayed by powerful chemotherapy type drugs they had invented. This has also led to preachers advocating

---

[349] http://www.nbc-med.org/SiteContent/MedRef/OnlineRef/FieldManuals/medman/Appxa.htm

sexual abstinence and to bishops blaming African bigamy. The result is that in Africa some have called AIDS the 'American Initiative to Destroy Sex!'

To make matters worse, individual African countries have exacerbated these errors. Tanzania has said just finding one of the above symptoms is all that is required for an AIDS diagnosis and Uganda for a period allowed TB by itself to be defined as AIDS. As a result, their AIDS diagnoses soared.

In South Africa however, a positive HIV test is now required and, despite the Bangui Definition, TB itself is acknowledged to be the greatest killer in South Africa, particularly among younger adults. This is verified by the 2005 official South African statistics based on death certificate reports. They tell us that TB kills 4 times more people than AIDS in South Africa, and that 'flu, pneumonia, heart diseases and diabetes all kill more than AIDS. (AIDS is today credited with 2.7% of deaths in South Africa.)

However, according to these same South African statistics, diseases of poverty are increasing, with malnutrition growing as a major cause of death for children aged under four. As severe malnutrition produces AIDS-like symptoms, [350] these cases could be misdiagnosed as AIDS in future.[351]

Certain AIDS scientists have contested these official figures on the basis that deaths from TB are really deaths from AIDS. However, TB has been around for far longer than AIDS – and has long been a major killer. The same is true of malaria. According to the World Health Organization, there are more cases of TB and malaria every year in Africa than the total number of African AIDS cases reported since 1982. [352] (HIV test manufacturers warn that both malaria and TB bacteria can falsely test positive for HIV.)

Dr. Christian Fiala, a researcher of AIDS in East Africa, has reported: 'TB is very widespread in Africa. It's a bacterial infection that infects the lungs. TB is spread by coughing, and is highly infectious. The typical symptoms of Tuberculosis are fever, weight loss and coughing. This is exactly what is required for an [African] AIDS diagnosis.' The tragedy, he added, is that less than one hundredth of the money spent on chasing the AIDS virus is currently spent on fighting TB or malaria. (Not all TB cases are in the lungs – sometimes the bacteria multiply in other parts of the body.)

In South Africa, WHO calculates its AIDS epidemic statistics, not from a survey of the whole population, or from overall population statistics, but from the presence of 'HIV antibodies' in blood tests done on a few thousand pregnant women attending clinics – despite research findings that show healthy human placentas often contain retroviruses (seen by Electron Microscope) that falsely test as if HIV. [353]

On top of this the WHO computer team in Geneva has vastly increased their statistical allowance for 'error factors' when working out their estimates for the numbers of AIDS victims in Africa. While their field reports list around 70,000 a year of Africans

---

[350] Papadopulos-Eleopulus et al. *AIDS in Africa: distinguishing fact and fiction* World Journal of Microbiology and Biotechnology 1995, 11. 135-143

[351] 'While an increasing number of deaths are associated with lifestyle diseases (such as *heart disease* and *diabetes*) as the underlying cause, the dominant contributors to the growth in mortality are deaths associated with *tuberculosis*, and *influenza* and *pneumonia. Malnutrition* was among the ten leading causes of death among children aged under 4. Although there was fluctuation during the three years in the percentages of deaths linked to malnutrition, the numbers of deaths increased steadily.' South African Health Statistics. Published March 2005.

[352] WHO, 1998

[353] Panem, S. 1979. C Type Virus Expression in the Placenta. Curr. Top. Pathol. 66:175-189 – quoted in Eleni Papadopulos-Eleopulus, Valendar F. Turner and John M. Papadimitriou Is a Positive Western Blot Proof of HIV Infection? BIO/TECHNOLOGY VOL.11 JUNE 1993. This can be found on www.theperthgroup.com The retroviral protein p30 common to many retroviruses was also identified in human placentas by antiblot testing in Proc. Natl. Acad. Sci. USA Vol. 81, pp. 6501-6505, October 1984 Medical Sciences Detection and immunochemical characterization of a primate type C retrovirus-related p30 protein in normal human placentas (retroviral core protein/two-dimensional electrophoresis/immunoblot analysis) Lois B. JERABEK, ROBERT C. MELLORS*, KEITH B. ELKON, AND JANE W. MELLORS Research Division, The Hospital for Special Surgery, Affiliated with the New York Hospital-Cornell University Medical College

as testing HIV positive; their annual estimate for AIDS in Africa is calculated by multiplying these reported cases by an ever increasing error factor to account for 'under-reporting.' In 1996, WHO thus justified multiplying the number of registered AIDS cases by 12 times to get their estimate, but in 1997 put this up to multiplying by 17 – thus statistically producing a horrendous estimate. [354]

Dr. James Chin should know what the correct figures are. He reported in his recent book '*The AIDS Pandemic: the Collision of Epidemiology with Political Correctness*' that he 'was responsible from 1987 to 1992 for receiving and tabulating national reports of AIDS cases submitted to WHO in Geneva.'  He reported that there is 'gross overestimation of most national HIV prevalence estimates in SSA' (Sub-Saharan Africa). As for the Philippines, he tells how initially 'the minister of health multiplied the 50 detected HIV/AIDS cases by 1000 to derive an estimate of 50,000!' He concluded: 'If you knew how most HIV/AIDS numbers are generally "cooked," you would surely use them with extreme caution!' It is 'very clear that reported AIDS cases in most developing countries are totally unreliable and thus unusable as any meaningful measure.'

What then of all the 'AIDS' orphans in Africa?  A World Health Organization report, marked for 'restricted' distribution, explained 'there is confusion as to what is meant [in Africa] by the term "orphan." It can mean the absence of one parent, temporary or permanent (as Madonna found when she was introduced to her orphaned child's father). It is also presumed that most African orphans are so because of AIDS. However, a WHO report on AIDS in Uganda noted, 'no distinction made as to the cause of orphanhood, which in some areas included the effects of war.'[355] Uganda between 1966 and 1986 had an estimated million people killed in war. Many other wars have recently devastated Central Africa with over a million also killed in Zaire.

But, with a very large proportion of the medical funds available in Africa earmarked for fighting AIDS, doctors must be greatly tempted to use the lax standards of the Bangui Definition to declare most of their patients have AIDS, as this could be the only way for them to get the funds they desperately need. Likewise for patients, most will easily qualify under this definition, so they too may benefit from asking for help as an AIDS victim.

The practical consequence of blaming so many common illnesses on HIV, despite each having its particular cause, is that African governments are today under enormous pressure to re-allot their scant health funds away from the diseases of poverty to pay for expensive antiretroviral medicines. Today, if any African government shows reluctance to spend most of its health budget on antiretrovirals, Western interests accuse it of malgovernance. If any local doctor needs funds, he also knows what he must say.

Finally and more optimistically, it should be noted that, that, despite the widespread malnutrition, poverty and disease, the African population is far from shrinking. The US Bureau of the Census, in its International Database 2001, reports that between 1980 and 2000, during reportedly the worse years of the African AIDS epidemic, the population of Sub-Saharan Africa went up from 378 million to 652 million.

---

354  Peter Duesberg, Evidence to South African Presidential Commission on AIDS, 2000.
355
     From Dr Christian Fiala, an Africa based AIDS specialist.

# Chapter 15

# Gallo fights back

In 2006 I decided that it was time to seek advice and comments on my work from senior scientists. I thus copied it to some. As I had just been invited to South Africa to help with a film on diamonds and human rights. I thought I would be able to update my research on AIDS in that country while I waited to see what comments my work drew.

Before leaving, to aid in this review process and to make it easier for myself, I posted online some of my work-in-progress on AIDS and links to research sources, including government health websites and dissident scientists. I put these up expecting little reaction. After all, what harm was there in noting online that there was scientific dispute over the HIV theory of AIDS? I also put up my working drafts of two lengthy articles I was writing entitled '*HIVGATE*' and '*AIDSGATE.*'

At the same time I contacted a professor, Patrick Bond of KwaZulu-Natal University in Durban about the diamond film I was coming out to South Africa to help make, and thought there was no harm in mentioning that I was also working on AIDS. He had earlier been in touch with me about my work on the diamond industry, offering to help. He is an economist, the Director of the Centre for Civil Society in Durban, and holds academic positions in Canada and South Korea.

On learning that I was on my way to South Africa he immediately replied by email to say he would love to help, and as it happened, he would be available in Johannesburg immediately I arrived. I was delighted and flattered. But, a few minutes later, he emailed me back.

*Janine, I just looked at the AIDS section [on your website]. You probably know just how controversial the dissident position has become here; it's not uncommon for my dear activist friends in the Treatment Action Campaign to describe the government's policy as genocidal, based on his denialism. I'm so sorry, it's just \*such\* an important, life-and-death issue to the civil society forces I work with across SA, that I'm not really going to be able to devote time to anything at all that might imply endorsement of denialism.'*

Much to my dismay and shock he thus withdrew his offer to help in my fight to improve conditions for diamond mine workers. Now 'denialism' and 'denialist' are for me red-flag terms. These words were originally applied to those who denied that the Nazis massacred the Jews. I had heard some AIDS activists were deliberately using the same terms to tar by association any scientist critical of the HIV theory of AIDS, but I was amazed to find Patrick among them.

The insult is based on the view that it is morally reprehensible for anyone to publicly sow doubt about the role of HIV, since this might put AIDS patients' lives at risk by dissuading them from taking antiretroviral drugs. But what are scientists to do if their research indicates that AIDS is not caused by a retrovirus? Stay silent?

But no one at all had previously applied such terms to my work for simply reporting the existence of scientific dissidence. I was thus quite unused to it, so I replied:

*Patrick, this totally amazes me. In 30 years of investigative work, I have never had people not even reading my papers or discussing things with me before refusing to talk to me - not even the Oppenheimer family [who control De Beers]. I get on with everyone.*

*It clearly shows the emotional intensity about this issue in South Africa right now. I need to know about this - and why scientific inquiry into the AIDS papers that comes to critical viewpoints, is to be rejected out of hand. Have I got to make my scientific decisions based on faith?*

*This is really unhealthy. As I said, I read the evidence and posted it so others could read it. Why are you so sure you are right - and why will you not talk to anyone who disagrees? Please do talk about this. Honesty goes with openness. Every good wish, from a woman who still would like a level discussion on this.  Jani*

He responded:

*Jani, hi, I'm \*really\* sorry but the damage done to the progressive movement - and the society as a whole - by AIDS denialists is so intense and deep that your website material on this will not make any other kinds of interactions possible.*

Now I thought in the 'progressive movement' we must always be ready to question scientists and pharmaceutical corporations - and I knew this professor is a fierce critique of such corporations, as also is the South African Treatment Action Campaign (TAC) with which the professor had associated himself. They have quite rightly denounced the wickedly vast profits these corporations make from their drugs and have taken centre stage in forcing a very substantial drop in prices.

Zackie Achmat of TAC took, to the best of my knowledge, a particularly heroic role in bringing this about by publicly refusing to take the antiretrovirals he was prescribed until the price fell to levels that more people could afford.

But this does not stop me from having doubts about the long-term safety of powerful antiretroviral drugs. No doubt some people tolerate them well - and that they can act as powerful antibiotic and antioxidant agents against Candida and PCP, but I have seen just too many medical reports linking them also to dangerously increased risks, including of heart problems, similar to the heart attack Zackie Achmat most unfortunately suffered soon after he eventually started on antiretrovirals. [356]

Liver failure, never an AIDS-linked disease, is now the major cause of death among AIDS patients in the US and is a result of the toxic nature of these drugs.[357] All that is said of antiretrovirals, even by their advocates, is that they delay an inevitable death. I too want to see a real remedy - and thus I think all AIDS research should be taken seriously, even the research that points to other remedies than antiretrovirals.

I replied:

*Patrick, you have just managed to convince me single handedly that there is something very wrong here. If you are not open to discuss the science, if TAC is likewise, something is highly wrong here and needs looking into. It stirs my investigative blood! I would like to meet TAC at some stage - perhaps after filming is done.*

No reply came before I boarded my plane, so I presumed there would be no meeting.  But in curiosity I looked up Professor Patrick Bond's work on the Internet and found, with the exception of his scanty writing on AIDS, I liked his work very much.

But his writing on AIDS was quite different in character. The academic tone simply vanished. For example, when a spokesman for President Thabo Mbeki criticized the safety of a 'relatively inexpensive anti-retroviral treatment for pregnant, HIV-positive women', the Professor had responded, not with evidence to the contrary, but by saying that 'this was one of most insane reasons for not treating HIV+ pregnancies with antiretrovirals, and

---

[356] http://www.thebody.com/content/art8640.html  His doctor suggests the heart attack is not related to the drugs he had just started taking – although such problems are frequently reported. For example: McKee et al. 'Phosphorylation of Thymidine and AZT in Heart Mitochondria: Elucidation of a Novel Mechanism of AZT Cardiotoxicity' in *Cardiovascular Toxicology* 4(2):155-67:  'Antiretroviral nucleoside analogs used in highly active antiretroviral therapy (HAART) are associated with cardiovascular and other tissue toxicity associated with mitochondrial DNA depletion.'

[357] Brink's detailed reports on these drugs are well worth reading and are available on http://www.tig.org.za. Achmat and the TAC have a very different viewpoint and are at www.tac.org.za

for not taking AIDS seriously.' He added that it made some academics 'conclude that the SA government is genocidal.'

Now I knew something of the story behind this. The US has banned an antiretroviral drug, Nevirapine, as too dangerous to be used with pregnant American women, while also approving the same drug for the same use in Africa, perhaps because it is relatively cheap. When a US health professional was given this drug after a needle accident, so badly did the drug poison her that she had to have a liver transplant. I have also read medical research that reports such effects as 'mitochondrial disease in the offspring as a result of antiretroviral therapy.'[358]

Another article I found of Bond's spoke of President Mbeki's 'bizarre questioning of the link between the HIV virus and AIDS.' But I could not find any attempt to justify calling this bizarre. I had thought Bond fairly iconoclastic – and thought well of him for this. But – this was an ill justified slur.

Now I have widely read on this issue, and now know of a Nobel Laureate who questions if HIV is the cause of AIDS as well as of a number of other senior professors at major universities who think likewise. I thought, don't they disserve to be taken a bit more seriously? Surely the reader at least deserves to know why their views are so 'bizarre' that the layperson must not be told of their work?

I then discovered that Bond gave thanks to 'Julie Davids and Paul Davis of ACT UP Philadelphia, my houseguests last night, who helped with corrections,' in an endnote to one of his articles. This revealed to me that the professor was connected to people internationally who see antiretrovirals as our only hope to defeat the AIDS epidemic. ACT UP was started originally by gay males to support their demand for medical treatment against HIV, but in recent years ACT UP on the American east coast, while lobbying fiercely for the increased use of antiretroviral drugs, has equally fiercely attacked ACT UP in San Francisco for exposing these drugs as dangerous.

I also found the Centre for Civil Society that Bond heads has on its Advisory Board Zackie Achmat. When I looked at how the Centre was funded, I found on its list of benefactors such major Western institutions as the Ford and Kellog Foundations, so it is very well connected.

But why did Bond exhibit such defensiveness? It did not make him more credible to me. While engaged on other investigations, I have come to associate a reliance on tags and insults, on 'ad hominem' arguments, with people who are vulnerable if questioned, who are unsure of their ground.

But, had some people become so emotionally involved in the drive to spread antiretroviral drugs as an answer to AIDS, that they are exasperated with having the HIV theory of AIDS questioned and think it unfair to have to continually defend it? But, even if so, surely this does not justify inferring one's opposition is as guilty as those who deny the Holocaust?

So has emotion overwhelmed reason in South Africa? I began to fear I was coming into a quagmire where one gets pilloried for questioning the scientific establishment. On my arrival in South Africa, it didn't help my depression at these events seeing on the road from the airport a large sign proclaiming 'HIV loves sleeping around'. A similar picture dominated the cover of a magazine I picked up at a Johannesburg café. A photo of a young appealing woman was overlain with the headline 'Sweet Sixteen. HIV wants you!' If the local scientific debate was also to be at this level, then perhaps I had better keep my mouth shut on this subject while in this country.

But I was determined to learn more. In the absence of Professor Bond, I accepted the invitation of a specialist known to be a critic of the HIV theory, Dr. David Rasnick, to

---

[358] Expert Opin Drug Saf. 2006 May;5(3):373-81. Mitochondrial disease in the offspring as a result of antiretroviral therapy. Venhoff N, Walker UA. Department of Rheumatology and Clinical Immunology, Medizinische Universitatsklinik, Hugstetterstr. 55, D-79106 Freiburg, Germany.

spend a weekend with himself and his wife Terri at their home near Pretoria. (See photo of Rasnick below [359])

He turned up to collect me wearing a T-shirt that featured his face - along with those of eleven other leading local political or scientific dissenters – with a slogan naming them as 'The dirty dozen'. He was clearly proud of this shirt, produced by those opposed to their research. He felt it meant that they were having some effect. But for me it suggested that that a strictly scientific dispute was getting horribly politicized.

I hoped he would explain to me why he opposed the HIV theory of AIDS – and he did. He gave me the most intensive and mentally challenging personal scientific workshop that weekend that I have ever experienced. At the end he presented me with 3 CDs filled with his research, saying: 'If any scientist is unwilling to explain his theories and justify them, then don't trust him. Any scientist worth his salt will want to share.'

But to my surprise, I found the heart of his work is not AIDS but cancer research –

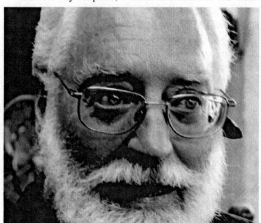

alongside Professor Peter Duesberg, his colleague at Berkeley, who is a Member of the US Science Academy, and, as the author of "Inventing the AIDS Virus,' probably the most famous of the AIDS dissidents. From what I learnt, their current work is revolutionizing our understanding of cancer. They have concluded the cause is not a defective gene or 'oncogene' – as they once suspected – but damaged chromosomes. Since I visited, they have published this research, receiving much scientific praise.

Professor Sam Mhlongo, a friend of President Mbeki and teacher of medicine, came for dinner that Saturday night with his wife Marie.[360] He had studied medicine in London and it was there, he said, that he had come to question the cause of AIDS – as also did President Mbeki. Both Mhlongo and Mbeki's heads were on Rasnick's t-shirt. But, what was particularly notable was that never once did I hear Mhlongo or Rasnick abuse their scientific opposition. Their aim, they said, was to get a level playing field for scientific debate.

I learnt that both of them were speaking next weekend at a day-long workshop on AIDS in Soweto. I shared with them some of my research and in response they invited me to speak at the same meeting. I am entirely a medical novice - but they said my research was of value.

Next day, when I pick up my email, I found that Professor Patrick Bond had finally conceded. He had emailed me after I got on the plane to say:

*Hi Janine, ok, I'll find some time on Saturday and try to brief you on this. It is, yes, perhaps the most serious problem here, with at least five million HIV+ people and a government unwilling to provide proper care, justifying its resistance by using Duesberg, Rasnick, Brink et al.*

But by the time I received this, I had already arrived in Johannesburg, had missed the professor, and had gone to see Rasnick to discover his views for myself.

---

[359] Photo by Janine Roberts

[360] Interview with Mhlongo http://www.virusmyth.net/aids/data/jsinterviewsm.htm

I was staying for the first few nights at a B&B in Melville, a suburb of Johannesburg inhabited mostly by white people, with their homes frightenly surrounded by razor wire and electric fences. But when I went down the street I discovered there were wonderful mixed-race cafes nearby.

This B&B was, I soon discovered, a great favourite among journalists and NGO people. Next day when I walked into the breakfast room a guest looked up with astonishment. He asked: 'You are not Jan Roberts?' He introduced himself as Jeff Atkinson from Oxfam. We had last met twenty years ago, in the late 1980s - when his NGO funded my anti-racism work. He explained he was in South Africa to help get cheap antiretrovirals to the people - as 'the government will not help.'

I am by now well aware just how hot this subject is, so I tried to be as low key as possible. I nevertheless wanted to engage him and to explore his views on AIDS. I thus said: ' I have come across a research paper by a top Harvard professor, Myron Essex, a quite conventional man. He reported the bacteria that cause TB can test as if HIV in the HIV test.'

Jeff reacted as if he had been stung. 'What do you mean, explain yourself? What do you mean?'

I replied that it surely was obvious. He repeated his question, his voice rising sharply.

Somewhat bemused I replied that this meant: 'If the HIV test on occasion detects an antibody against TB bacteria and not HIV, this means antiretroviral medicine would be entirely inappropriate for that patient. What they would need would be drugs against their bacteria infection.'

This gets me nowhere. My mention of the inappropriate use of antiretrovirals seems to mean that he can put me into a slot – that of a woman misled by the crazily stubborn deniers of the HIV doctrine! I tell him I am quoting Professor Essex, a member of the US Government's Task Force on AIDS – but it is no use. He rolls his eyes and says something like; 'So that is what you think'

I think, what else can I say without stirring up a pointless confrontation with a man who is otherwise an ally.

I mention the loose rules for AIDS diagnosis given by WHO for Africa - how it expressly says persistent diarrhoea, intermittent fever and a persistent itch (dermatitis) is all an African needs to be diagnosed with sexually transmitted AIDS. He looks blankly at me. It seems he has never heard of this. But when I say 'the theory' of HIV and AIDS, he interjects: 'The THEORY of HIV'! She says 'The Theory.'' He sits back as if he has delivered a killer blow. It seems I should have said 'the Doctrine'.

At this point a London Times correspondent staying in the house, joins in the conversation. 'My wife would sort you out if she were here. She would love to. I would enjoy watching it.' It turned out that his wife was currently writing a report on AIDS for an international agency.

It made me feel very much the outsider. It seemed it is now fashionable among the great and good, among journalists and NGOs, to wear the HIV/AIDS theory as if it is a Bob Geldof endorsed fashion accessory that puts one among the saints.

As I left, I was asked where I was off to and I replied: 'Soweto.' I do not say what I planned to do there. I don't want to pour oil on the fire. I was in fact off to the Soweto workshop on AIDS. It will be in the main Community Hall - the very place from which Nelson Mandela and the ANC had led the anti apartheid movement.

I found Soweto very different from Johannesburg. A population over 3 million - some say six. As I entered I saw little sign of razor wire and no electric fences. Unexpectedly, it was a more relaxed place, with clean streets, built on the other side of the gold mine dumps that line the southern side of central Johannesburg. Professor Sam Mhlongo acted as my tour guide. He told us that the one hospital we passed had to serve the entire Soweto population of six million - and that unemployment rates were savage. He was one of the founders of PAC, a more militant ANC. They started it at this same community hall. When I entered, I was surprised to find two solid rows of seats filled by men and women in red uniforms, with the words' Traditional Healer' across their chests. They were the herbalists and doctors of the people. Most Africans trust them more than they do the western trained doctor.

Professor Sam Mhlongo told me he was surprised to discover that many of these doubted the HIV theory of AIDS, and had continued to treat the symptoms of illness rather than use blood tests to find invisible symptoms.

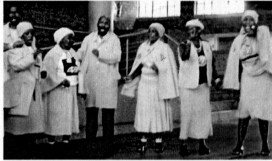

The healers started the proceedings with a greeting dance and then the first speaker was from Living Positively, for people found HIV positive. She said they were glad to be able to discuss the science - and needed to know more. A translator accompanied most talks - for English was the second language, or third, for most present.

Mhlongo told how President Mbeki soon after coming into office had asked his chief medical officer if he had read Professor Duesberg, Professor De Harven or the Perth Group on AIDS, only to be told that he had never heard of them. Mbeki later asked Sam: 'What can I do if they will not read?'

Mbeki in 2000 formed a 'Presidential AIDS Advisory Panel,' with two thirds of the invited members prominent scientists who believed HIV caused AIDS, and one third prominent scientists who were not so convinced. Among those invited were Dr. Robert Gallo, Professor Luc Montagnier and Professor Peter Duesberg.

The end result was a report that described crucial experiments that could prove once and for all if HIV caused AIDS or did not. When I asked Sam what happened to this much needed research, he replied, 'The report went to Cabinet, and it voted in favour of funding these experiment.' 'Have they then been done? I asked. 'No', he said, 'Their funding has been blocked lower down.' I asked how, and he shrugged. It seemed it was still at an impasse.

When Rasnick spoke, he passionately declared the HIV tests should be banned, since they were based on very poor science and misleading. He went on to describe the science behind these tests and the health statistics for South Africa, concluding that there was no statistical evidence to support the view that large numbers were dying of AIDS.

I finished up my own brief talk by holding up the altered draft of the Popovic scientific paper that is still widely cited as proving HIV to cause AIDS. (See Appendix below) Everyone could see that it was covered in handwritten changes. For me, this original paper reveals it was not simply a disagreement between scientists. All science is based on trust that the foundation research is documented in honest and accurate papers. If this work is inaccurate, or worse – fraudulent, it undermines the validity of the work based on it. Afterwards one of the most senior of the traditional healers present, a woman, made a point of personally thanking me for this information.

I then travelled to visit diamond mineworkers living in shanties next to lucrative diamond mines. Whenever I mentioned to them AIDS, they were keen for more information, saying they were given very little. I found among them little of the emotion, and none of the outrage, that accompanied the subject when I spoke of it to people in NGOs. They seemed genuinely interested in what I knew.

I did not have to say much for an animated discussion to begin. Once I had presented the research that showed TB bacteria and fungi test positive in the HIV test, they realized the implications. They all knew that TB was by far the biggest killer in their country – and quickly concluded that it might be this that the HIV test was picking up. On the same 2006 trip to South Africa I also met with Professor Emeritus of Occupational Health, Tony Davies. He told me that TB bacteria can be found in all adult humans – but this does not mean they are all ill with TB! Other factors seem to be required to make the bacteria dangerous.[361]

I then learnt from the mineworkers, and from Professor Davies, just how dangerous is the dust in the diamond mines. The owner of these mines, De Beers, claims that it is harmless and thus will not spray water to suppress it, as normal in other mines. But Davies told me that, when 200 retired miners from the Premier Diamond Mine were tested, every single one was found to have asbestosis. This was not surprising as diamonds are sometimes found in mines in Chrysolite or white asbestos – with De Beers' mines reported by scientists to be thick in asbestos fibres, something that I documented in my previous book 'Glitter and Greed.'. Yet very few know of this danger. It has been kept hidden for decades.[362] De Beers' reports say the dust is not a danger. It seems to link the TB to AIDS, inferring that working conditions in its mines are irrelevant. I now had to ask – were the TB bacteria multiplying in lungs that are already critically damaged by toxic dust?

What I had learnt in South Africa has made me ask, 'What do we need to resolve the AIDS crisis?' Is it a Galileo? Are we sure that we don't have such a person among the dissident ranks? I have now read closely-argued paper after paper on AIDS by senior specialists that cast doubts on the claimed role of HIV – but all such reports seem to have been either ignored by the media or dismissed casually as 'denialist.' Their suggested remedies are ridiculed for not blaming HIV and thus are not tested.

Until AIDS is cured, we surely cannot afford such a luxury as ridicule. We need to consider every theory seriously put forward. Our media should report this debate. Right now we cannot afford to tarnish the reputations of dissident scientists with undeserved and utterly unscientific insults.

When I returned to the UK, I anticipated a quiet period in which I could finish two lengthy articles on AIDS that had been commissioned by the *Ecologist* magazine – as well as completing a chapter on the toxic deadly dust in diamond mines for a new edition of my book on the blood diamonds.

I looked forward to seeing the staff of *The Ecologist* again. Their managing editor, with his health editor, had generously wined and dined me the day before I went to South Africa, telling me to be sure to tell Africans that their magazine would definitely publish my articles on AIDS. They paid me an advance. I was assured repeatedly that the *Ecologist* was not scared to take on the AIDS establishment! After all, they had already published my work on polio and pesticides.

I really appreciated being reassured that day – for I had submitted these articles to them a year earlier and had suspected that the delay in publishing them was due to the managing editor being nervous about challenging the liberal establishment.

But I was now in for a great shock. The managing editor's attitude was dramatically different from the moment I walked in the door. He said my drafts were utterly unworthy of publication. I was absolutely roasted and it was entirely unexpected. My self-pride was

---

[361] This also made me wonder about TB in cattle. Is it right to test them simply for the presence of TB bacteria? Could they have these bacteria without being ill. Were some other factors required to make them ill?

[362] Roberts, Janine. *Glitter and Greed: The Secret World of the Diamond Cartel.* Second Edition 2007, Chapter one. The Disinformation Company, New York.

at stake. My work has been published prominently in magazines and major newspapers over twenty years. Never before had I run into such trouble.

I then learnt that heavyweight experts had contacted the Ecologist in my absence, telling the editor that they should not publish me. It seems that someone had shown them the draft articles I had put up on my website during my African trip. I wondered if this had come about through my correspondence with Professor Bond?

But I weathered the storm, or so I thought. We parted with a written assurance from the managing editor that he would not be deterred from publishing my articles. Some weeks later he wrote to say that he would personally edit the articles – and would definitely be publishing 'powerful versions' – but I was sure that behind the scenes nervousness still ruled. I was thus not surprised when he failed to find time for them before he left the magazine some months later.

He, however, did provide me with copies of two of the emails sent to the Ecologist. The first was addressed to Zac Goldsmith, the owner and editor.

*Dear Zac Goldsmith,*

*Two weeks ago I sent your editorial staff an email asking them if they intended to publish two articles by Janine Roberts called HIVGATE and AIDSGATE. I've not yet received any reply.*

*In case you are still undecided about whether to publish these articles, I thought you might appreciate a more detailed explanation of why I think you should not do so.*

*In the first 14 pages of HIVGATE, Roberts discusses at length four papers written by Robert Gallo and his colleagues in 1984. Gallo's own conclusion was that these four papers 'suggest that [HIV] is the primary cause of AIDS' or 'provide strong evidence of a causative involvement of the virus in AIDS'. Even in 1984 this conclusion was well supported by epidemiological studies of gay men, hemophiliacs and other groups that very strongly suggested an infectious cause. Though nothing in science is ever certain, more than twenty years of research since that time have put the case beyond all reasonable doubt.*

*Leaving aside Roberts' personal opinions about what Gallo and Popovic did or did not do in 1984, it should be stressed that, though they may be historically interesting, these four papers are certainly not necessary for demonstrating that HIV causes AIDS, any more than the 'Principia Mathematica' or the 'Origin of Species' is necessary today to support the theories of gravitation or evolution. It is misleading for Roberts to suggest otherwise.*

*After finishing with Gallo, Roberts moves on to a discussion of HIV testing. Here she says that someone is not confirmed HIV positive until they have had two confirmatory tests. This is true. However she then suggests that these two tests are the p24 test and the viral load test. This is entirely false and misleading.*

*HIV testing in the UK generally consists of a series of three antibody tests. The first of these is designed to be highly sensitive (to minimize false negatives), while the third is highly specific (to minimize false positives). Someone will only be diagnosed with HIV if they test positive on all three antibody tests. Neither the p24 nor the viral load test is ever used for confirmation.*

*The p24 test is among those used to screen blood because it can detect HIV infection sooner than an antibody test. The p24 test may also sometimes be used to test babies (though I believe the PCR test is now more common) because these may retain their mothers' antibodies to HIV for the first few months of life, even if they are not themselves infected, which makes antibody testing unreliable in babies. Roberts' claim that the UK uses the p24 test as 'an official confirmatory test for all' is simply not true.*

*The viral load test is used for monitoring progression of HIV disease and responses to antiretroviral treatment. It is not used for diagnosis. The genetic sequences detected by the viral load test are derived from the genome of isolated HIV. Numerous strains of HIV have been isolated and have had their nine genes sequenced. These nine genes belong to the virus and code for HIV proteins - they are not found in the human genome.*

*Viral load in the blood is a surrogate marker for the progression of HIV disease. As Roberts notes, even counts of 10,000 or more may correspond to quite low concentrations of virus in the blood. However this does not mean that the virus is not present in much higher concentrations elsewhere in the body, or that it is incapable of doing harm. Numerous studies conducted all over the world have found a clear association between viral load and progression to AIDS and death.*

*In her next section Roberts returns to antibody testing and suggests that many test results are false positives. Here she picks selectively from mostly very old studies and ignores the vast mass of literature confirming that HIV antibody tests are among the most accurate in medicine. While it is true that every diagnostic test produces occasional false positives, the proportion found in HIV testing is tiny. Roberts fails to explain why scientists are able to isolate HIV or detect its genetic material in virtually everyone who tests positive and in virtually no one who tests negative. Nor does she try to account for soaring HIV prevalence rates worldwide since the early 1980s, which follow the pattern of other transmissible diseases and correlate with AIDS diagnoses and deaths.*

*The subsequent discussion of antiretroviral treatment is ridiculous for the way it neglects to mention countless studies that have consistently found such treatment to be highly beneficial. If the drugs don't work then why do people who take three drugs fare so much better than those who take only two (as repeatedly demonstrated in large-scale, controlled studies)? Why is recovery after initiating drug treatment associated with a fall in viral load to undetectable levels? Why do people who take the treatment intermittently fare worse than those who take it continuously? How come doctors can predict whether the drugs will be effective by testing a sample of cultured HIV from the patient for drug resistance? Why has the rate of AIDS diagnoses and deaths plummeted in every industrialized country since triple drug therapy was introduced in 1996-1997?*

*Nobody denies that the drugs can cause some very nasty side-effects. But sadly they are the only thing we know that actually works against HIV/AIDS. And they really are highly effective.*

*Roberts says, 'But what happens if antiretroviral drugs are not administered? Extraordinarily, there are practically no studies published on this'. This is, of course, completely untrue. Several very extensive monitoring studies have found the average time from HIV infection to AIDS diagnosis, in the absence of treatment, to be around ten years. Only a very small minority do not develop AIDS within twenty years.*

*Roberts says, 'These drugs do not target HIV itself - they are not designed to do so; and, despite their name, they do not directly target retroviruses.' Again this is not true. NRTI and NNRTI drugs target a retrovirus protein called reverse transcriptase, while protease inhibitors and fusion inhibitors were specifically engineered to target HIV's unique form of protease and gp41 (an HIV surface protein) respectively.*

*Robert says, 'The drugs must soon start to seriously damage the cells of our immune system, since these also reproduce quickly - thus doing the very damage blamed on HIV. As they interfere with DNA, they can also produce cancer.' This is another lie. If Roberts had taken the trouble to read the full text of the article she cites here, she'd have seen it does not support her argument at all.*

*Need I go on?*

*To finish her article in typical fashion, Roberts' presents an analysis of the evidence for heterosexual HIV transmission that ignores most of the relevant studies and misrepresents the rest.*

*In conclusion, HIVGATE is simply not good scientific journalism; nor does it contain anything new. It appears to have been mostly cobbled together from various well-known 'AIDS dissident' websites such as VirusMyth.net and AidsMythExposed.com (which Roberts believes to be a 'large knowledgeable forum'). As such it is littered with false statements, misrepresentations, critical omissions and some quite basic misunderstandings.*

*And AIDSGATE is just as bad.*

*Anyone who has studied the scientific literature or worked with people with HIV/AIDS will recognise these articles for what they are. My concern is that some non-experts could be confused by what appear at first glance to be science-based arguments. At its worst this type of misinformation can kill by dissuading people to take medication that saves lives.*

*I don't think it is in anyone's interest to publish these articles. It certainly won't do The Ecologist's reputation any good.  Sincerely, Rob Noble (AVERT).*[363]

Much of his email was misleading. For instance, he was completely inaccurate on the official UK HIV testing protocols. The UK government health websites currently explicitly call p24 testing one of the primary confirming tests that they recommend. In fact the p24 test and the HIV blood test are now combined as one test in the UK. (See the chapter 'Targeting the Real Enemy' below.)

Then, a few days later the *Ecologist* received an email from Professor John Moore of Cornell University in the States. I recognized his name. He had taken the lead in defending the polio vaccine from accusations that it might have spread HIV.

*Dear Mr Ram,* [the managing editor] *I have become aware that The Ecologist intends to publish an article from Ms Roberts that takes the position that HIV is not the cause of AIDS. Ms Roberts has a habit of promoting this view, which runs contrary to all the established scientific facts. You may wish to consider the strongly negative response that the scientific community took to another article from a card-carrying AIDS denialist, Celia Farber, that was recently published in Harper's Magazine in the USA.*

*That article was riddled with errors of fact, to the extent that a rebuttal document and associated commentaries have been posted on the Internet at www.aidstruth.org* [A brand-new website that he had just taken a lead-role in setting up . [364]]. *Harper's Magazine is, I understand, publishing several protest letters as partial acknowledgment of its errors (the magazine's and the article's).*

*Ms Roberts' article is in the same genre as Ms Farber's. I urge you to read the material on the above website and decide whether a reputable magazine like The Ecologist truly wishes to publish an article that runs so counter to scientific truth. The reputation of your magazine in the wider arena of ecology depends upon it publishing articles that are solidly based in science; you should not compromise that reputation by giving space to Ms Roberts to promote her unscientific views on a subject that is not central to the general philosophy of your magazine.*

*Yours sincerely, John P. Moore, PhD Professor of Microbiology and Immunology, Weill Medical College of Cornell University, New York'*[365]

All this I found quite amazing. Quite contrary to what he said, I have never before written on this subject. He seemed to mistake me for a twin of Celia Farber, a writer well known in New York, who has written much on this topic but whom I had not met. I also knew that her publisher, Harpers, stood by the recent article she had contributed on AIDS.

I wrote to the Ecologist in response, suggesting that they publish both the criticism and my defence as a follow-up to my articles:

'*The only real response I feel I should give is to say to my readers - please check the text of these emails against what I actually said in my articles. I think you will find I am being constantly misquoted.*

'*To the first attack by AVERT - I would point out that prior to the publication of the 4 Science Articles, all the research indicated that most cases of AIDS were among the*

---

[363] From AVERT - Averting HIV and AIDS World-wide 4 Brighton Road, Horsham, West Sussex, RH13 5BA, United Kingdom  Tel +44 (0)1403 210202 Fax +44 (0)1403 211001 info@avert.org

[364] The website AIDStruth.org states in 2008: 'Two factors led Moore and like-minded thinkers (who now number 11) to take off the gloves and hit back with AIDSTruth.org , which went online in March 2006.' One of these two factors was Farber's critique in Harpers. The other was the TAC controversy in South Africa.

[365] From: 'John P. Moore' <jpm2003@med.cornell.edu>Date: Thu, 06 Apr 2006 08:56:38 -0400To: <editorial@theecologist.org>Subject: Articles by Janine Roberts

*heavily drug-taking section of the Gay community - with a 90% correlation with those who took nitrite inhalants and 60% correlation with other sniffed recreational drugs - and with the AIDS diseases that killed most people being all related to the respiratory tract.*

'*It is disingenuous to say 'leaving aside Roberts' views as to what Gallo and Popovic did ' - airily dismissing this as irrelevant. I am saying what they did is highly germane. They committed major scientific fraud. The evidence for this is clear and given in my article - and significantly bypassed by this response. Gallo forged the very scientific paper that is heavily cited in the HIV test's patent, that is the scientific basis for this test. These papers are still cited by the health authorities as trustworthy - and are cited in many thousands of papers.*

'*As for the confirming HIV tests, this is a periphery matter not germane to my argument, but you would not know this from his email. I was citing directly from the UK heath authorities. I did not say the p24 test is a usual confirming test but that it is mostly used with babies, I added to this that, since p24 is a common protein not specific to HIV, its presence cannot indicate the presence of HIV, thus making this test totally useless. He misses this important point entirely - and perhaps deliberately.*

'*As for the HIV tests, I would dispute his assertion that they are incredibly accurate. I note that they are tested against the presence of particular proteins - such as p24, not against the virus itself. If these proteins are not unique to HIV, then the test will not work, not matter how well they find these proteins. I also quoted major studies dating from the 1980s right through to the 2000s - not just early studies as he alleges.*

'*On antiretrovirals - may I call his attention to the existence of several scientific studies that show cancer is a known side effect of taking them. I believe the manufacturers acknowledge this in their literature - although, as I said in the article, liver disease is now in the West the major cause of death among those being treated - and a well-known long-term side effect of antiretrovirals. I would however appreciate it if he would provide citations for the numerous studies that he claims show practically all the HIV positive will die of AIDS within twenty years if they do not take these drugs. I am not aware of them.*

'*He also states 'Roberts says, "These drugs do not target HIV itself - they are not designed to do so; and, despite their name, they do not directly target retroviruses." Again this is not true. NRTI and NNRTI drugs target a retrovirus protein called reverse transcriptase.*'

'*I am amazed at this. Every cell of our body possesses reverse transcriptase - this is established cellular biology - as taught to children in our schools. This illustrates precisely the kind of poor science found today in many AIDS studies. If the antiretroviral drug targets reverse transcriptase, it can target our cells or the reverse transcriptase released whenever a cell of our dies - as they do in large numbers when we are on these drugs (Glaxo Wellcome acknowledges that body wasting is a known side effect of these drugs)*

'*I do not deny the existence of AIDS as such - for damaged immune systems are the root cause of many illnesses. However many factors can do this damage - and do.*'

I later learnt that Moore was also engaged at this time in a 'debate' with the Perth Group of scientists who have long questioned if HIV is proven to cause AIDS. They wrote to him stating: 'Let us make it clear that we are not AIDS denialists. That is, we do not deny that in 1981 a syndrome involving a high frequency of KS and a number of opportunistic infections was identified in gay men and subsequently became known as AIDS.' They explained why they disagreed with the HIV theory, citing 73 academic references. But Moore only answered with 2 rude and ungracious notes. He said first that they had said "absolutely nothing that is of any conceivable interest to me ... All you will receive from me is my continued contempt, and derision.' When they again asked for a reasoned reply, he wrote back: 'I despise you and your fellow AIDS denialists, and I regard your level of "scientific analysis" as pitiful and laughable. [signed] John Moore.'[366]

I then astonishingly received an email addressed directly to me, from Dr. Robert Gallo himself.

---

[366] The full correspondence is at http://www.theperthgroup.com/latest.html

**From:**      gallo@umbi.umd.edu
**Subject: HIV/AIDS**
**Date:**      27 April 2006 18:06:16 BDT
**To:**        janine@janineroberts.plus.com
**Reply-To:**            gallo@umbi.umd.edu

*Dear Ms. Roberts,*

*Since you obviously have a built-in bias about the causative role of HIV in AIDS and about me, I am not surprised that you didn't interview me nor find out what in the end happened to S. Hadley's report. Even Congressman Dingell 'disavowed it', and he was going after numerous scientists during that period, and clearly not trying to find anyone free of wrong doing. Even though I'm sure you won't read it I suggest you should take a look at the history myself and Montagnier did (The discovery of HIV as the cause of AIDS. New England Journal of Medicine. 349:2283-2285, 2003.).*

*I'm sure it also doesn't bother you that Montagnier and I have written the history of these events twice, the last being in the New England Journal of Medicine in 2003. We have zero differences of views in the history, not even one comma. I think we are the ones who know the facts and not you and Ms. Hadley who had fed a reporter and some others the nonsense you willingly and I think eagerly swallow. You may not understand that Ms. Hadley is not a scientist, was bent on finding wrong doing, (note there were hundreds of millions of dollars involved in the patent we won for the U.S., and much of that money went to U.S. lawyers representing the French group). I have my thoughts about Ms. Hadley's relationships with these people. Most of us also find Ms. Hadley to be a quite unusual person. Let me leave it at that and the fact that she was ultimately disqualified as a 'qualified' witness.*

*Of all your libelous, vicious untruths the most bizarre is that the Secret Service found evidence of 'forgery' in our books. This is a Hadley fantasy. The Secret Service openly denied any significance of Hadley's putative 'findings'. Moreover, if we were of that kind of people who would do forgery, do you believe we would be stupid enough to then hand over our books? Be aware that in those days no one was even required to keep such records, and if one did, holding on to the books was usually not longer than three years. Hadley was doing her unprofessional work some 6-7 years after those events.*

*I'm sure you do not care but people suffered a great deal in that period. Scientists like Nobelist David Baltimore and his associates and collaborators; the great cancer physician – Bernie Fisher; Popovic, myself, and many many more scientists during Hadley's witch hunts and, of course, our families. Needless to say medical research from many groups was stopped for 4-6 years. This is the true scandal – not the issues you consciously or unconsciously have so distorted. Your writing is as vicious and slanderous as anything I have witnessed. One hopes in vain that if you do not understand the issues or history, you would at least have some human decency and correct what you wrote.*

*Sincerely,*

Robert C. Gallo
Director
Institute of Human Virology
University of Maryland Baltimore
725 W. Lombard Street
Suite S307
Baltimore, MD 21201
phone: 410-706-8614
fax: 410-706-1952
email: gallo@umbi.umd.edu
www.ihv.org

I was not only amazed to receive this – I was astonished by what Gallo had chosen to object to. He did not object to what I wrote about the last minute changes he made to the Popovic paper, nor did he object to my citations from the devastating conclusions of the Office of Research Integrity (ORI) or from the Inspector General's investigations into his work, but only to my mention of what the Secret Service had discovered in his papers.

After receiving this, I thought it best to check what the Secret Service had to say, to make sure I had not made any errors. I have previously investigated many intelligence operations. This has given me contacts I can call on when needed. Within three days, I had the former Head of the Secret Service on the phone, Larry Stewart, the man who had led their investigation into Robert Gallo's HIV research.

He confirmed that they found convincing evidence that many of Gallo's laboratory documents were 'fixed' prior to being presented as evidence `– and were thus fraudulent.

But I was not the first to cite these Secret Service findings. They are also presented in some detail in John Crewdson's 2003 book, *Science Fictions,* as Gallo surely must have known. If he had solid legal objections to my brief mention of the Secret Service findings, then I am sure he would have taken it up earlier with Crewdson.

Crewdson detailed how the Secret Service's forensic laboratory had proved that laboratory records presented as evidence by Gallo were fraudulently created, not on the date stated, not when the experiment was done, but later. This was particularly obvious in one document dated 1984 that reported the use of 'HIV' – years before the virus was given this name. [367]

As for Gallo saying 'Moreover, if we were of that kind of people who would do forgery, do you believe we would be stupid enough to then hand over our books? Gallo had no choice. He had to produce his records in 1985-6. He was legally forced to do so by lawyers acting for the French (thus within the three year period he mentioned); then later these same records were retrieved by the NIH and the Congressional Investigation.

But I was most surprised by his defensiveness. It seems that 23 years after he published his research, he still feels highly vulnerable to challenge.

However, much more pleasurably, the drafts of my AIDS articles had another most unexpected consequence. They led to my being invited to a gathering of 'AIDS dissident' scientists in New York in the summer of 2006 under the auspices of the 'Rethinking AIDS' group. [368] It was called to consider what to do about the refusal of the medical establishment to even consider alternative theories on AIDS.

I expected to meet with a certain amount of paranoia, created by scientific persecution, but I could not have been more wrong. The atmosphere was relaxed, and easy. I met for the first time with Professor Peter Duesberg of Berkeley, a legendary 'dissident' who was the first scientist to describe the genetic codes of retroviruses. (See photo) He was affable, white haired, and quick with his questions. He probed my knowledge gently, asked me

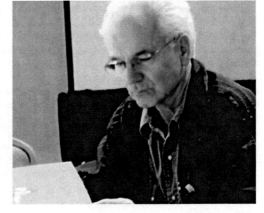

[367] Crewdson, John. *Science Fictions* (page 507-8)
[368] http://www.rethinkingaids.com/

where I stood on the major issues dividing even the dissidents. [369]

I also met with the well-known New York journalist Celia Farber for the first time. As I mentioned, she is the author of a substantial Harpers' article on the problems of the HIV theory– that had caused her to be attacked even more than I had just been. From what they said, it was probably because of the impact of her article that they came after me. They did not want another such piece to appear. But, I was grateful to see that several professors of medicine had leapt to her defence.

On the second day of this gathering, there was a conference phone call from lawyers defending an Australian, Andre Parenzee, who was appealing a conviction for potentially infecting three women with HIV, one of whom later was positive.' His defence team bravely intended to argue that HIV had never been proven to cause AIDS and, perhaps more discreetly, that, since there was legitimate scientific dissent to the theory that HIV caused AIDS, Parenzee could not be reliably convicted.

This court action provided Robert Gallo with another opportunity to defend his theories – this time in February 2007 by video link from the USA to the South Australian Court of Criminal Appeal. The significance of this case was such that it had prompted the prosecution to gather as powerful a team as possible.

After Gallo was sworn in as a witness, he was asked about the early days of AIDS research. He explained that in 1984: 'I was called from Europe to come back to a press conference I did not know would be called, because the Secretary of Health had got hold of our papers that were to be published ...When she got wind of what was in these papers she felt compelled to publish it.'

I was surprised. He was stating on oath that he had no part in the calling of this press conference – or in his papers getting to the Secretary of Health. But the historical records document otherwise. He gave these papers to the Secretary of Heath's department on March 30th, the same day that he gave them to the journal. He had then briefed the press – thus forcing the hand of the Health Secretary. He must have known that patent applications are only valid if applied for in advance of press reports. The Secretary of Health thus had to swiftly apply for a patent for the HIV test, in the course of which she would have to make public the first of the four *Science* papers before it was peer-reviewed as it was the basis of the patent.

As for the earlier French research with HIV, the account he now gave was both at variance with historical records, and with what he had previously admitted to governmental investigators. The French did not succeed, he now said, because they had a 'technical difficulty'. This is not what the NIH concluded. He claimed he discovered how to grow the virus before the French 'in the spring of 1983'. He testified that he had 'isolated HIV' from '48 different patients.' All these claims had been scornfully dismissed as false by these governmental investigators. But he now got away with it – for the Defence did not know of all the contradictions and the Judge was inclined naturally to believe the great expert.

Gallo then rejected the claim that all that he had found were 'endogenous retroviruses' produced naturally by human cells. 'That is utter nonsense and, if it were true, molecularly it is simple to distinguish HIV from endogenous retroviral sequences, they are night and day, it is like a giraffe to a gorilla.' He was not asked to cite any papers to establish this.

Later, when he was asked: 'I want to put to you the suggestion that's been made in this court, that in effect the whole argument that HIV exists rises and falls on the first experiments conducted by Montagnier?' Gallo exploded. He scornfully replied: 'That's silly of course. You know that. I mean everybody knows that sitting in the courtroom.'

He then made an extraordinary claim.

'Scientifically, by 1991 Luc Montagnier acknowledged that what he sent us was the wrong virus, that is – it was a contaminant in his lab. That occurred with an accidental mix up of his original culture, which is a strain of HIV that cannot grow. What we grew was his contaminant, by an accident, in our lab. That also happened in his lab.' In other words, when he secretly tried to grow the French virus, it was not really the French virus. This was an excuse that had earlier been investigated and disallowed.

He finally in frustration had burst out with: 'Stop focussing on the Montagnier paper. The world did not end with the Montagnier paper!' 'Why you are still focused as if the world stood still when he published? I know what I published. Let's deal with what I published.' 'What people want you to forget is that we published 48 isolates and not one was a contaminant of his lab.' Gallo knew the judge and defence council would not be aware that the earlier US governmental investigations had concluded that this claim was false, that none of these 48 were proven to contain the virus.

He then spoke of his 'co-worker Popovic, whose paper was being attacked for what I would call very slight things.' 'Nobody ever in that group (ORI) charged anyone with misappropriating a virus, that was innuendo.' 'The first science paper is the continuous production in the viruses; the technical break-through that led to savings of countless lives on earth. That's the first paper.'

He was asked about the US government investigations of this work and incredibly claimed 'we were totally vindicated as you must know, because you're a man... after all the sound and fury, one would have expected some culpable evidence of wrongdoing. Period! This is not the case – period! I would be glad for you to have that for your records.'

He also testified under oath: 'Just know this: no scientific committee ever found me guilty of a single thing, ever. There was political pressure in an office in Washington by a powerful congressman [John Dingell] that was paralleling some of the worse stages of American history in the past, in some respects. [An apparent reference to the McCarthy witch-hunt for 'communists'.] That congressman went after some scientists, nothing happened.' Gallo conveniently forgot about the successful criminal prosecutions of his co-workers – and how narrowly he had himself escaped prosecution before being pushed out of the NIH.[370]

He then testified about Congressman Dingell: 'His office, not him, apparently put some pressure on people that were lawyers, such as yourself, in an Office of Research Integrity in Washington DC having nothing to do with science.'

This sworn testimony was astonishingly misleading. The reports damming Gallo were written by eminent scientists under the Office of Research Integrity. It was probably the most eminent investigation into scientific error ever held.

Yet, Gallo now continued to testify: 'No scientific review body found me guilty of anything. Lawyers, for a few weeks, did, then dropped it all when my colleague [Popovic], who did the work that was being contested, went forward and it was reviewed by objective people, by scientists, retrovirologists, molecular biologists - a host of people brought into a room like you're in and, over a considerable period of time, evaluated the whole thing and found him totally innocent as well and they dropped anything with me.' 'I went through an inquiry and investigation by scientists, nobody found me guilty of anything. Amen.'

My mouth was agape. He had just reversed under oath the verifiable historical record. It was scientists, not lawyers, who had indicted him. (I extensively quoted them in the ORI indictment *'Offer of Proof.'*) They had a list of about 100 scientists who could testify in support of their indictment. As for his claim that scientists had cleared him, it

[370] John Crewdson. *Science Fictions* Little Brown and Co. 2002 pp 515-517.

was a panel of lawyers, not scientists, who had cleared Popovic of 'intending' to deceive – and who would then have judged him if the case had proceeded.

Gallo next had unpleasant innuendos to make about Suzanne Hadley who had headed both the OSI and Dingell Investigations. He muttered quite nastily in Court; 'She had other problems also that I will not go into, but if I were on trial...'

He added: 'We were not found guilty of anything. I have documented every single one of the 48 isolates we claimed we have.' Hadley reported that these were fraudulent. He was clearly still bitter.

He was then asked about the claim the Perth Group of scientists made, that he did not find HIV, only the activity of reverse transcriptase (RT), an enzyme present in every healthy cell.

He briskly dismissed the idea that the RT found in retroviruses was of the same kind as that found in a cell. He could not possibly have made this error! 'Nobody but the dumbest of the dumb could confuse a retrovirus reverse transcription by innumerable parameters from the reverse transcription process' found in cells. 'I told you before. You would have to be really stupid to confuse the two; beyond stupid.'

This surprised me. It was in his scientific papers. They reported the activity of RT as such. There was no mention of any difference between retroviral and cellular RT.

He was then asked how he came to believe that HIV is spread by sexual transmission. It was easy, he replied: 'One population [heterosexual] doesn't have any HIV at all; another population [gay] has plenty. Of course it had to be oral sex.'

He argued it must be obvious that their 1984 papers were accurate, for when they appeared, the medical establishment stopped funding experiments designed to look for other causes of AIDS. 'Let me put it this way, in '83 people were looking for the cause of AIDS, in '84 the scientific community no longer looked at the cause of AIDS.' He gave an example of research into other possible causes of AIDS that was previously funded to the tune of $40 million dollars but which, he said, was 'terminated' when their 1984 papers appeared.

He moved on to discuss more recent science, claiming that there was only one human retrovirus: 'the only endogenous retrovirus particles known are HERV-K; human endogenous retroviruses K. They make particles  … they can't be transmitted.  They are irrelevant to everything you are talking about.'

I was astonished that he got away with this. There are countless scientific articles published on other kinds of human retroviruses than HERV-K – and many papers that describe how retroviruses pass genetic codes from cell to cell – a process impossible if they cannot 'transmit.' For example:  Katsumata and Yoshika in 1997 reported: 'Endogenous retroviruses and those related genes are thought to be originated from integration of infectious retroviruses to germ cells or evolved from transposable genetic elements.' [371] Professor Shapiro has also recently reported on how cells produce retroviruses to move genetic codes from cell to cell in a continuing process of cellular evolution.[372]

But to return to Gallo's court testimony: when asked if HIV had been 'purified', he confidently replied that they had done this. 'We succeeded in putting 6 of the 48 isolates into permanent culture, meaning in a leukaemic cell line ... The virus came out in great quantities and forever thus making purification already accomplished.' He was totally rewriting the *Science* papers.

---

[371] Katsumata, K., and T. Yoshiki. 1997 [Endogenous retroviruses in autoimmune diseases]. Nippon Rinsho. 55(6):1475-81.

[372] James A. Shapiro *A 21st Century View of evolution* Department of Biochemistry and Molecular Biology, University of Chicago, Chicago, IL 60637

For him, this 1982-4 experiment meant it had become scientifically unnecessary to isolate HIV. 'In fact doing isolation tests now would add time, labour and astronomical costs.' It is also, he said, no longer necessary to electron microscope the virus. 'You don't need micrography any more. You are wasting time and money.' `

In any case, he added, all viruses are identified the same way nowadays. 'This is not unique to HIV... it is done by serology [finding antibodies], not by virus isolation.' He added; 'If more sensitive tests for the presence of the virus are needed, then PCR may be used to find if a viral genetic code sequence is present. However, PCR can only be used as 'a component of evidence. You couldn't use it to prove necessarily a virus [is present].'

As for confirming what proteins came from HIV, for Gallo this was not a problem. He said the genes of HIV encode these proteins, and that these codes never, never, are present in 'normal' human DNA. He gave no confirming evidence for what again was a controversial claim.

When he was asked in Court – how HIV could cause AIDS when antibodies to it are only found in a minority of AIDS patients, in 30.2% of adults with Kaposi sarcoma and 47.6% with opportunistic infections; he pointed out that it was the same for all viral-caused illnesses. 'The viruses cannot be found in all cases. Let me ask you and your witnesses this question: what percentage do you think you can isolate of any virus from any disease, other than in a peak of an acute viremia?'

But, identifying the presence of a virus is one thing. Saying what it does is quite another. He continued: 'we still do not know exactly how polio works. We are still working on a new leads on how influenza causes influenza. There are many ways that HIV leads to impairment of the immune system and some of them are still mysterious.' There may be also 'factors to promote aggression.'

He was finally asked again about the images of HIV published in his 1984 papers. This time he became very rattled. 'Did you listen to anything I said? I told you here is a picture of RF [a sample from the patient RF]. Look at the paper. You see RF, that is us.' But he had no answer when the Defence Council pointed out that his paper reported no electron microscopy was done on the sample from patient RF.

When Gallo was asked to explain why it was hard to take such images, he explained: 'If there is a lot of cellular debris there, it will degrade virus particles and change morphology. If you cultivate it too long the [HIV] envelope will fall off. You won't see knobs if you have minimal production.' Without these knobs, they cannot attach to cells or invade them. Unfortunately Gallo was not asked to how this delicate virus then survives inside us, mixed with so many cells.

With this his evidence came to an end. No further questions were put to him.

## TURNING A DISASTER INTO VICTORY

In all this, Gallo was remarkably defensive. Yet he has had remarkable success since 1994. He was then at a very low point. He was being forced out of the NIH, according to one of the senior scientists involved, Dr. Sam Broder of the NIH, who reportedly stated: 'Believe me, Bob is going to leave here one-way or another. I'm going to tell Bob it is time to retire. And if he doesn't, other things are going to happen. As far as I am concerned, the books can be closed if Bob leaves. But the implications of his leaving will be clear. Bob has beaten a rap. There will be no ticker tape parades.' He then told Gallo: 'You have degraded the institute. You've degraded the public and you have degraded the reporters by lying to them. I have not forgiven you for this. People are dying of real diseases and this is not a game.' [373]

---

[373] John Crewdson *Science Fictions* page 515.

Broder later told Suzanne Hadley: 'Frankly Suzanne, it was a Nobel Prize run. You guys do not talk about this but I was there and I know. And frankly, he almost got it and if he had, he would be invincible.'[374]

The following year Gallo set up his Institute of Human Virology in Baltimore despite some outraged opposition. The *Baltimore Sun* reported on the 11th April 1995: 'Four government scientists have launched an aggressive campaign to withhold state funds for a virology institute in Baltimore from Dr. Robert C. Gallo, renewing claims that the researcher took too much of the credit for major AIDS-related findings. The scientists say that a number of documents, computer disks, and tapes of a British television report show that Gallo committed serious ethical lapses.' One of these scientists was Dr. Suzanne Hadley, who had headed up both the OSI and Congressional investigation teams. The others were also government-employed scientists.

But it seems this challenge was too late. The Maryland Governor had already pledged some $9 million in 'taxpayer dollars' to the planned institute. Since then Gallo has continued to head this Institute and it is where he still works.

His institute in 2008 is launching an appeal for 'philanthropic' funds to endow a permanent Professorial Chair 'in honour of Dr. Robert Gallo' because' 'unleashing his intellect and his passion on some of the world's most intractable afflictions, Dr. Gallo has done more to advance the field of research, in general, and AIDS in particular than any single scientist in the world.' The Institute states: 'The chair's first occupant will be IHV's first visionary, Dr. Gallo.'

What cannot be disputed is that he is the first with his claims. Gallo did not hesitate to tell the Australian Court that he was 'the most referenced scientist in the world between 1980 and 1995.' He boasted 'I was third in the world in impact factor for, I think, the last 25 years' according to the US National Academy of Science.

He would have by July 2007, he said, a total of '27 honorary degrees from universities around the world.' He already held 'the United States' most prestigious prize … the Albert Lasker Award: I've won it twice.' He also had 'Germany's prestigious award – the Frederick Stohlman Memorial Award' and many other awards, some shared with Luc Montagnier, all for work on HIV.

Clearly the multiple charges of scientific fraud had done little to damage his reputation. All is forgotten. He is now feted for discovering HIV and cited for this by virologists and universities around the world.

As for his institute, employing in 2008 around 200 scientists: 'We have enormous involvement with the developing world, especially Nigeria, but including six other African countries, Guinea (sic) in South America and Haiti… by next year in Africa we'll be treating over 100,000.' They were now establishing 'sister institutes; there is one now in Nigeria' and next year one in Mexico.

The chairman of its Scientific Advisory Board is someone we came across earlier. He is Hilary Koprowski, described here as 'the discoverer of the first vaccine against poliomyelitis which was based on oral administration of attenuated polio virus.'

I knew very well just how influential Gallo is. In 2005 his Institute recommended that people be prescribed an intensive and expensive course of antiretroviral drugs if they fear they might have been infected with HIV, say after a night when a condom broke. A year later this became official CDC policy for the USA and for the countries that follow the US lead.

His institute is now developing tests that are likely to label many more people as HIV positive. These are based, not on symptoms of illness, but on finding small fragments of genetic code in the patient's blood that he says come from HIV. Thus a fragment that partially encodes p24 might suffice in future by itself for an HIV diagnosis – despite this

---

[374] Ibid.

protein being in every healthy cell in our body. Thus every one of us is in danger in future of being put on antiretroviral chemotherapy.

When asked about his future research plans, he reported that he was now 'interested in the mechanism of how the virus causes the disease.' This was extraordinary – for it infers that he does not know this despite his earlier claims. He confirmed this by adding that these 'mechanisms' are 'just starting to be unravelled at this point of time.'

He was also continuing to try to develop the HIV vaccine promised in 1984. He explained the delay. 'The antibodies are only specific against the virus you use to make the vaccine, but HIV is highly variable, another horrendous problem for vaccine development.' It seems HIV's genetic code cannot be clearly defined. HIV has so many different forms that 'I don't even keep track of them. We're now getting combinations; there are so many different forms ... Even within an individual with one virus strain, there are micro variants ad nauseam, just endless more variants.' [375]

'This is a disease that science is keeping up with but you have to keep fighting to keep up with it because treatment is life-long and in combination. Life-long treatment is, for most diseases of man, as you know, almost invariably associated with problems of side effects or problems with drug resistance by the microbe in question, so we have a major interest in that as well.'

Today the IHV boasts that it is 'The only academic institution in the world selected by the International AIDS Initiative (IAVI), a group funded by the Gates Foundation, to test the most promising vaccine candidates being evaluated today.'

So it seems this is a field that will absorb the rest of Gallo's life, but, with his more sensitive tests about to appear, I think I can safely predict that his work will make more and more of us test positive with his lucrative HIV test and thus perhaps to spend the rest of our lives on powerful and expensive antiretroviral drugs. [376]

---

[375] Most of the potential 'HIV vaccines' on trial in 2008 are based on inserting a few proteins said to be part of HIV, such as P24, into the shells, 'capsids,' of other viruses and exposing volunteers to these. These trials have only shown either no increase in immunity to AIDS – or even an increased risk of being tested HIV positive as in a Merck trial abandoned in 2007. See *The Continuing HIV vaccine saga'*, http: www.medimmunol.com content 4 1 6. Significantly, none use inactivated or attenuated HIV itself, perhaps because it remains as difficult as Gallo found it in 1984 to isolate and grow?

[376] According to WHO in 2007, an estimated 80% of the 'HIV infected', living in low or middle-income countries, do not know of their infection and their approaching AIDS. Statement made at Sydney CIS 2007 conference.

# Chapter 16

# Searching for fragments

Robert Gallo was joined in his testimony in the Adelaide Court by some of the top AIDS science brains in Australia. [377] Together they told how they were solving the problem that has bedevilled HIV science since 1984 – of how to find HIV itself, as a whole virus, in AIDS patients   This problem, they claimed, was now bypassed. They no longer had a need to find HIV in AIDS patients, no need to isolate HIV, not need to purify it so it can be studied – for modern techniques now meant that HIV can be proved present by finding a tiny fragment of genetic code in the unsorted chaos of a cell culture.

How did they know for certain that a fragment, less than a fortieth of the size of HIV's genome, is from HIV?  Not by studying the whole wild virus it turned out. They reported that scientists have painstakingly assembled out of the milliards of fragments of genetic code found in the blood of AIDS victims, a whole viral genome from which they could clone a retrovirus – one that they were sure was identical to HIV. [378]  By studying this manufactured clone, they believed they had found the exact genetic code of HIV – and thus learnt how to recognize any fragment of it  – an enormous achievement – especially given Gallo's testimony in 2007 that HIV's genome is rapidly and constantly mutating into 'so many forms that I cannot keep track of them.'

But before they gave this explanation to the Court, they were asked about Gallo's claim that he was the first to isolate the 'wild' HIV as found in nature. Surprisingly they did not find this question too easy to answer, despite being experts who jointly had over 80 years of experience in AIDS research.

Dr. David Gordon, the Chair of the Clinical Drug Trials Committee at Flinders University, was sure, 'the virus was first isolated by Montagnier and he published that in 1983,' but Professor Elizabeth Dax of the University of Melbourne was equally convinced that it was isolated by someone 'in 1985', while Professor Martyn French of the University of West Australia, replied 'in 1983, by Gallo and Montagnier.'

However, collectively they gave the prosecution much strength. The financially impoverished Defence team, led by barrister Kevin Borwick, working without fees, were only able to bring to Court two Defence experts, medical physicist Eleni Papadopulos-Eleopulos and Dr. Val Turner, both at the Royal Perth Hospital, a teaching hospital of the University of Western Australia. They had long maintained that HIV was never truly purified and isolated and were certain this also meant its genome and proteins were still not reliably identified.

Eleni Papadopulos-Eleopulos has researched AIDS nearly as long as Robert Gallo. She had submitted for publication a scientific paper suggesting a non-viral cause for AIDS around the same time as Robert Gallo submitted his May 1984 papers. Her training in physics and radiation gave her another viewpoint to that of the virologists – for she was an expert on the damage done to cells by toxins. She has since formed with other scientists the Perth Group, with their papers and articles on AIDS freely available on their website.

---

[377] Rex. v PARENZEE [2007] SASC 143 In the South Australian Supreme Court. Permission to appeal.

[378] Letter from Gallo to Jun Minowada, dated 29th March 1984

[379] As a group they have been influential despite being frequently subjected to abusive attacks because of perceived 'scientific heresy'.

The Court thus wanted to know from the Prosecution's experts what they thought of the Perth Group's view that HIV has never been successfully 'isolated' and 'purified' from all contaminants.

It was immediately evident that for these experts, the verb 'to isolate' had an entirely different meaning from that held outside of virology. It did not mean obtaining a pure sample of a virus free of all contaminants. This they had dismissed as totally unnecessary, saying getting such a sample was an expensive difficult task that modern technology made totally irrelevant.

One of them, Dr. Gordon, testified that it was ridiculous to ask them to do this with HIV, when no virus at all, not flu, not measles, has ever been so isolated! When the Judge asked him: 'Do you need to purify a virus in order to identify it?' His answer was: 'No – not with any virus in fact. I would [question] has any virus ever been purified? The issues are exactly the same with any virus.'

His words made me pause. He seemingly was contradicting himself. He had earlier said that Montagnier isolated HIV in 1983. Now he was questioning if any virus had ever been isolated! What was the truth of this?

He then added 'acceptance of the Defence experts' arguments would lead to the conclusion that no viruses or virus diseases (such as measles, mumps, polio, hepatitis B and C, smallpox and many others) exist at all. ... All the issues, such as antibody testing and virus isolation, these would apply to every single virus. That is impossible.'

No disease viruses have ever been isolated or purified? From what he was now testifying, the issue was essentially not about a particular virus, but about virological theory itself, and the scientific methods it employed to identify the presence of any virus.

This was a great surprise for me – first because I thought this debate was solely about HIV, and secondly because I had understood that only if a virus were isolated from contaminants, could we identify its parts with surety. It now seemed that I was out of date. He with the others was testifying that no virus was purified – it instead was 'isolated' only in the sense of finding a tiny straw of code, less than a thousandth of a whole virus, within a haystack.

This perplexed me. How could a virus be analysed when not separated from other things? How could its parts thus be identified with surety? But, his words reminded me of the government scientists from whom I had learnt that it is literally impossible to remove all contaminants from vaccine cultures. I thus started to understand just what a difficult task virology had set itself in trying to separate out and analyse a virus that is less wide than a light wave.

When Gordon was asked how they detected the presence of HIV in a cell culture, he replied: 'A sample [of fluid thought likely to contain the suspect virus] is added to a cell line that is able to be infected with that particular virus and then the presence of that virus is detected by several methods – either by a change in the appearance of these cells, by their death, or the release of a particular protein from the virus that can be tested for, or by the detection of [part of] the genetic sequence of the virus.' I was again surprised. None of these tests were designed to find the virus itself. All the evidence for its supposed presence was entirely circumstantial.

But, apart from the detection of the genetic code, these experts were testifying that they still used exactly the same methods that Popovic had used when carrying out the final HIV-hunting experiments of March-April 1984. Not one of his tests was for the virus itself. Cellular illnesses were looked for instead.

---

[379] www.theperthgroup.com

Dr. Dominic Dwyer, a Senior Medical Virologist who previously worked at the Institut Pasteur in Paris, expanded on Gordon's testimony[380]. He started by saying that 'the terms virus isolation and virus culture are used interchangeably.' When we try to grow HIV, 'we take lymphocytes we get from the blood banks, as we know they are HIV antibody negative; we stimulate them with compounds such as PHA ... you add a clinical sample [from the patient being tested] and away you go.' His presumption clearly was that any resulting damage to the cells is caused by the sample from the patient, not by PHA.

He then told how they similarly produce other viruses. For example 'with flu, we use other things [than PHA] like trypsin, an enzyme, to make the cell permissive [to enable the cell culture grow the virus in question.]' This was fascinating. The established theory is that a virus infects cells and this makes these cells to produce more such viruses. But he was now emphasizing that an important part of this virus-production process in the lab. is exposing the cells to different toxic chemicals!

Trypsin I knew as a chemical that breaks down proteins. Phytohemagglutinin (PHA) is a mitogenic chemical that forces cells to divide and causes red blood cells to clump together[381] It thus seems that cells have to be chemically stressed to produce viruses – or alternatively to produce RT activity, or to fall ill or die, all of which these specialists took as signifying the presence of viruses. After all I had learnt from studying the polio epidemics, from studying other illnesses blamed on viruses, I had to ask in some amazement, were toxicology textbooks totally banned from virology laboratories? They added a toxin and then blamed the resulting illness solely on a virus.

Dwyer was then asked in court: 'How do you know what you have in there [in the culture] is virus and not some contaminant caused by the cells?'

He answered: 'that's a very good point because you can have contaminants that come out of cell cultures. You see that a lot. ... We need to check the cell lines before we add clinical material to them to make sure they don't have other things in them, like mycoplasma or foamy virus... ... Viruses like some of the herpes viruses, HHV6, HHV-, they arose unrecognised out of cell cultures.'

But he assured the Court: 'Because we have been doing this for a long time, we know how to look after the cells; because of the tests we do on the material that is produced from the infected cultures, we know that it is not something other than HIV.'

He was then asked what tests they did to ensure that only HIV is present. He replied: 'We look to see what the cell lines are looking like. ... The virus will often cause cytopathic effects. In other words, because their cells are infected they look as although they're going to die, and they are dying... in fact sometimes they all clump together and they take on a very bizarre shape.'

Gallo and Popovic had mentioned the same in the first of the four 1984 *Science* papers. They said that the cells clumped together after they added mitogenic chemicals. Gallo suggested this clumping was a reliable test for HIV but it was then found that this effect was produced by the cancerous T-Cells used for the culture, not by the virus.

Gordon went on to say that they look for similar phenomenon in all cell cultures, including cultures growing samples from patients with flu. If the cells start to look sick, then they theorise that the germ they are looking for is present. This is not just for HIV or flu virus. 'This is a principle for all the viruses we culture.' He stressed this: 'Again that is the same principle that we use right now for other things – like influenza cultures or measles cultures. You look what the cells look like. If they have a cytopathic effect [if the cells get ill or die] then you have the various measures of the viruses in them.'

But he then qualified this by saying that the appearance of cellular illness 'doesn't say HIV is causing that effect.' They needed to do another test to discover if it were HIV.

---

[380] At the Institute of Clinical Pathology and Medical Research in Sydney, Australia

[381] Nucleic Acids Res. 1977 August; 4(8): 2713–2723.

'We also do a control culture,' ... growing 'the same' cell culture without putting in the 'clinical sample' of cells from patients. If the cells do not fall ill this time, the cause of the illness must be in the 'clinical sample' from the patients. So far well and good – but what is in this sample that might make them ill?

He had already said that the sample is not pure. Do they study the sample to prove it contains whole 'HIV' viruses? This would be logical – but it is not what happens. Dwyer continued: 'We do other tests. In the case of HIV we look for the production of the p24 antigen which we know to be an HIV antigen – or we look for RT activity, or you can look for genetic sequences of HIV in that cell – which [test] you chose depends entirely on the cost to your laboratory.' 'Should you so desire, you could even do an EM [electron microscopy] – although that is not at all the normal thing to do with viral replication.'

But the electron microscope can only prove particles look like HIV; that is, if it has been proved that HIV has a unique shape, for which no evidence was produced in court. So, do the other indirect tests he mentioned work? Dwyer said they did, because: 'There is a p24 that is unique to HIV [and] the RT of retroviruses is somewhat unique. There are certain parts of the genome [the encoding for the p120 protein] that are essential for viral replication that do not change.'

I was surprised by what he said of p24. Gallo had at one stage claimed this protein 'must' come from former HIV particles as he had found it in AIDS victims, but it is now known to be a normal constituent of healthy cells. I was also aware that Gallo similarly claimed that RT was unique to his virus and that the official scientific investigations of his work proved this to be erroneous.

From Dwyer's testimony, Gallo was fortuitously rescued from error only by the later discovery that p24 from HIV, and RT from HIV, had unique genetic code features that made them different from the common kinds. Professor Dax similarly testified in court: 'HIV p24 has a different sequence to a non-HIV p24.' But, this meant to my mind, that HIV surely must have been isolated, for how else could the unique features of its proteins and enzymes be identified?

Another of the Prosecution witnesses, Dwyer, was not so ready to say that HIV had never been isolated. He stated: 'When you are the first identifier [of a virus], you are required to use these more traditional methods of virus culture and microscopy and so on.' He then went on to say that, since this earlier traditional work had been done successfully, there is now utterly no need to isolate HIV, or any other known virus. 'In fact most of the laboratories around the world have given up doing virus isolation as a diagnostic step.' As for purification, 'we don't do that for any form of virus isolation, whether it be for measles, rubella, influenza.'

He explained they now put their trust in a cheaper technique that we have already come across, PCR or Polymerase Chain Reaction. This enables scientists to match genetic code fragments against primers made from previously identified codes. He testified of this – 'it does not require a great purification step', 'it is pretty cheap, it is extremely reliable and robust' but 'the downside is that you have to know the genetic structure to begin with.'

There I thought was the rub. As I found out earlier, the PCR test can only reliably identify a genetic code fragment as belonging to a certain virus if it is an exact match for a code that has been previously proved unique to that virus.

But one by one the scientists present for the Prosecution swore by PCR –testifying it is the technique they use all the time to look for HIV. They said they did not have to match much of HIV's genetic code to prove that it was present. Generally a tiny snippet, perhaps a 40$^{th}$ of the whole, was enough.

Professor Martyn French similarly testified: 'In routine clinical practice we don't do that [purify]. ... 'That was something that was done many, many years ago in research. In routine clinical practice we only isolate virus particles, not the whole virus.' They now 'use RT PCR' '(Real Time PCR).

This again confirmed the crucial nature of the earlier research– and possibly the critical nature of the flaws in this research that I had earlier discovered. This expert was surely testifying that 'many years ago' the whole genome of HIV must have been sequenced and identified? But when Dr. French was asked: 'Do you know of any published paper that purports to prove that HIV particles have been purified,' he replied; 'I cannot cite you a paper. No.' For me, this made it more and more perplexing.

The Court then moved onto other topics. A recent research paper by a Dr. B. Rodriquez et al. was mentioned that was published in September 27th 2006 issue of *The Journal of the American Medical Association.* This concluded that HIV is not responsible for more than 5-8% of the loss of CD4 immune cells that is necessary to cause AIDS: stating ' across broad categories of HIV RNA levels, only a small proportion of CD4 cell loss variability (4%-6%) could be explained by presenting plasma HIV RNA level.' Therefore he concluded that something else must have killed these cells.

French was now asked what he thought of this research. He accepted its validity and commented: 'It would be more correct to say that AIDS is caused by factors in addition to HIV... this is something we have known about for many years.' 'HIV is necessary but it is not sufficient.' He then continued: 'What we now believe is happening in patients with HIV is that the virus replication stimulates the immune system and activates it. The virus does in itself destroy some cells, but one of its main actions is to stimulate the immune system.'   So HIV does not cause AIDS by killing our immune cells, despite this being what we have been told for years.

Instead HIV is now said to give us AIDS mainly by 'stimulating our immune system.' I had thought stimulating this system a good thing. I now had to resist the urge to see the new theory as saying that HIV tickles us to death. But seriously, this dramatic volte-face shows how utterly baffling HIV's relationship to AIDS has proved to be for over 20 years.

French said the Rodriquez's paper helped explain why there was no obvious relationship between the number of CD4 immune cells in a patient and their 'viral load' of HIV. 'Everyday ... you can see a patient who has a low viral load and advanced CD4 cell depletion, and you can see the opposite.'

His final point was that 'some of the best evidence that HIV exists, and is the cause of AIDS, is that antiretroviral therapy has led to a dramatic drop in the amount of disease and death.'   However, he also acknowledged that there were some HIV positive people who did not require antiretroviral treatment. He called these 'long-term non-progressors' or 'elite controllers.' To these he added the '10% of the population' that did not get AIDS because they had CCR5 gene deletion – the gene that codes for 'a protein molecule that the virus uses' to infect cells.

Another witness, Professor Elizabeth Dax, was the director of the Australian National Serology Laboratory with responsibility for 'the quality of HIV, hepatitis and blood-borne viral testing in Australia' She also stated she was not a virologist – but, from what she said, like many virologists she had anthropomorphised this tiny bundle of proteins and minimal code called HIV.  She called it 'the cunning virus' because it coats itself in healthy human proteins to make it look like part of us – 'one of its clever ways of escaping the immune system.' Also she said this tiny particle 'is very clever at mutating ... another mechanism to escape the immune response.'

She explained that fortunately this devious virus cannot change all of its code. This made it possible for them to recognise it by PCR testing – for example, by finding a fragment of DNA that encoded p24. She concluded with: 'I think this is the gold standard [test for HIV] these days, it's the genetic code.'

As firm evidence that HIV really has been detected, she then produced electron microscope micrographs 'of HIV', but when the judge asked: 'Can you tell us where those photos come from?' she replied: 'No, I can't tell you exactly what the source is... We don't know electron microscopy ... I took those photos off the Internet.' They were of retroviral or vesicle shaped particles scattered among cells. No proof of their HIV status was presented.

But – returning to PCR, I had a niggardly but serious worry. If no isolation was done, how and when was the genetic code of HIV accurately determined? None of the evidence presented to this court had so far explained this. I knew Gallo and Popovic had not published its genetic codes in their famous May 1984 *Science* papers.

Dr. Gordon then helpfully testified that a few scientists have managed to accurately and fully sequence HIV – by cloning it, not by isolating it. He told the Judge this could be done without any need to isolate the virus: 'I might just draw your attention to the fact you can take the genetic material of the virus in a laboratory, you can artificially make the virus and put this into a cell line, and you can produce infectious virus particles.' So it was easier to make than to find them.

Another witness for the Prosecution, Professor Peter McDonald, similarly testified. 'So basically that's evidence that you can take the whole gene sequence, put it in an uninfected cell culture, and then cause more virus to be produced. And that has become pretty much the standard for producing large amounts of virus.'

At first sight, this felt like a clinching argument. They were saying that they could be certain they had identified HIV's genetic codes correctly, because they could clone it in the laboratory from genetic code fragments they found scattered in cultures. They said its RNA has been repeatedly assembled and used to make cloned HIV by different labs throughout the world who had all came up with the same sequence, one that encodes a viable retrovirus – an event that is extremely unlikely to happen by chance.

But then I thought – how can we be sure that the result is the same virus as HIV? They could not test it to see if it causes AIDS in humans. Nor could they easily compare it to 'wild' HIV – since they did not have a pure sample to compare it against.

Putting together the genetic code of HIV must thus have been like assembling a giant jigsaw puzzle without having the original picture. But I wondered if the scientists involved had a template in their mind, a model of an infectious retrovirus, to which they tried to fit the fragments, discarding all those that did not fit – thus making a cloned 'HIV' that was in fact an artefact? I also wondered, when they find the bits do not quite fit, if they have been inclined to blame this on the jigsaw pieces 'mutating?'

Then I found a paper by Gallo and Hahn, published in late 1984, that described their production of 'the first infectious molecular clone of HIV-1.' They said they created this by cloning an assembly of 'proviral DNA' in a phage (bacterial virus) and then in E. Coli bacteria. They then inserted this bacterial/DNA assembly into mammalian cells. They claimed this became an HIV complete with reverse transcriptase! I just could not see this working; for how could they prove the offspring of such a mutant marriage to be HIV? But then I have much to learn.

The cells they thus poisoned with a bacterial/DNA concoction might well have produced endogenous protective retroviruses – or, being very ill, made poorly constructed retroviruses. Another paper pointed out that the cloned HIV produced in the laboratory had proved to be more deadly than real HIV. [382] How then could they say that they had made clones of 'real HIV'?

---

[382] Dufton M. Mwaengo and Francis J. Novembre   Molecular Cloning and Characterization of Viruses Isolated from Chimpanzees with Pathogenic Human Immunodeficiency Virus Type 1 Infections
Journal of Virology, November 1998, p. 8976-8987, Vol. 72,
No.11 http://jvi.asm.org/cgi/content/full/72/11/8976

But did they yet know what the real HIV does? Their easy acceptance of the 2007 Rodriquez paper, that found HIV cannot be killing more than 5% of the T-cells said to be typically missing in AIDS cases, reveals that, at this late stage, they are still trying to resolve what exactly their so-hard-to-find HIV does to cause AIDS.

Professor Peter Duesberg at Berkeley, the best known of the 'dissident' scientists, accepts that a virus known as HIV has been cloned and sequenced – but holds this is incapable of causing AIDS. He is an expert in this field, holding the international credit for being the first to sequence the genetic code of a retrovirus. He thus disagrees with Papadopulos-Eleopolus, the witness for the Defence who maintained that the HIV has not been isolated. She had asked: 'How can one claim cloning of something before there is proof that it ever existed?'

Duesberg answered her challenge thus: 'Cloning is isolation, and is in fact the most rigorous isolation science has to offer for retroviruses,' for, he explained, fragments of genetic code can be extracted from impure cultures without any need to purify. He did this in 1975 before PCR was invented. At that time he broke up viral particles and cells with detergent and discovered some genome codes that seemed to have remained entire. He later said the whole retroviral genome was provably found, since, when it was added to a cell, it produced a retrovirus complete with its enzymes and proteins.[383] But was this product HIV?

He argued this must be HIV since its genetic codes are found in the 'HIV positive' and not the 'HIV negative.' As proof of this he cited an experiment in which 'HIV specific DNA,' as present in the cloned virus, was found in 403 out of 409 HIV-positives and in none of 131 HIV-negative people. [384]

This is a powerful argument – but its accuracy is linked to that of the HIV test and thus to the proteins it uses being proved unique to HIV – something that the inventor of this test never did confirm. Also Duesberg does not conclude from this that HIV or its clone is the cause of AIDS. He suggests that it is a fellow traveller. But I have then to ask; is it then proper to call this clone HIV? Virology always names viruses for the illnesses they are thought to cause. If this clone has not been proved to cause AIDS – then what is it?

I went back to the research papers and found Montagnier reported his cloning was based on the 'genomic DNA of LAV-infected T lymphocytes.' [385] He was thus using as his source the DNA of a blood cell. We now know that the DNA of a blood cell will encode normal non-pathogenic retroviruses.

Could it simply be that the scientists assembling the clones tested them for the inclusion of the codes for the proteins used in the HIV test, presuming these had to be from HIV. I found it hard to believe that they assembled the virus without having some kind of blueprint in mind. If they had – then of course their clones would test positive as Duesberg had reported. They would have been selected to be so!

But in practical terms, the difference between Duesberg and Papadopulos is not so great. From their different standpoints, both conclude that HIV is not the cause of AIDS and that cellular damage from drugs, malnutrition, and other factors, can increase the incidence of the key 'AIDS indicating' diseases without any need for 'HIV.' (More about these theories later.)

---

[383] Peter Duesberg, Continuum Feb./March 1997 'Such infectious nucleic acids initiate replication of virus in uninfected cells from which new virus particles are subsequently released.'

[384] Jackson JB, Kwok SY, Sninsky JJ, Hopsicker JS, Sannerud KJ, Rhame FS, Henry J, Simpson M and Balfour HH Jr.: Human immunodeficiency virus type 1 detected in all seropositive symptomatic and asymptomatic individuals. J. Clin. Microbiol. 28:16-19 (1990).

[385] **Molecular cloning of lymphadenopathy-associated virus**. MARC ALIZON, PIERRE SONIGO, FRANÇOISE BARRÉ-SINOUSSI, JEAN-CLAUDE CHERMANN, PIERRE TIOLLAIS, LUC MONTAGNIER & SIMON WAIN-HOBSON *Nature* **312**, 757 - 760 (20 December 1984);

There is one last thing to report from the Australian court action. Unexpectedly, right at the end, a Nobel Laureate scientist entered the fray. It happened like this. Professor Peter McDonald of Flinders University was so indignant at the attacks on the credibility of the PCR test that he thought to immediately consult Dr. Kary Mullis, who won a Nobel Prize for inventing this test.

He thus emailed him while the Court was still sitting – only to receive a reply that concluded: 'Prosecuting people based on an unproven hypothesis would seem to be unfair and rash.' 'A nucleic acid segment very similar in size and terminal base could easily, in a cursory examination, be mistaken for the sequence in question. If this happened in the course of a normal scientific finding, somebody would finally notice it. Papers are retracted all the time. I am not aware of the nature of the evidence you are considering, but when it comes to legal issues, retractions don't necessarily make up for the original mistake, and if I were to offer advice to the courts system of Australia, I would plead that they realize that the AIDS/HIV issue is what is not settled scientifically, not the effectiveness of PCR.'

Dr. Mullis is one of the eminent scientists who have dared to question the HIV theory. He reported that he was astonished when researching AIDS to find that the evidence underlying the HIV theory was lacking. He states that his invention, the PCR test, is misused in HIV research; that it is a method for studying genetic code fragments, and matching them to similar fragments, not for identifying viruses as the cause of AIDS or of any other illness.

He has said: "Human beings are full of retroviruses … We don't know if it is hundreds or thousands or hundreds of thousands. We've only recently started to look for them. But they've never killed anybody before. People have always survived retroviruses. … The mystery of that damn virus [HIV] has been generated by the $2 billion a year they spend on it. You take any other virus, and you spend $2 billion, and you can make up some great mysteries about it too.' [386]

Why McDonald got in touch with Mullis is something of a mystery, for the views of this Nobel Laureate were attacked earlier during the Court Hearing, when the Defence Counsel asked Prosecution Witness Dr. D. Cooper: 'Who founded polymerase chain reaction (PCR)?'

Cooper had responded: 'One of the AIDS Denialists. He won the Nobel Prize for it. I can't remember his name. It escapes me right now. He won a Nobel Prize for that discovery.'

Counsel: 'Can you remember what he had to say about the use of his technique for the diagnosis of HIV?'

Witness: 'No, I can't remember it.'

Counsel: 'Can't remember it or don't want to remember it.'

Witness: 'Sorry I can't recall what he said because it is just wrong.'

But despite this obvious prejudice, Judge John Sulan in his final judgement explicitly rejected the Nobel Laureate's statements, incredibly calling them 'not supported by research.'

The Judge also ruled that he had no need to consider the issues raised by the two scientists called from Perth as Defence Experts, as their knowledge of AIDS was solely gained by studying the scientific literature over the past 24 years rather than by carrying out their own experiments. He said of Dr. Val Turner, that he was not an Expert as he did not treat AIDS patients (he treats emergency patients) and since: 'His opinions are based on reading scientific literature, studying of scientific literature, and spending a considerable amount of time thinking.' It made no difference to the Judge that Turner, like Papadopulos-Eleopulos, had authored a number of widely reviewed scientific papers

---

[386] Quotations from interviews by Celia Farber published in Spin in July 1994

on the subject. Many a Nobel Laureate would be banished as a court expert, if Judge Sulan's strange rules for expertise were universally followed.

As for Papadopulos-Eleopulos, he dismissed her as 'not independent' since 'she is motivated to create a debate about her theory.' He added: 'I consider that her knowledge is limited to her reading. She has what one might describe as a textbook understanding of the science of viruses, but she has no depth of knowledge or understanding and she simply relies upon written material.' I do not know if she has experimented with AIDS patients, but the judge seemed very strangely unaware of the well-established place there is in science for critical reviews of published material. Such studies frequently appear in peer-reviewed scientific journals, for good science can only be built on a deep understanding of what has come before.

The judge particularly questioned the relevance of her expertise in medical physics as he could not link this to virology, This betrayed that he had not read her original paper on the cause of AIDS, for it seems it was her knowledge of how radiation or chemicals can damage cells that led her to consider non-viral causes of AIDS.

She was belittled by the judge in his conclusion for only teaching in a hospital, albeit one linked to a university. It was not mentioned that this was an extremely distinguished hospital, with two doctors in the same department as herself having won Nobel Prizes in 2005!

He, however, had no difficulty in accepting that the Prosecution Experts really were experts. He accepted their description of the scientific opposition as 'Denialist' without any question. He quoted extensively in his final judgment from a website put up just a few months earlier to defend the HIV theory from a critique written by a journalist, Celia Farber – and astonishingly he even rebuked the Defence Witnesses from not quoting from the same website! [387] Yet this site introduces itself in scarcely a neutral fashion by saying: 'The purpose of this website is to expose the denialist propaganda campaign for what it is, in order to prevent further harm being done to individual and public health.' It then went on to directly attack her.

The Judge finally ruled that, as he had found that the scientific discord over HIV was between expert and non-expert, the case presented by the Defence was invalid and no reason for an Appeal.

However, while this judgement seems very ill based, I was highly intrigued by the case for the Prosecution. Their experts had insisted again and again that they could not have got HIV wrong, for if they had, then they must have got other viruses wrong, such as polio, measles and mumps, as they analysed them all in the same way. They said this was clearly ridiculous – but it made me wonder.

What if they were right? I had looked at poliovirus and HIV in some detail, and found much flawed science. But was the same also true of the research into measles, mumps, rubella and 'flu? Was there something deeply wrong in the normal practices of contemporary virology?

I was being forced to look still more deeply, at the cell and why it made viruses in the first place – for one thing we do know for sure, is that no virus exists that is not made by a cell.

But first there were some other issues I needed to examine.

---

[387] www.AIDStruth.org

# Chapter 17

# Targeting the real enemy with the blood test

Naturally, my thoughts had to turn to the HIV test, since it had come up so frequently in the Australian Court action. The science underpinning its claims to great accuracy was clearly of great importance. The UK Health Department claims that the statistical correlation existing between positive test results and the risk of getting AIDS is definite proof that HIV causes AIDS. [388]

The HIV test does not seek to detect HIV itself, as one might be forgiven for presuming. In late 1985, shortly after it was released, it was reported 'there was and still is no procedure that can detect the presence in blood samples of the HTLV-III [HIV] virus.' [389] Again, this is a terrible dilemma that has always plagued HIV science: the virus cannot be readily found in patients, so something related to it like an antibody is looked for instead.

I went back to the original research on which the HIV test is based and found its patent extensively quotes from and relies solely on the discredited 1984 Popovic paper. There have been only minor changes to this test since. Probably the most significant is the replacement of the natural proteins claimed to be from HIV that it used as targets with synthetic proteins made in their likeness.

If the UK authorities are right about this statistical correlation, I had to ask – how did our scientists get AIDS science right after such a bungled beginning? Since the HIV test was invented, it is estimated that the US has spent some $190 billion dollars on AIDS research without finding a cure or a vaccine. One might have reasonably expected this investment would at least have ensured that any flaws in the original research were corrected – but was it instead good money thrown after bad?

The blood test technically is known as an 'ELISA,' It often involves diluting a sample of the patient's blood 400 times then exposing the result to the 'HIV proteins' provided in the test kit. If enough antibodies in the blood adhere to these proteins, this produces a colour change that indicates a positive result. If these antibodies are present in the right numbers to produce the designated colour change, then it is presumed that the patient's immune system encountered HIV earlier, creating these antibodies as a defence against it. The test thus depends for its accuracy both on the accuracy of the technician's judgement and on the proteins used for the test being previously proved unique to HIV – and the antibodies found being previously proved not to adhere to anything else.

I was thus very surprised to discover that Gallo had sent the 'HIV proteins' needed to make this test off 'in January and February 1984 ... to contract facilities for large-scale production' of the HIV test! [390] This was before Popovic had carried out the crucial

---

[388] Unfortunately it makes this claim without presenting sources or the relevant statistics. The website reference is later in this chapter.

[389] Chicago Tribune (CT) - December 15, 1985; Page: 10. http://www.aegis.org/news/ct/1985/CT851203.html

[390] The Staff Report of the Dingell Congressional Inquiry 1994. Part IV. EVENTS LEADING TO THE APRIL 1984 HHS ANNOUNCEMENT. Section A. Last sentence.

experiments now credited for identifying HIV! At that time Gallo simply did not have any proteins that were proved from HIV. This astonished me, for, if the US Congressional Staff Report that supplied these dates was accurate, this seemed to be clear evidence of fraud! The Congressional Investigation Staff Report stated 'by Dr. Gallo's own testimony, it was not until February 29, 1984, that "the critical serology" ... was performed.'[391]

Gallo must have been supremely confident in their uncompleted research to send off untested proteins to manufacture the HIV test. How could he have been so confident? Was it through an extraordinary act of divination or inspired guesswork – or because he believed he could subsequently alter Popovic's research papers to fit?

Going by the dates, Gallo probably took these proteins from the plasma sample sent by the French. But, even if HIV proteins were present, they would have been mixed with proteins from many sources. There was no way that they could not be. The sample had never been fully purified – as both Gallo and Montagnier have since verified. The latter has even said that the sample did not contain particles that looked like retroviruses![392] At that time they simply did not have the tools to purify their sample. If we cannot purify important vaccine cultures with all the tools available today, how could Gallo have achieved this back in 1984?

Thus it is difficult to see that he had any scientific basis for his HIV test patent. But then I had to ask myself – why are we still using it? Why is it now said to work perfectly? Surely the correlation with increased risk of AIDS means the correct HIV proteins must have been since identified and put to work?

When I checked the historical documents, I was not surprised to find that the blood test immediately proved seriously inaccurate. In 1985 Dr. Robert Chapman, the medical director of a major blood centre, reported that two-thirds of the blood donations that had tested positive for HIV (antibodies) the first time they were checked, did not test positive when they were again checked![393] Dr. Bernard Turnock, Director of the Illinois Department of Public Health stated: 'We now feel that [only] half the individuals (confirmed as HTLV-III [HIV] antibody positive with the test) are carrying the virus.'

Then there is the issue of the original critical PCR tests used to identify genetic codes as from HIV – of which we have heard much in the previous chapter. Much to my surprise I now discovered that, when Gallo supplied third party contractors with the proteins needed to make the HIV blood test 'in January and February 1984', he had also arranged for them to deliver to his laboratory supplies of HIV, 'The contractors in turn provided MOV [another name for LAV or HIV [394]] to the molecular biologists at the LTCB, who used it, among other things, to develop the first cDNA probes for HIV,' for

---

[391] As Above.

[392] Dr Val Turner of the Perth Group reported: 'In an interview published in late 1998 which Montagnier gave to the French journalist Djamel Tahi, Montagnier was asked why he and his colleagues did not publish electron micrographs proving that the 1.16g/ml band (the "purified virus") contained isolated HIV particles. Montagnier answered: No such proof was published, because, even after "Roman effort", at the density of 1.16g/ml they could see no particles with "morphology typical of retroviruses". He gave similar answers to repeated questions, including "I repeat, we did not purify", that is, isolate HIV. See http://www.virusmyth.net/aids/data/dtinterviewlm.htm. The original text, as transcribed from the videotape of the interview at the Pasteur Institute in July 1997 is as follows. Montagnier was asked, "Pourquois les photographies du EM publiées par vous, proviennent de la culture et non de la purifcation?" Montagnier's reply was: "Il y avait tellement peu de production que c'était impossible de voir soit dans un culot de virus à partir d'un gradient. Il n'y avait pas assez de virus pour faire ça. Bien sûr on l'a cherché, on l'a cherché aussi dans les tissus de départ, de la biopsie également. On a vu des particules, mais elles n'avaient pas la morphologie typique des retrovirus. C'était trés différent... relativement différent. Donc avec la culture il a fallu beaucoup d'heures pour trouver les première images. C'tait un travail de romain".

[393] Chicago Tribune December 15, 1985.

[394] The Congressional Staff report states: 'they performed all of these experiments with the IP [Institut Pasteur] virus, first under its own original name ("LAV"), then under two different names -- "MOV" and "HTLV-IIIb."'

use with the PCR technique invented in 1983. [395] This suggests that these vital PCR probes were based on DNA found in fluid samples provided by Gallo before he discovered what caused AIDS!

I need to emphasize just how important this is so please forgive me if I repeat this. The PCR technique relies on the accurate prior identification of genetic codes, To use it to detect the presence of HIV genetic codes, the codes it uses as primers must be previously proved from HIV and unique to HIV. [396] Likewise for the HIV blood test – the proteins used must be proved to be from HIV and nothing else. It now seems that Gallo was so desperate to beat the French, and to possibly win a Nobel Prize, that he cut corners, used untested material, and thus based his HIV test and his vital cDNA probes on guesswork. Those who then used his test were in fact his victims.

It is thus no wonder that Gallo panicked in mid-March 1984 when he saw Popovic's draft paper and realised that he had not proven any virus to cause AIDS. It was not only the publication of his *Science* papers that this put in jeopardy. Gallo had hinged everything on Popovic's success with the French virus. What if it now came out that he had already started to mass-produce the blood test before the critical experiments had been successfully concluded; before he had any evidence that the proteins and genetic codes he planned to use for his patented tests came from HIV?

It seems there was only one thing that was certain in his results. It was his report that only 20% to 50% of the AIDS patients he tested had proved to have antibodies against the proteins he used for the HIV test. No surprise – he had not proved these were from HIV.

Today, whenever the medical industry tests the HIV test's accuracy, they extraordinarily do so by assessing its accuracy in finding antibodies, rather than in detecting the presence of HIV itself. I have searched the medical literature, but have failed to find any experiments carried out to test the reliability of the HIV test against the actual presence in the patient of the entire virus, of HIV itself,

I have instead found that HIV scientists compound this error by testing the PCR technique's accuracy in finding HIV genetic codes by contrasting its results with those of the antibody blood test, again not against finding the virus itself. This is like matching a fingerprint found on a glass with one found on a knife – and forgetting to match these with the fingers of the suspect.

There is also little use of electron microscopy in all this. They could have filtered blood serum to remove all particles larger than retroviruses, and then centrifuged and imaged this to see if any retroviruses seem to be present and then tested these to see if they cause AIDS. This method is not used it seems, because the virus is, as Gallo reported, extraordinarily hard to find in fresh cells from AIDS patients, even with the electron microscope. [397] But even if retroviruses were imaged, it still would be extremely difficult to show that any of these causes AIDS, given how long it is supposed to take.

I had long accepted the validity of the HIV test, but when I tried to think it out logically, it seemed to me that there is something very odd about using an antibody test to identify the presence of a virus – for antibodies are said to remove viruses – and to persist

---

[395] The Staff Report of the Dingell Congressional Inquiry 1994. Part IV. Events Leading To The April 1984 HHS Announcement. Section A. Last sentence.

[396] Professor de Harven kindly commented on my text as part of its pre-publication checking. He wrote on this: 'It is even more crazy than what you explain here! PCR so-called measurements of 'Viral load' are made on homogenates from leucocyte nuclei [from normal human blood]!!! No surprise it is full of human DNA, therefore with plenty of retroviral sequences, since an important percentage of the human genome is analogous to retroviral genome! PCR measurements of the so-called viral load were NEVER done by FIRST trying to isolate retroviral particles from the blood! TOTALLY CRAZY !!! Correlation has NEVER been observed between p24 measurements and PCR viral load... They should go hand in hand, but they don't!

[397] Professor Etienne de Harven, an expert on the use of EM, told the author that he regards the neglect of electron microscopy in HIV research as most remarkable. He regularly used this procedure to image retroviruses.

in the blood, giving us continued protection, long after the virus is defeated and removed. When this test (an 'ELISA') is used to detect rubella antibodies, antibody presence is interpreted to mean the patient is protected from rubella – on the basis that the antibodies have destroyed the viruses! All childhood vaccines are designed to help produce antibodies to protect us. So how did Gallo reverse this common paradigm? When did he prove that his HIV antibodies don't protect us? Why is their presence now said to equate to HIV's undefeated presence? When I surveyed the scientific literature I found Gallo reported in July 1985 that: 'Despite these extensive studies, there are no reports of protective effects of HTLV-III [HIV] antibodies.'[398] Surely this finding should have called into question whether these antibodies were present to fight HIV? If I am to be utterly cynical, it seems Gallo made a test for these particular antibodies solely because he could find them in blood from AIDS patients. He then told the world that the detection of these antibodies was enough to prove that undefeated HIV was present – even if it could not be found and thus his thesis could not be proved!

The antibodies they found might well have been present against other targets than HIV. I have searched the literature but can find no evidence of him trying to prove that they were unique to HIV. Alternatively, they might be total failures – antibodies that are useless against their target. Gallo apparently opted for the latter option without considering the former, as that would have meant failure for him in his hunt.

He instead suggested that HIV antibodies were ineffective because the virus hid itself so well in our cells that, despite the virus stimulating the production of antibodies, these could not find it. He based this on what he thought to be the nature of retroviruses. He believed they invaded cells to incorporate their genetic codes into the cell's DNA in a devious hidden sexual fusion that perpetuated their own kind. Once incorporated, he held they mimicked our natural DNA– and thus were not visible as foreign entities to antibodies. This cunning behaviour, he theorized, made futile the body's efforts to defend itself. Many other theories have since been evolved to explain how HIV evades antibodies, but his was the original theory.

The method he had developed for testing for HIV also ruled out the development of a normal vaccine – for vaccines give us antibodies and thus would make us all test positive! In any case, why use a vaccine to produce antibodies that are useless?

But, the UK Heath Authority currently states on its website that ample evidence for the HIV test's validity now exists, in the form of 'a statistical correlation'. It argues that the test's results prove HIV causes AIDS, since 'those who are HIV infected are far more likely to become ill or die.' But the advice it gives to doctors is still grimmer. It says the HIV test detects not a greater risk, but inevitability. If it is 'positive', if you have these antibodies, you will get AIDS. [399]

Thus the HIV test looks for 'HIV antibodies' that are useless against HIV, and it is terrible news if they are found  – but what exactly are these 'antibodies'?

Antibodies are said to be the smallest of warriors, molecules created by certain white blood cells (the 'B-Cells') to mark foreign molecules for destruction. They do so by being individually designed to stick onto particular surface feature of these molecules.

For Gallo's blood test to work, the features his antibodies attach to must be unique to HIV. If identically shaped features are on other molecules from different pathogens, as sometimes happens, then the same antibody will be effective against all of them – and be created in reaction to any one of them.

So – when did Gallo say these HIV antibodies proven to only target a surface feature on a protein certainly unique to HIV? Again I had to turn back to the research published in the May 1984 *Science* papers, as this is still the basis for this test.

---

[398] Nature, 1985 Jul 4-10;316(6023):72-4.

[399] These statements are from the UK Health Protection Authority's current website - http://www.hpa.org.uk/infections/topics_az/hiv_and_sti/hiv/hiv_causes_aids.htm

What I found in these papers was a simple argument. It said 'extensive accumulation of p24 and p41 [two protein molecules] occurred in the virus preparation' made from 'sera from people with AIDS or pre-AIDS', This was followed by a truly amazing assumption. It said these proteins were so plentiful in the serum, 'they may be considered [HIV] viral structural proteins.' Gallo and his colleagues reported no experiment to verify this. Similarly, other proteins floating loose in the patients' blood serum were said to be parts of HIV on the same basis, that they were plentiful in AIDS patients' blood.

Nowhere in this research could I discover any evidence of an attempt to prove these proteins unique to a particular virus. On the contrary: the supposedly authoritative *Science* papers perplexingly report that the same proteins are also found in two retroviruses that do not cause AIDS! Even more puzzlingly, they state 'p24 ...(is) not detectable in most AIDS patients'! How then could they say finding p24 is the same as finding HIV?

These papers argue instead that these proteins are proved to be from HIV because antibodies 'proved to be against HIV' attack them, and that these antibodies were 'proved to be against HIV' because they attack these proteins – an entirely circuitous argument!

It thus seems that the theory underlying the HIV test fails at the first hurdle – on the basis of the very science quoted in the HIV Test patent – as well as by the way Gallo sent off the proteins to be used for his HIV test before this research had come to a conclusion.

But, all this only makes the more puzzling the UK Health Authorities insistence that they had proved positive HIV test results correlate with a real risk for developing AIDS. After this seemingly mistaken and bungled science, how could this test turn out to be accurate?

## WHAT THE HIV TEST REALLY TELLS US

Earlier in this chapter I mentioned there were two possible explanations for why the antibodies detected with the HIV test are useless to protect us against HIV. One was that the antibodies were really against something else entirely; the other was that these antibodies could not find HIV as it hid itself inside our cells.

HIV science chose the second alternative as a focus for its research – but this route has in over 20 years produced no remedy or vaccine. So –perhaps it is time to consider the alternative – that the antibody detected is there for another purpose than attacking HIV?

I asked myself: what do we know about the illnesses that started the AIDS epidemic, the 'opportunistic infections'? Was it at all possible that the antibodies detected with the HIV test are present to fight, not HIV, but these very real illnesses? If they are, couldn't this explain a correlation between positive results and a risk of getting AIDS – without requiring the presence of HIV, without proving it the cause of AIDS?

Fungal Pneumonia (PCP), alongside severe Thrush, was long the major cause of death in AIDS cases in the West. These fungal infestations still affect over 70% of Western AIDS patients. So, could these antibodies be present to mark fungi for destruction?

In Africa those diagnosed with AIDS often have TB, a disease in which mycobacteria play a major role. Was it possible that the antibodies found with the HIV test are also able to attack these mycobacteria?

Could I go one step further? Could the 'HIV antibodies' found with the test be produced against both mycobacteria and fungi? This at first seemed a highly unlikely hypothesis – for it was just too obvious. Surely this possibility would have been checked when AIDS was first investigated? Then I came across scientific research that showed this is exactly what is happening!

Much to my amazement I have learnt that over a decade ago it was scientifically established that these antibodies directly attach to proteins of both mycobacteria and fungi! For me, discovering this was like finding the final missing piece in a jigsaw. It explained why Africans and Westerners tested positive with the same HIV test despite often suffering with very different opportunistic diseases.

The primary research on mycobacteria is in a paper produced by a scientific team that included Myron Essex of Harvard, a colleague of Gallo in the US Government's AIDS task force, and a co-winner with him of the prestigious Lasker Award.[400]

A paper he co-authored on leprosy, a disease linked to mycobacteria, states 'leprosy patients and their contacts show an unexpectedly high rate of false positive reactivity of HIV-1 proteins on WB (Western Blot tests) [83.6% patients; 64.1% contacts] and ELISA (the HIV Test) … Sera from 63.6% of leprosy patients and 23% of their contacts were repeatedly positive for HIV-1 by ELISA.'

The paper then went on to consider other widespread illnesses linked to mycobacteria, such as TB, saying 'HIV antibodies' also attack TB mycobacteria, giving a false positive result with the HIV test.

It explained that the antibodies found with the HIV Blood tests (both the ELISA and Western Blot) target a 'carbohydrate-containing' feature on the surface of Mycobacterium Tuberculosis and other mycobacteria. The paper concluded: 'ELISA and WB may not be sufficient for HIV diagnosis in AIDS-endemic areas of Central Africa where the prevalence of mycobacterial diseases is quite high'.[401] It warned that even the contacts of TB patients are liable to falsely test positive for HIV.

Other scientists later confirmed and extended this finding. They reported the carbohydrate structure targeted by the 'HIV' antibody is also on molecules from fungi, including the thrush fungus better known as yeast![402] This to my mind is enormously important. It shows why the HIV test can detect a risk for AIDS without HIV being present, in both TB-infected Africa, and among fungi-infected Western AIDS victims.

Also, as countless millions of otherwise healthy people are infected by yeast[403] and minor fungal infections are everywhere, I wondered if this could explain why so many more people test positive than get AIDS; in the UK over twenty times more. A positive HIV result thus might indicate no more than a need for an antifungal medicine.

As for mycobacteria, they are everywhere, even in tap water, but they are normally harmless, even if sometimes they can test as if HIV. Gallo in the 1980s detected 'HIV' in Haiti at a time when mycobacteria-linked TB was prevalent there, as it is a disease strongly associated with poverty and poor living conditions. TB was also at that time treated with large doses of antibiotics, which are very immune suppressant.[404] The same reasons may explain why 'HIV' is now detected among Blacks living in poor conditions within the USA.

At a recent AIDS conference, Professor Papadopulos-Eliopulos of Western Australia presented a transparency contrasting the results of tests for 'HIV antibodies' on leprosy, TB and AIDS patients. The results were indistinguishable from one another. All the samples tested as if positive for 'HIV.'

When I looked at how HIV-positive patients are medically treated today, I found anti-fungal and anti-mycobacterial medicines are commonly prescribed alongside

[400] Kashala O, Marlink R, Ilunga M, et al. Infection with human immunodeficiency virus type 1 (HIV-1) and human T cell lymphotropic viruses among leprosy patients and contacts: correlation between HIV-1 cross-reactivity and antibodies to lipoarabinomannan. J Infect Dis 1994;169:296-304.

[401] Kashala O, et al. J Infec Dis. 1994;169:296-304.

402   Muller WEG, Schroder HC, Reuter P, Maidhof A, Uhlenbruck G, Winkler I. (1990). Polyclonal antibodies to mannan from yeast also recognize the carbohydrate structure of gp120 of the AIDS virus: an approach to raise neutralizing antibodies to HIV-1 infection in vitro. AIDS 4:159-162.

O'Riordan DM, Standing JE, Limper AH. Pneumocystis carinni glycoprotein A binds macrophage mannose receptors. Infect-Immun 1995;63:779-784.

[403] Matthews R, Smith D, Midgley J,. Candida and AIDS: Evidence for protective antibody. Lancet 1988;263-266.

404   *The Coming Plague*. Pp. 515-6.

antiretrovirals, and even given priority over antiretrovirals on the basis that the antiretrovirals interfere with the former's effectiveness. Could this explain beneficial effects from this treatment, despite the absence of a retroviral infection?

When I dug deeper, I found the antibodies detected with the 'HIV test' are now known to target even more molecules. Today the test manufactures warn that 'false-positive' results may occur after a recent flu or tetanus vaccination as well as during malaria, kidney failure, rheumatoid arthritis, herpes, hepatitis and even pregnancy! [405]

This is not a problem that is now fixed. These reports are current. The Indian Government lists online the following as falsely producing a positive HIV test.

'- *Multiple pregnancies*
- *Multiple transfusions*
- *Antibody to gammaglobulinemia (HLA-DR4)* (a common arthritis risk [406])
- *Hypergammaglobulinemia* (low antibody numbers)
- *Antipolystyrene antibodies* (sensitivity to polystyrene)
- *Chronic alcoholism*
- *Hepatitis*
- *Hepatitis immunisation*
- *Technical error etc.'*

Also, a medical work published in 2005, co-authored by Professor Elizabeth Dax, whom we came across as an 'Expert' in the 2007 Australian trial, reports: 'Among the medical conditions that are suspected or occasionally known to produce false-positive screening test results are as follows:

• *Malaria*
• *Syphilis*
• *Pregnancy*
• *Hypergammaglobulinemia, renal failure, liver disease*
• *Some parasitic diseases and viral diseases (e.g., influenza)*
• *Auto-antibodies (autoimmune diseases)*
• *HIV vaccination (becoming a major cause)*
• *Transfusions (usually multiple)'* [407]

The UK government gives other risk factors for a false-positive test: 'Most mistakes in HIV laboratory diagnosis arise from procedural errors such as mislabelling, misplacing specimens in a rack or microplate, cross contamination due to carry over on a pipetted tip or by a splash, faulty transcription of results or bad communications.'

The relationship between pregnancy and falsely testing positive for HIV is particularly disconcerting in South Africa, as I have noted, since WHO bases its estimates for national HIV infection rates there on tests done at antenatal clinics. Malaria is also common in Africa, and as it also falsely tests positive, this again means more and more Africans are being wrongly told they have sexually transmitted HIV.

I have also come across research that very surprisingly reported: 'Normal human serum contains natural antibodies reactive to carbohydrate structures of HIV (glyco)proteins' – meaning that these so-called 'HIV' antibodies are so common that we may all naturally have them! [408] Intriguingly, this suggests that the molecules we call

---

[405] 'transfusions, transplantation, or **pregnancy**, autoimmune disorders, malignancies, alcoholic liver disease, or for reasons that are unclear...' (Archives of Family Medicine. Sept/Oct.2000). 'liver diseases, parenteral substance abuse, hemodialysis, or vaccinations for hepatitis B, rabies, or influenza...' (Archives of Internal Medicine, August 2000).

[406] http://www.bmj.com/cgi/content/full/311/7021/1665 - this risk is found more prevalent among senior academics!

[407] Constantine, Saville and Dax *Retroviral Testing and Quality Assurance, Essentials for Laboratory Diagnosis*

[408] Tomiyama T, Lake D, Masuho Y, et al. Recognition of human immunodeficiency virus glycoproteins by natural anti-carbohydrate antibodies in human serum. Biochem Biophys Res Commun 1991;177:279-285. Its Medline

antibodies are not necessarily present solely to help identify foreign molecules. They could also have other functions entirely.

But then – why do we all not test positive in the HIV test? We all have fungi and mycobacteria in our bodies even when not ill. But I have looked at how the test is performed and have found, I think, the answer. It may lie in the stipulation that blood samples must be diluted 400 times before being tested. This is a highly unusual requirement. When syphilis antibodies are tested for the same type of test (an ELIZA), no dilution at all is required.

This requirement aroused the suspicion of an AIDS researcher, Dr. Roberto Giraldo, who consequently tested his own blood repeatedly, without and with dilution. He found without dilution, he was HIV positive, and with dilution, he was HIV negative.[409] Could it be that without dilution, so many of us would test positive for 'HIV' that the results would be rejected as unbelievable?

In July 2006 the BBC reported the Bill and Melinda Gates Foundation was about to fund research 'to isolate a large number of antibodies from humans and animals, including llamas, to see if they can neutralise HIV.'[410] But – the HIV test is said to work by finding such an antibody! So why are they now looking for it elsewhere? This was getting even more confusing.

## WHAT THEN OF THE OTHER HIV TESTS?

If our blood tests positive in the HIV test, then the sample of our blood is sent for confirmatory tests. Could one of these reliably detect HIV?

In the US the Western Blot test is used for this purpose, but it too only looks for antibodies. For this test the blood sample is separately exposed to the various 'HIV' proteins used. It thus produces a separate reading for each. However, there is no agreement on how the results of a Western Blot should be read. Some countries require for a positive result that 2 proteins test positive, others demand three or four. This means that with the same results a patient could be reported positive for HIV in Europe – but be HIV negative in Australia – then HIV positive again in Africa. In the UK the Western Blot is looked on with some suspicion (perhaps also due to its cost), so two other tests are mostly used – although it's said that one test can suffice if the first is strongly reactive. [411]

---

synopsis reads as follows: Biochem Biophys Res Commun, 1991 May 31;177(1):279-85 Recognition of human immunodeficiency virus glycoproteins by natural anti-carbohydrate antibodies in human serum. Tomiyama T, Lake D, Masuho Y, Hersh EM. Teijin Institute for Biomedical Research, Tokyo, Japan.

Anti-carbohydrate antibodies were isolated from Human immunodeficiency virus (HIV) negative human serum by affinity chromatography using yeast mannan followed by protein A. The purified mannan-binding IgG (MBIgG) bound to HIV glycoproteins gp 160, gp 120 and gp 41 in Western blot. Immunofluorescence revealed that MBIgG bound to HIV/IIIB-infected H9 cells but not to uninfected H9 cells, suggesting that carbohydrate structures recognized by MBIgG are specifically expressed on HIV-infected cells. MBIgG did not neutralize infectivity of HIV. These results show that normal human serum contains natural antibodies reactive to carbohydrate structures of HIV glycoproteins propagated in human cells. PMID: 2043114 [PubMed - indexed for MEDLINE]

[409] Interview with Dr Rodney Richards - 'HIV Tests' Can't Tell You Whether You Have HIV by Mark Gabrish Conlan  *Zenger's Newsmagazine* Oct. 2001

[410] BBC Report Gates gives $287m to HIV research 20 July 2006, 03:49 GMT

[411] UK rules for testing for HIV December 2003,
http://www.hpa.org.uk/cdph/issues/CDPHvol6/No4/6_4guideline1.pdf.
'In England and Wales the prevailing approach is to employ two different tests following the initial reactive screening test.... In many countries laboratories employ a two-test algorithm that examines repeatedly EIA screen reactive specimens by western blot, but in England and Wales, the prevailing approach has been, and remains, to employ at least two different tests following the initial reactive screening test, as recommended by WHO, or an additional screening test with a line immunoassay (LIA)
One of these can be a Western Blot and tests for p24, Igm anti-HIV and viral nucleic acids to determine whether the individual from whom the specimen is collected is truly infected with HIV.' But 'when the first specimen was unambiguously anti-HIV positive, a single strongly reactive test on a follow-up specimen may be considered sufficient to confirm the diagnosis.'

One such confirmatory test can be the 'p24'. This tests for antibodies to the p24 protein. But recent biology research has discovered that p24 plays a key role in the creation of vesicles that our cells use as transports. P24 is a normal part of healthy cells. [412]

Nevertheless the p24 test is routinely used to screen blood supplies and to test babies for HIV infection. It is becoming a key HIV test used alongside the ELISA. The latest versions of the HIV blood test have the p24 test built into them –as p24 is said to be detectable 'earlier after infection' than antibodies. Both tests are thus done at the same time. 'The advent of 4th generation assays, usually in the form of a combined anti-HIV antibody assay (using recombinant and/or synthetic antigens) with an integral test for HIV p24 antigen has been shown to close the diagnostic window by a further 5 to 7 days.' [413]

I suspect that this is because p24 is easy to find. This is not surprising, given the official AIDS Vaccine Clinical Trials Group has reported; 'The presence of p24 band was common among low-risk, **uninfected** volunteers. In another experiment, p24 was detected in 70 of 100 **HIV-negative** and healthy people [414] - while, in yet another experiment, p24 was found only in 24% of 'HIV positive' people! [415]

Whatever the truth of this, Philip Mortimer, a top UK government expert, has reported; 'Experience has shown that neither HIV culture nor tests for p24 antigen are of much value in diagnostic testing.' [416] It is thus disturbing, to say the very least, that, despite it not being 'of much value,' the UK approved it as an HIV test for infants.

Another test, the Viral Load, is often used to see how soon will the HIV positive require antiretroviral drugs – and to monitor the effects of these drugs. But like the others, this does not look for HIV itself. Nor does it count viruses. It uses PCR to look in a sample of our blood for tiny fragments of genetic code said to come from HIV.

Detecting the correct genetic code in our blood is not an easy task, when each of our cells contains 5 feet of DNA, with much of this coming from retroviruses; for, when our cells naturally die, a vast amount of this retroviral code is fragmented out into our blood and thus can be picked up by PCR. If we suffer from body wasting, a common AIDS symptom, then large numbers of such cells will die – giving us a higher load with utterly no need for these retroviral code fragments to come from HIV.

In contrast, a virus contains a length of code some thousandth of a millimetre long – and PCR can only identify a tiny fragment of this by matching it!   PCR multiplies any error in the identification by over a million times – so prior very accurate identification of fragments as certainly from HIV is absolutely vital to this test's validity. [417]

There is no clear correlation between having a high 'viral load' and having AIDS. When I looked at a scientific study of 47 'HIV positive' patients who had refused to take antiretrovirals and remained healthy, I found 30 of these were reported to have viral loads 'higher than 10,000 copies/ml and 3 had viral loads higher than 500,000 copies/ml.' [418]

---

[412] Jutta Rötter, Roland P. Kuiper, Gerrit Bouw and Gerard J. M. Martens Cell-type-specific and selectively induced expression of members of the p24 family of putative cargoreceptors Journal of Cell Science 115, 1049-1058 (2002)

Also Chis Kaiser 'Thinking about p24 proteins and how transport vesicles select their cargo Proceedings of the National Academy of Science, USA' *PNAS* 2000;97;3783-3785

This information is current as of March 2007

[413] UK government regulatory health website, February 2007.

[414] Genesca et al. (1989)

[415] Delord et al. 1991. (quoted in Papadopulos-Eleopulos et al. 1993b, pages 697-699)

[416] Mortimer, P.P. 1989 The AIDS virus and the AIDS test. Medicine Internationale 56, 2334-2339.; Mortimer, P.P. Parry, J.V. & Mortimer, J.Y. 1985 Which anti-HTLV-III/LAV assays for screening and confirmatory testing? Lancet II, 873-877. Refer also footnote 236 in Rebuttal of NIH case http://www.robertogiraldo.com/reference/Johnston_NIH_Rebuttal_March2003.pdf.

[417] Using a technique called Polymerase Chain Reaction (PCR)

[418] Candotti, Daniel et al. Status of long-term asymptomatic HIV-1 infection correlates with viral load but not with virus replication properties and cell tropism. *Journal of Medical Virology* Vol 58. 3. Published 1999

Many events, even vaccinations, may sharply increase the numbers of relevant code fragments in your blood. A medical paper reported that 'increases in HIV RNA [genetic material] levels in blood of as much as 300-fold have been observed within two weeks of routine immunizations against influenza, tetanus, or pneumococcus.'[419] Again, this strongly suggests that this RNA can come from other sources than HIV.

There is finally another test used after 'HIV' diagnosis. This is to measure the damage thought done by HIV. It is called the T-Cell Count and may be ordered immediately a person is found 'HIV positive'. Again, this does not look for HIV. It counts the number of CD4 'Helper T-Cells' in a microlitre sample of blood. It is now said that if you have less than 350 of these present, this is a definite sign that you are starting to get AIDS.

But healthy people typically have a wide range of T-cell numbers– from 237 to 1817 in one study.[420] Also, the relationship between these numbers and the efficacy of our immune system is not so easy to determine. A recent study of 'HIV+' people found many remained 'free of illnesses and of AIDS over three years after their CD4 counts fell below 200'. The CDC itself estimated in 1993 that up to 190,000 Americans had levels this low without showing evident signs of illness.[421] In any case, the CDC does not regard the number of T-Cells present as critical to an AIDS diagnosis. It stated in 2002: 'If a person has been diagnosed with an AIDS Indicator Disease, then that person meets the 1993 AIDS Surveillance Case Definition, regardless of the CD4 count.'

Many factors can cut the number of T-Cells. An article published in *Science* in December 2004 reported that 1 part per million of benzene fumes can cut the CD4 cell numbers in blood by 15 to 18%.[422] Other studies indicate that nitrate inhalant drugs and crack cocaine can dramatically cut the number. Even the stress from being told that you are HIV positive can lower the number.

A study of patients in intensive care in hospitals concluded that low levels of CD4 cells need not involve HIV and are no measure of severity of illness: 'Our results demonstrate that acute illness alone, in the absence of HIV infection, can be associated with profoundly depressed lymphocyte concentrations. Although we hypothesized that this depression would be directly related to the severity of illness, this relationship was not seen in our results. The T-cell depression we observed was unpredictable and did not correlate with severity of illness, predicted mortality rate or survival rate.'[423] In short, no relationship was established between the severity of illness and the numbers of T-Cells.

The 2006 Rodriquez paper cited by the Prosecution in the above Australian HIV trial established that HIV could not be killing 95% of the CD4 cells lost in AIDS cases and concluded: "The results of our study challenge the concept that CD4 cell depletion in chronic HIV infection is mostly attributable to the direct effects of HIV replication. Future efforts to delineate the relative contribution of other mechanisms will be crucial to the understanding of HIV immunopathogenesis and to the ability to attenuate it.'[424]

How then is HIV causing AIDS? This we are told is still a mystery. Robert Gallo testified at the 2007 Australian trial that in future he planned to focus on trying to establish how the virus is linked to AIDS. When asked about his plans, he said he was 'interested in the mechanism of how the virus causes the disease.'

---

[419] Saag MS et al. HIV Viral load markers in clinical practice. Nat Med. 1996 Jun;2(6):625-9.

[420] Ram Yogev *Antiviral treatment of pediatric HIV infection.* P 152

[421] See 1993 CDC Redefinition of AIDS.

[422] Nathaniel Rothman et al. *Science* 2nd December 2004.

[423] Feeney C et al. T-lymphocyte subsets in acute illness. *Crit Care Med.* 1995 Oct;23:1680-5

[424] JAMA September 17th 2006 paper  - link to full text at http://www.duesberg.com/articles/index.html

# Chapter 18

# But Antiretroviral Drugs help AIDS patients?

For the past 20 years the only medical treatment provided officially for AIDS is antiretrovirals; drugs designed, not to cure, but to extend the life of those with AIDS.

All the research aimed at actually curing AIDS has seemingly failed. Thus Dr. Anthony Fauci, the director of the US National Institute of Allergy and Infectious Diseases, was quoted on July 23rd 2007 as saying at a major world AIDS conference: 'As for a cure, let's just stop talking about it' and 'So far we haven't even come close to truly eradicating it in anyone, and I think we should just stop talking about it.'[425] For him, HIV's ability to integrate itself into the genetic makeup of human cells means it is practically impossible to eliminate.

As for vaccines, in 2007 the Merck anti-HIV vaccine trials were abandoned when it was found that its recipients were more likely to get immunodeficiency disorders than if they had not taken it. It turned out that this vaccine was based on an artificially constructed virus made by putting 'HIV' proteins into the emptied shell of a cold virus. But, normally vaccines use weakened or killed samples of the virus said to cause disease. Why did they not do the same with HIV? Because it was too dangerous, answered Merck. But was it because they simply could not find enough 'wild' HIV to weaken or disrupt?

It is often said that HIV is hard to find because retroviruses hide within our cells. But this is not something special to HIV. All viruses cease to exist shortly after they enter a cell. The cell immediately takes them to pieces. With retroviruses, their genetic code is absorbed into the cell's own DNA. The genetic codes of other viruses go elsewhere, often into the cell's cytoplasm. Thus vaccines are developed, not from viruses within cells, but from fluids from laboratory cell cultures that contain the requisite viruses. Did Merck find an HIV laboratory culture too dangerous to use because, in this case, the fluid would be from a culture of cancerous blood cells? There was of course the alternative of 'cloned' HIV constructed artificially in the laboratory. But, as I have reported, this has been found to be more dangerous than natural HIV, as well as probably prohibitively expensive to use for a vaccine.

Antiretroviral drugs are designed to stop our cells from making retroviruses including HIV. Since retroviral codes become an intrinsic part of the cell's nucleus, these cannot be directly attacked within cells without critically damaging the rest of the cell's DNA.[426] These drugs are designed to try to skirt around this problem, by not directly attacking this code, but by hindering the natural processes our cells use to absorb or make retroviruses. A problem with this is that our cells use these very same processes to carry out other essential functions.

These anti-viral drugs also face another major problem. Viruses cannot be killed as such since they are already 'dead!' (More about the biology of viruses later.) This is

---

[425] Associated Press report of 27 July 2007. Fauci was appearing as one of the keynote speakers at the Fourth International AIDS Society Conference on HIV Pathogenesis and Treatment

[426] After 26 years, how does HIV really cause AIDS? Report on the 4th International AIDS Society Conference, July 2007

another reason why these drugs are designed to attack viruses indirectly – by trying to block the entrances that cells might use to absorb them, or by trying to make the cell unable to make them. 'Thus, for the most part, anti-viral agents will also be anti-cell agents.'[427]

I found this strange on reflection. Not only are viruses very hard to isolate, not only is HIV itself near impossible to find in its reported victims; but all viruses are near impossible to directly attack. There is not a single drug that can directly target them. Antibiotics cannot touch them. It made me start to suspect that we may not have properly understood them?

The first licensed anti-viral drug was idoxuridine (1963). It tried to stop virus production by attacking the ability of cells to synthesize DNA. The drug failed. It was reported: 'It is toxic because it lacks specificity, i.e. the drug inhibits the cell's DNA polymerization'[428] In other words, it makes cells critically ill and stops them reproducing.

The first antiretroviral drug was AZT, invented in the 1960s as cancer chemotherapy – but rejected for that purpose as too dangerous. It is now prescribed against HIV, along with other antiretroviral drugs, to delay 'inevitable' deaths. The HIV positive are thus kept on them for life; although ironically, if they had been prescribed them as chemotherapy for cancer, they would have been kept on them for as short a period as possible to avoid serious side effects, as it would be still hoped that they would recover.

Patients are now prescribed a 'cocktail' of three such drugs, with the combination varying as side effects or immunities develop, until their AIDS reaches a near-terminal phase when 'salvage therapy' is prescribed involving a cocktail of 4 to 7 antiretrovirals.[429] It seems 'cocktails' are safer than large doses of one such drug because it is easier for our bodies to tolerate a mixture of challenges.

I wondered if their effectiveness against AIDS was the proof I was searching for that proved a retrovirus the cause of AIDS. Gallo might have got his science wrong – but don't the results achieved with these reveal that eventually HIV scientists did get it right?

The Nobel Laureate, Walter Gilbert, despite having earlier cast doubt on the HIV theory of AIDS, has since testified: 'Today I would regard the success of the many antiviral agents which lower the virus titres and also resolve the failure of the immune system as a reasonable proof of the causation argument [that HIV causes AIDS].' [430]

These drugs are, as their name indicates, not just against HIV, but against all retroviruses, even those normally made by our cells, the ones we presumably need. The reason is that HIV itself, including its genetic code, is extraordinarily hard to detect in human cells. In the HIV positive, less than one in 100,000 of their CD4 immune cells normally show any 'signs' of possible HIV infection. As HIV cannot be singled out, it is presumed that the loss of natural retroviruses is worth the cost of stopping HIV.

But, when I looked at specifically how the drugs are designed to work, I was surprised and somewhat horrified. Their manufacturers report that, to stop virus production, these drugs are aimed against the cell's most basic operations, such as making DNA! This did not make sense. I knew that many patients now have lived on these drugs for years without dying. How could this be? Was it that they are now given very weak doses?

---

[427] http://pathmicro.med.sc.edu/lecture/chemo.htm

[428] As above.

[429] By giving three or more antiretrovirals together, this also minimalises the cells' ability to produce mutations in retroviruses, a possible from of cell defence – and a great frustration to those trying to keep track of the virus.

[430] This was immediately after his admission that his efforts to dose patients with CD4 cells to counter the effect of AIDS had 'failed because the virus in patients didn't have the high affinity for CD4 that the lab-grown virus had.' This to my mind suggests that the cloned HIV virus he was working with is not the same as the putative wild HIV.

AZT is marketed today as 'Retrovir' or 'Zidovudine,' and is one of a class of drugs known as the 'Nucleoside RT Inhibitors' (NRTI). These target the bone marrow cells that make our red blood cells, and are meant to hinder their ability to use RT – the reverse transcriptase enzyme vital to our cell's ability to make new cells. The drugs supply to our cells a useless look-alike ('analogue') of thymine, one of four basic building blocks ('nucleosides') of DNA. If the cells are fooled into using this to make DNA, the process is stopped. The drugs are thus known grimly as 'Terminators.'

How could such a drastic termination be in the slightest bit healthy? Surely it weakens the patient by stopping the replacement of dying cells, thus causing chronic body wasting? So, where is the scientific evidence that this medicine is ultimately safe? No use looking to see if patients recover on it. They are all reported to die of AIDS. But did this impeding of DNA formation make them live for longer?

When I looked for the safety trial AZT must have had before it could be released, I discovered disquietingly that, when it was first developed as chemotherapy against leukaemia, it was rejected for that purpose as too dangerous, since it killed the blood cells it was meant to save.

In 1987, after the US government came under great pressure to release an anti-HIV medicine, it was decided to see if AZT might stop HIV, perhaps because AZT attacked blood cells and HIV was said to infect blood cells! The US health authorities gave it a three-month safety trial but this went seriously wrong when patients in the placebo group, eager to get any drug that could provide a cure, insisted on moving to the group taking AZT. Despite this wrecking its safety trial, making it prove nothing, the need for a drug against HIV was judged to be so urgent that it was still released. Within two years, one third of the patients given AZT on this trial were dead. [431] Today the dose given of AZT has been sharply cut to prevent the deaths that initially resulted from its use.

But, does it still kill blood cells? When it was first released, medical reports said a third of the patients put on this drug soon afterwards required blood transfusions.[432] But, surely by now it has been made safer? When I went to check, I was horrified to find many patients still develop serious anaemia and require blood transfusions. For example, a recent medical report stated: 'In a retrospective evaluation of medical records of 32,867 HIV-infected persons followed in nine cities in the United States ... use of ZDV [AZT] either currently or in the past 6 months was associated with anemia...A total of 41.5% of those with a history of ZDV in the past 6 months and 27.7% of those without such history were anemic at baseline, [there was a] strong statistical associations between worsening parameters of HIV disease and increased likelihood of anaemia.'

Another major study reported: 'For this study, 1278 patient charts were screened, and 758 were included in the study...Of [these], 30.3% (230) were anemic ... Anemia was significantly more prevalent in patients who were currently being treated with HAART regimens containing zidovudine [AZT].' And another study: "We found that 78.2% of the patients with mild or severe anaemia at baseline had received zidovudine [AZT]" [433] A study of 'preterm infants' on AZT found that 'slightly more than half developed anaemia severe enough to require a transfusion.' [434] Today the manufacturers of this drug warn it can kill both white and red blood cells – which is ironic given that HIV is supposed to kill the same cells. Other antiretroviral drugs have since been associated with anaemia 'typically occurring within the first three months of therapy.' But patients are told that

---

[431] A full account of this trial is given in Peter Duesberg *Inventing the AIDS virus.* Pp 314-324.

[432] Walker RE et al. Anemia and erythropoiesis in patients with the acquired immunodeficiency syndrome (AIDS) and Kaposi sarcoma treated with zidovudine. Ann Intern Med. 1988 Mar;108(3):372-6

[433] Mocroft A et al. Anaemia is an independent predictive marker for clinical prognosis of HIV-infected patients from across Europe. AIDS. 1999 May 28;13(8):943-50.

[434] Capparelli E et al. Pharmacokinetics and tolerance of zidovudine in preterm infants. J Pediatr. 2003 Jan

HIV has killed their white blood cells, and that is why they are being prescribed AZT!

Other antiretroviral drugs have also been released without the long-term safety studies and placebo trials mandatory for other drugs, on the grounds that this remains an emergency with no space for time-consuming precautions. A study in *Lancet* in 2000 reported; 'the severity of the HIV epidemic led to accelerated licensing of many antiretroviral agents, often with very little known about long-term safety'.[435]  Today antiretrovirals are still regularly released without long-term safety tests. If they are tested, it is usually only to compare one antiretroviral drug with another. They are rarely tested against placebos as noted below.

Alarmingly, the side effects of these drugs proved difficult to distinguish from the symptoms of AIDS itself.  Thus GSK (GlaxoSmithKline) bluntly warns: 'Prolonged use of Retrovir [AZT] has been associated with systematic myopathy [body wasting] similar to that produced by HIV'.  Their warning is reinforced by a medical reference work *Drug Information for the Health Care Professional* (1996). It reports; 'it is often difficult to differentiate between the manifestations of HIV infection and the manifestations of Zidovudine (AZT). In addition, very little placebo-controlled data is [*sic*] available to assess this difference.'

Despite these drugs frequently being labelled as 'life-saving' in the media, the scientific literature is absolutely full of reports like the following; 'Mitochondrial toxicity of some nucleoside analogues, when used alone or in association, is now well established.' They damage human cells by 'inhibiting mitochondrial DNA synthesis.' [436] Since the mitochondria produce the energy our cells need, the result is a severe lack of energy, body wasting and a greater susceptibility to infections – all symptoms readily observed in AIDS patients.

Likewise the manufacturers warn that the drugs often supplied to HIV positive pregnant women carry a real risk that the children they are carrying will suffer brain damage.[437] There is even a cancer risk.  In September 2005 the CDC reported; 'Data regarding the potential effects of antiretroviral drugs on the developing foetus or neonate are limited. Carcinogenicity and mutagenicity are evident in … **tests for all** FDA-licensed NRTIs.' (Yet they are still licensed!)

The more one reads the scientific literature, the more depressing it gets. The symptoms of AIDS, if not present already, 'often appear shortly' after these drugs are prescribed. A medical study found; 'opportunistic infections, AIDS-associated malignant conditions and other non-infectious diseases ... often appeared shortly after the introduction of HAART.' [438] (HAART being Highly Active Anti Retroviral Treatment or 'Cocktails'.) This is precisely the opposite of what the press usually reports.

Also, critically, as far as I can discover there is little experimental evidence backing the claim that these drugs are responsible for keeping people alive for longer. One highly reputed study actually concluded: 'In our study the observed improved survival cannot be ascribed to HAART.' [439]

PCP is deadly disease; a major killer in AIDS cases, and another research paper concluded that it frequently strikes soon after antiretrovirals are prescribed: 'Among HIV

---

[435] Carr A, Cooper DA. Adverse effects of antiretroviral therapy. *Lancet.* 2000 Oct 21;356:1423-0.

[436] Walker UA et al. Toxicity of nucleoside-analogue reverse-transcriptase inhibitors. *Lancet.* 2000 Mar 25;355(9209):1096.

[437] Stéphane Blanche: Mitochondrial Toxicity Resulting from the Treatment of Pregnant Women and Infants Hosp Necker, Paris, France

[438] DeSimone JA et al. Inflammatory Reactions in HIV-1-Infected Persons after Initiation of Highly Active Antiretroviral Therapy. Ann Int Med. 2000 Sep 19;133(6):447-454.

[439] Morris et al [28: Morris A, Wachter RM, Luce J, Turner J, Huang L. Improved survival with highly active antiretroviral therapy in HIV-infected patients with severe Pneumocystis carinii pneumonia. AIDS 2003; 17: 73-80.

positive patients, PCP manifesting acutely during the initiation anti-retroviral therapy is a well-recognized phenomenon.'[440]

A recent study concluded; 'It is safe to conclude that a cure is extremely unlikely with the current approach to treatment...There is growing concern about the long-term toxicity and adverse effects of therapy, including liver damage and mitochondrial toxicity caused by nucleosides, the most studied anti-HIV drugs. After drugs are approved, fewer organized efforts are made to monitor them for long-term toxicities...the quest for HIV treatment is fuelled by the expensive, technologically oriented approach used in wealthy countries.' [441]

But, if so, then how could these drugs be so widely called 'lifesaving'? How come that they could be featured with Bono on the cover of Vogue in the summer of 2007 as both life transforming and life-saving?

Shockingly, the antiretrovirals provided for the Third World are sometimes so damaging that they are banned in the West! In 2007, Dr. David Cooper reported in Sydney to the largest of all annual international conferences on AIDS, that: 'In the developing world we are giving out the most toxic combinations of drugs, which are not being used in the developed world. We are rolling out these bad regimens, because they are cheap.'

But we still have to look at the other two major classes of these drugs, called the 'Non-Nucleoside RT Inhibitors' and 'Protease Inhibitors', for these are prescribed as part of 'HAART' cocktails along with the above 'Nucleoside RT Inhibitors'.

'Non-Nucleoside RT Inhibitors' attach drug particles to the enzyme RT within cells to prevent it from working, thus hoping to stop cells from making retroviruses. One of these is Nevirapine. In 2002 President Bush made this the centrepiece of US aid to Africa, despite the CDC having warned, on the 5th January 2001, that 'healthy health care workers stuck by needles' should not be given this drug as 'Nevirapine can produce liver damage severe enough to require liver transplants and has caused death." [442] Nevertheless, this drug is still prescribed to pregnant mothers and others in Africa, with strong support from pro-antiretroviral activists and some international agencies. As previously mentioned, this drug has also been linked to serious heart disorders and was unfortunately prescribed to the pro-drug activist Achmat of TAC shortly before he had a heart attack. Another prescribed to him was Stavudine (d4T), a drug reported to cause liver poisoning in 6% to 14% of those taking it.[443] Despite these dangers, he is still continuing his campaign to have these drugs made more widely available in the firm belief that they are protecting him and others from inevitable death from HIV.

There is now a battle royal in South Africa between the Treatment Action Campaign (TAC) headed by Achmat and the Treatment Information Group (TIG) [444] headed by the magistrate Anthony Brink, who, after extensive research, has found that the scientific evidence for these drugs' grave toxicity is now so strong that their prescription may well be a major reason why 6,000 South Africans have died taking HAART since 2004. He concludes that their prescription is criminally irresponsible.[445]

Extraordinarily, the Professor who invented AZT, Richard Beltz, wrote to Brink to say, 'you are justified in sounding a warning against the long-term therapeutic use of

---

[440] http://www.pubmedcentral.nih.gov/articlerender.fcgi?artid=539247

[441] Henry K. The case for more cautious, patient-focused antiretroviral therapy. Ann Int Med. 2000 Feb 15;132(4):306-311.

[442] Sha BE, Proia LA, Kessler HA. Adverse Effects Associated With Use of Nevirapine in HIV Postexposure Prophylaxis for 2 Health Care Workers [second case]. JAMA. 2000 Dec 6.

[443] http://www.medscape.com/viewarticle/413244

[444] Treatment Information Group (TIG)

[445] http://www.tig.org.za/pdf-files/openletter_gsk.pdf Also see http://www.tig.org.za/pdf-files/openletter_gsk.pdf for a description of AZT known side-effects.

AZT, or its use in pregnant women, because of its demonstrated toxicity and side effects. Unfortunately, the devastating effects of AZT emerged only after the final level of experiments was well underway. ... Your effort is a worthy one. I hope you succeed in convincing your government not to make AZT available.'[446]

Today: 'Liver disease has become the leading cause of death among HIV patients at a Massachusetts hospital.'[447] This is also true at many other hospitals. In 2002, at the 14th International AIDS Conference in Barcelona, Dr. Amy Justice of Pittsburgh University produced one of the first surveys of the main cause of death in AIDS victims, based on the records of nearly 6,000 AIDS patients in the US. She reported that today 'the most common cause of death among HIV positive people is liver failure'. These patients were all on antiviral medicines – and liver disease is often highly related to exposure to toxins. When asked if she felt these drugs were involved in their deaths, she replied she did. 'It is the dark side of these drugs.'[448]

Another study grimly reported; 'A comprehensive retrospective review of more than 10,000 adult AIDS patients participating in 21 different AIDS Clinical Trials Group (ACTG) studies [confirms]... that antiretroviral therapy is associated with a high rate of severe hepatotoxicity [liver damage], regardless of drug class or combination.'[449]

Others of these drugs are called 'Protease Inhibitors,' because they target the protease used by our cells to enable the creation of more cells - again an absolutely essential part of life. They have their own very damaging side effects. A study noted: 'Hyperlipidaemia [high levels of blood lipids] at degrees associated with cardiovascular morbidity, occurred in 74% of protease-inhibitor recipients.'[450]

Some of the mechanisms producing these side effects have only recently been discovered. The July 16th 2007 early edition of the *Proceedings of the National Academy of Sciences* reported that HIV protease inhibitors can block a cellular enzyme that helps our cells make the vital scaffolding that supports their nucleus. 'We show, for the first time, that certain HIV protease inhibitor drugs directly inhibit an enzyme called ZMPSTE24, which is important for generating the structural scaffolding supporting the cell nucleus,' said Catherine Coffinier. These grave side effects are not rare. They occur in up to one-third of the patients taking these drugs.

Health professionals unsurprisingly – for they do read these reports – do not have the confidence in these drugs expected of their patients. In September 2005, the CDC reported; 'as a result of toxicity and side effects among health care professionals, a substantial proportion have been unable to complete a full 4-week course.'

But today many of their patients feel so hopeless about what they understand to be an incurable epidemic, that they will embrace, and feel safer, with anything that modern medicine and their doctors endorse.

These drugs nevertheless remain the major Western answer to the AIDS epidemics – although none are claimed to be cures. Dr. Anthony Fauci, Head of the National Institute of Allergy and Infectious Diseases, admitted in 2000. 'There is no hope for a cure for AIDS with the current drugs.'[451]

---

[446] Professor Richard Bletz to Adv. Brink, 11 May 2000.

[447] Liver disease raises questions for AIDS patients. Reuters. 1999 Nov 19

[448] www.lhealsd.org/organfailure.html

[449] High Rate of Severe Liver Toxicity Associated With Antiretroviral Therapy. Reuters Health. 2001 May 23.

[450] Carr A et al. Diagnosis, prediction, and natural course of HIV-1 protease-inhibitor-associated lipodystrophy, hyperlipidaemia, and diabetes mellitus: a cohort study. Lancet. 1999 Jun 19;353(9170):2093-9.

[451] 'There's no hope for a cure for AIDS with current drugs', the head of the National Institute of Allergy and Infectious Diseases (NIAID), Anthony Fauci, said at the 13th International AIDS Conference. 'Eradication is not possible,' Smith M. Current drugs no match for AIDS epidemic: Fauci. *Biotechnology Newswatch*. 2000 Jul 171

But none of this explains why AIDS patients on these drugs are so widely reported to be living longer and healthier lives? Are these reports false? Surely they cannot all be? Many of us know someone on these drugs who is seemingly doing OK.

This conflict is enough to confuse anyone researching this subject – and long perplexed me. When I first learnt how these drugs worked, that they are designed to inhibit normal healthy processes of cellular life, I thought taking them must be a quick death sentence – and so they sometimes proved in early days. But the reality today is, they are reported in the media not to be rapidly killing all the patients on them. Some patients report health improvements – at least in the short term. Had I overlooked something very important?

Was it because the drug doses given today are more carefully monitored, with drugs being changed whenever 'viral loads' go up and CD4 counts down? This surely must be reducing their damage. The reason given for such treatment changes is normally that the virus has acquired 'resistance' to the drugs, not that the drugs are causing undesired side-effects.

Some reports of initial success come from bacterial infections being rapidly cleaned up, as they will also inhibit the production of DNA in bacterial cells, thus killing them off quickly. Secondly, CD4 numbers may well increase initially, as our cells produce them as a defence against toxins. They will make as many as possible before being overwhelmed.

The artificial nucleosides supplied with AZT need to be 'triphosphorylated' by our cells before they can be used to build DNA, but there is now fierce controversy over whether sufficient are so changed for the drugs to work as designed. Does this failure protect us from them? Protease Inhibitors reportedly may also inhibit some of the damage done by other antiretrovirals. But I feel these factors alone cannot explain why these chemotherapy-type drugs are not always accompanied by immediate grave side effects.

Professor James Umber put forward in 2007 a theory that might explain this. He explained that antiretroviral drugs produce Nitrogen Monoxide (NO) – as do other drugs including Poppers, This gas prevents cell death if the antioxidant glutathione, a normal constituent of our cells, is also present. (Thus also producing a low 'Viral Count'). But, if we continue to take these drugs over a medium to long-term period, the NO uses up all the glutathione, and then the damaging effects of Nitrogen Monoxide poisoning will be unleashed, creating such notorious AIDS symptoms as body wasting. [452]

But, while not doubting the relevance of the above important research, I have come to think there is another, more fundamental, reason why people on the antiretroviral drugs are now surviving longer than they did on AZT when it was first released.

## WHAT IF ANTIRETROVIRALS ARE NOW GIVEN TO HEALTHIER PEOPLE?

The widely held belief that 'antiretroviral drugs are staving off death from AIDS' is totally dependent on the assumption that the people prescribed these drugs are about to get AIDS. But, what if this belief is ill founded?

An examination of the 2007 UK official health statistics brings surprising results. They report that, although some 70,000 have been found HIV positive since 1984, less than 800 have been diagnosed with AIDS, less than 3% of those found HIV positive. Nevertheless 38,000 of these HIV positives have been prescribed HAART, meaning that nearly all were prescribed them despite not having AIDS. Likewise, despite the epidemic now being over twenty years old, extremely few of the HIV positives have gone on to get AIDS. [453]

---

[452] J. Umber, Professor of Chemistry. Nancy, France See next chapter.

[453] http://uk.gay.com/article/5516

The time to prescribe these drugs in the West is now decided, not by symptoms of illness, but by the regular monitoring of the 'HIV positive' to discover if they have less than 350 (200 officially in the UK) CD4 T-Cells in an extremely minuscule 1000th of a millilitre blood sample. At this point antiretroviral drugs are prescribed. Yet some 61% of people with 200 or less CD4 cells per unit had no visible symptoms of AIDS illness, according to the CDC in 1997 (the last time they published this statistic). The CDC in 1993 estimated that up to 190,000 untreated Americans had levels this low without showing signs of illness. [454]

In Africa, there are entirely different diagnostic rules for AIDS diagnosis. Under the WHO guidelines, Africans normally need to have symptoms of illness to be diagnosed with AIDS – so they are not healthy when they start on antiretrovirals, unlike in the West. Thus they survive for much less time on these drugs.

But in the West, although many have no outward symptoms of AIDS when prescribed these drugs, the diagnosis will immediately ensure that they are worried sick by being told that these drugs can only delay AIDS, that their life expectancy on the drugs may not be more than three to five years, although more is hoped for – and that they are ill because of shamefully poor sexual hygiene. Such fear and anxiety can by itself suppress their immune systems – and diminish their ability to survive on these drugs without constant medical supervision.

But what happens if antiretrovirals are not administered? Extraordinarily, I could find few studies on this, perhaps because it has been considered unethical to delay giving antiretrovirals, or to have a control group put on placebos? However, a recent study of 'HIV positive' people who had refused these drugs revealed that many remained 'free of illnesses and of AIDS for at least three years after their CD4 counts fell below 200'. [455]

## ANTIRETROVIRALS FOR THE HIV NEGATIVE.

The CDC in January 2005 recommended that immediately a person suspects they may have been exposed to HIV though 'unsafe sex', that they are put on a 'cocktail' of these drugs for 28 days. They recommend starting this treatment within 72 hours of the incident so the drugs can prevent the virus from infecting them. [456]

The CDC did not pull any punches. They recommended an immediate short intense courses of triple cocktails including AZT on the 'assumption that the maximal suppression of viral replication ... will provide the best chances of preventing infection.' [457]   (In all there are 65 'mights' and 22 'possibles' in its statement authorising this drastic treatment.)

Lisa Grohskopf of the CDC explained; 'The new guidelines are designed for use in specific situations, such as an occasional lapse in safer sex methods, a broken condom, rape or one-time sharing of needles.' Ronald O. Valdiserri of the CDC added, in language reminiscent of the moral push of the W. Bush Administration, 'the drugs are not a substitute for abstinence [and] mutual monogamy.' [458]

Unfortunately, this decision means in future the manufacturers of these chemotherapy-type drugs will be able to drive up demand simply by building on our fear and paranoia. [459] Although the CDC says, seek guidance from your doctor if you are not sure about the risk, a broken condom suffices in its judgement. This is likely to lead to a

---

[454] See 1993 CDC Redefinition of AIDS.

[455] As above.

[456] A CDC statement reported by the BBC on Radio 4 on 22nd January 2005.

[457] www.cdc.gov/mmwr/mmwr_rr.html

[458] The CDC has also followed a Bush agenda in withdrawing funding in 2004 it previously gave for AIDS prevention among Gays

[459] www.cdc.gov/mmwr/mmwr_rr.html

vast increase in the use of these drugs – some of whose effects, if their manufacturers are to be believed, cannot be distinguished from AIDS itself.

## HIDING THE SIDE EFFECTS OF ANTIRETROVIRALS

It is supposed to take HIV up to 10 years to destroy the immune system. The antiretroviral drugs can do the job much faster.

In what looks like an attempt to hide that antiretroviral drugs may themselves help bring about AIDS, the HIV orthodoxy has made the complex of illnesses caused by these drugs an illness in its own right! They have named it as Immune Reconstitution Syndrome or IRS. Extraordinarily this supposedly 'new' syndrome has the same associated illnesses as AIDS – as revealed by this list. [460]

| IRS = Anti-retroviral drugs plus one or more of these diseases | AIDS = one or more of these diseases with or without a positive HIV test. |
|---|---|
| Kaposi Sarcoma<br>MAC<br>TB<br>Cryptococcus<br>Fungal Pneumonia PCP<br>Cytomegalovirus<br>Histoplasmosis<br>Herpes<br>Leukoencephalopathy<br>Leprosy<br>Meningitis<br>Lymphoma | Kaposi Sarcoma<br>MAC<br>TB<br>Cryptococcus<br>Fungal Pneumonia PCP<br>Cytomegalovirus<br>Histoplasmosis<br>Herpes<br>Leukoencephalopathy<br>Leprosy<br>Meningitis<br>Lymphoma |
| S. A. Shelburne, et al.,<br>Medicine 81: 213-27, 2002 | CDC HIV/AIDS Surveillance<br>Report, year end edition, 1997 |

'IRS is common and will become more so as HAART is rolled out worldwide;' was the conclusion of a recent scientific paper. [461] It added that IRIS seemed to damage the immune system, for it was accompanied by many signs of bacterial infection.

Another paper reported: 'Fever was the initial manifestation of the illness [IRS] in all [108] patients. It occurred within 2 weeks of starting ZDV [AZT] therapy and was often profound, with temperatures of >40C occurring in some patients. Patient 4 was hospitalized for 5 weeks because of severe and protracted fevers. No cause for the fevers was demonstrated despite extensive investigations ... three patients developed mycobacteraemia [despite not having this infection earlier] 8-25 months after commencement.' [462] Again, it seems that the drugs damage the immune system – making possible diseases commonly associated with AIDS

And another report said: 'It is now also evident that the development of HAART associated immunity can lead to a variety of new clinical manifestations. These have been collectively termed as immune reconstitution inflammatory syndrome (IRIS), immune restoration or immune restitution disease and immune reconstitution

---

[460] Dr David Rasnick. Personal communication with author.

[461] Lipman, Marc; Breen, Ronan: 'Immune reconstitution inflammatory syndrome in HIV. HIV infections and AIDS'; Current Opinion in Infectious Diseases. 19(1):20-25, February 2006

[462] French MA et al. Zidovudine-induced restoration of cell-mediated immunity to mycobacteria in immunodeficient HIV-infected patients. **AIDS**. 1992 Nov;6(11): 1293-7.

phenomena...Paradoxical hypercalcaemia and acute renal failure following initiation of anti-tuberculosis therapy and HAART add to the more commonly described fever, worsening of lung infiltrates, new Lymphadenopathy and swelling of tuberculomata...'

'In a retrospective series based in London, we demonstrated the occurrence of active tuberculosis as an IRIS-like phenomenon in a group of individuals who had recently commenced HAART. [463] This occurred at a median of 37 days, and affected 3% of such patients starting antiretrovirals... The number of clinical conditions associated with credible IRIS phenomena continues to grow. A full description of these is beyond the scope of this review.'

When pressed, some doctors will grudgingly admit most of this but still say the benefits of taking the drugs outweigh the harm. Yet I could not find a single controlled clinical trial that proved people taking these antiretrovirals live longer than do a contemporary similar group of HIV-positive people not on these drugs.

The FDA must know these drugs are not proved to increase survival time, for it requires all manufacturers of antiretrovirals to supply a package slip insert stating clearly that these drugs are not proved to increase survival. The insert for Glaxo's Ziagen drug astonishingly says: 'At this time there is no evidence that Ziagen will help you live longer or have fewer of the medical problems associated with HIV or AIDS.' Merck's protease inhibitor insert is no more encouraging: 'It is not yet known whether Crixivan will extend your life or reduce your chances of getting other illnesses associated with HIV.' The disclaimer for Boehringer Ingelheim's Viramune (also known as Nevirapine) reads: 'At present, there are no results from controlled clinical trials evaluating the effects of Viramune [on] the incidence of opportunistic infections or survival.' I would like to ask, how do our media then justify claiming these drugs are proved to be life extending? Don't they read these inserts? I fear the spin put afterwards on these drugs by their manufacturers and the government departments funding them is proving most deceptive.

The UK government's Heath Agency reported in 2007 that 4.7% of the deaths of the HIV infected were of those who refused antiretroviral treatment. It did not mention the converse; that 95.3% of the deaths were of those who were on antiretrovirals.

It also stated that 30% of the deaths of the HIV positive had 'undetectable viral loads' – in other words, presumably no HIV infection? Also 'about half' had CD4 cell counts above 200 cells/mm3 – so presumably did not have AIDS. Conservatively it then concluded that one third of deaths were not due to HIV.

According to a recent investigation on the BBC, some antiretroviral drugs are scandalously 'safety tested' by major drug companies on uninsured American children in certain children's institutions. If the children are reluctant, and remember many adults drop out of using these drugs because of their serious side effects, the powerful drugs are forcibly administered to the children through surgically inserted stomach tubes. The excuse is that this experiment is to 'save' them, even if they were not clinically ill beforehand. This was documented in a powerful film called 'Guinea- Pig Kids' transmitted on the BBC in December 2004. This was based on the work of investigative journalist Liam Scheff who discovered the Incarnation Children's Center in New York was subjecting orphaned HIV positive children to these trials. [464]

---

[463] Lipman M, Breen R. Immune reconstitution inflammatory syndrome in HIV. Curr Opin Infect Dis. 2006 Feb;19(1):20-5.

[464] This use of children was documented in an outstanding investigation by Liam Scheff in 2004. His work then appeared as a 2004 documentary shown on the BBC; 'are The Guinea-Pig Kids'. It's transcript is available on http://www.acftv.com/pdf/BBC_This%20World_Guinea_Pig_Kids_Transcript.pdf. One caution I must make, the producers described the drugs used on the children as 'experimental' when they were in fact mainstream anti-retrovirals such as AZT and Nevirapine. This is not an error made by Scheff, as can be seen in his earlier excellent article. It should be noted that the TV program was later officially faulted for not saying that the expert it employed had previously come to the conclusion that HIV does not cause AIDS, but it was not faulted for saying that these drugs were forcibly administered, were part of a drug trial, and made the children ill!

This centre stated on its 2003 website that '34 children are currently participating in 7 clinical trials.' It then listed the antiretroviral drugs being tested on the children, mentioning particularly AZT and Nevirapine – two whose many dangers are described above. The Center's children were being 'recruited' into anti-retroviral drug studies organised by Glaxo Wellcome (now GSK) and other major pharmaceutical companies. Apparently, issues of 'compliance', that is, of refusing the drugs, were being treated at local hospitals. Since then Russian children's homes have also been implicated.

Because of the controversy this caused, I went to US governmental sources to verify the records for myself. I found that currently, as of April 2008, there are 15 clinical antiretroviral drug trials that use children from the Incarnation orphans home. One is to 'evaluate the safety and immunogenicity' of drugs on children from one month old who had at the start of the experiment no, repeat no, symptoms of AIDS. Other trials tested on the children the relative safety of AZT and other drugs. One ongoing experiment is subjecting children from 4 years old with experimental cocktails that combine 7 antiretroviral drugs, over twice as many as normal for adults, as a 'Salvage Therapy' for 'Advanced AIDS patients,' using 'higher than usual doses!' The medical notes for this trial state: 'Doctors are seeing many HIV-positive children who did not get good long-term results from the current anti-HIV drugs. Some doctors believe anti-HIV drugs fail because drug levels in the body are too low. In this study, doctors will give patients 7 drugs, some at higher doses than normal. Since it is very important that patients on the study take all of these drugs, doctors will make it as easy as possible.' [465] The drugs are mostly administered in the children's home. They do not say if these children are the victims of other trials, which they may well be, but one can take it from the above that they are approaching death. The official website for the trial lists Incarnation as a participating institution, along with several hospitals and medical centres.

So, apparently the exposure on the BBC has proved useless. These trials are still going ahead at full steam and are still organised by major pharmaceutical firms who are still experimenting on orphaned children from Incarnation, a Christian home in New York.

In fact, similar trials were earlier carried out in London, at the Great Ormond Street Hospital for Sick Children and others around the world, particularly the PENTA I Trial of 1992 that targeted 300 'HIV positive' infants with no AIDS symptoms prior to entering the trial. It tested them to see if giving them powerful AZT would prevent them from getting AIDS – in the utter presumption that they were doomed to AIDS otherwise. As it happened, most of the children selected for this were Blacks. Dr. Nicholson, the editor of the *Bulletin of Medical Ethics* with whom I had met when I started on this journey, stated: 'What on earth is the use of continuing with a trial to find the correct time to start AZT in HIV-positive children when you haven't conclusive evidence that AZT does the children good at any stage?' A similar trial in the USA, in which AZT was given to HIV positive pregnant women, was halted when their children started to be born with too many toes and fingers. [466]

Today most of the $6.5 billion spent annually on AIDS research in the US goes on expanding medical establishments, employing ever more scientists, and developing the vastly profitable antiretrovirals. By 2003 the annual US market for these was worth around $15 billion and expanding.

GlaxoSmithKline made in 2003 over $317 million from AZT sales alone. This drug has now brought the company over $2.5 billion in total. The same company also makes 'Trizivir,' a 'cocktail' of three Nucleoside RT Inhibitors including AZT. When it was launched several deaths occurred within a year. The company told the Financial Times: 'clinical trials have indeed shown that it has a potential for side effects ... patients have

---

[465] http://www.clinicaltrials.gov/ct2/show/NCT00001108?term=incarnation+trials&rank=8

[466] See Joan Shenton ,*Positively False* pages 185-192. 1998 I B Tauris & Co. London.

died from using it.' [467] In its first two years of use, this cocktail brought the company about $350 million in revenue. Its 2006 US price was $1,170 for a month's pills, making it one of the most expensive.

The 'Sydney Declaration,' issued at the 2007 4th International AIDS Society Conference, demanded that all governments 'allot 10% of all resources towards AIDS research.' The conference justified this tremendous demand on the grounds the current drugs are neither completely successful nor safe and thus new ones are needed.

I will finish with the testimony of a person who believes these drugs gave him AIDS.

*'I was 'diagnosed' in 1989. I was prompted to test after my partner at the time decided to get the test and it came back positive. Mine was positive also - CD4 count 462... 'I had no symptoms, but was told; 'Unfortunately, the virus is already destroying your immune system. You must start AZT immediately... Later, I was told I would start to get sick in about 18 months, and then I would get very sick within 2 years - and die.*

*'All I remember for the first several months or so is sleeping, throwing up, an unimaginable nausea, and an unending headache. I got weaker by the day. I lost a lot of my hair.*

*'After a year I thought 'Well, if I only have another year, I'm not spending it like this.' So I stopped the pills.*

*'I slowly got better over the years - I may have made a full recovery that time, I don't know. I started living again, though, for sure. Oh...my CD4 count NEVER went above 500 during the whole experience.*

*But he remained HIV positive. 'In '97, I started 'the cocktail'. Sounded nice enough. It consisted of Crixivan, Epivir, and Zerit (instead of AZT because according to my Doc I had had a 'bad' reaction to AZT.)*

*'Before I knew it I had moderate/severe lipoatrophy (fat loss) and myopathy (muscle loss). My arms had stretch marks at the biceps area and looked like shrivelled balloons. I remember my arms always being tired because I held my body up with them when I sat down due to the fact that I sat on bone.*

*'My face was the worst: hollow cheeks and temples and no fat anywhere. When I smiled, the skin looked like someone pulling back curtains on a stage. I looked extremely shrivelled up and old for my age. My eye sockets were hollow, my eyes looked sunken in. I always looked kind of scared, like an animal caught in a car light. Eventually, I knew it was the 'meds', but was terrified to stop.*

*'After three and a half years I had had enough. I figured I was the living dead already, so what the hell - again I threw out the meds. By now it was Crixivan and combivir (which is AZT and something else, maybe Epivir - yeah back to AZT because unfortunately I had a worse reaction to Zerit than I had to AZT).*

*'Then - nothing. I held my breath - waiting for IT. Oddly, I began to feel better. I got stronger - and calmer. Around a year and a half after stopping, I was rubbing my eyes and realized the skin on my face was thicker. I thought about it and realized I had been sitting down without the use of my arms for a while without realizing it.*

*'It's been 3 years since I stopped the meds. I can still see scars from that time; my body is not the body I used to have. But it's better. I'm back at the gym.* ' [468]

---

[467] Kibazo J. Glaxo plays down Ziagen fear. Financial Times. Aug. 21, 2000

[468] He remains unidentified, as requested, to protect his privacy

# Chapter 19

# What then could cause AIDS?

By now I had travelled a long distance from thinking there was no reason to question that HIV causes AIDS. I was increasingly perplexed by how academics could assure us with one breath that 'HIV is definitely the cause of AIDS' and feel able to say next minute, despite some 25 years of research: 'We still do not understand exactly how HIV infection leads to progressive immune deficiency [AIDS].'[469]

If the scientific orthodoxy is wrong, it is a fearful thing. But the original research it relies on now seemed to me so flawed that I was surprised that anyone was still citing it. Likewise the HIV test was not as reliable as I had once presumed. So, I had to ask: was there anything else that could cause AIDS?

Logically, I had to start with the major clinical symptoms of AIDS. So I went back to the original diseases defined as AIDS-indicating; that is to fungal pneumonia (PCP), Candida and Kaposi Sarcoma. The first two were the original killers, and are still major 'AIDS-Indicating' diseases in the West. Outside the West, TB is the major killer in AIDS cases. What did these three have in common?

In AIDS cases, all three are mainly respiratory tract infections. The first two involve yeast-like fungi that normally live harmlessly in all of us. The third involves bacteria that are also in most of us. So, what happens with AIDS? What makes these grow massively out-of-control?

For a start, the cause is unlikely to be a general breakdown of the immune system. If it were, then much more common illnesses would mostly be inflicting the victims, like 'flu, measles and mumps. No, this is far more specific.

Fungi, as can be observed in woods, normally feed on dead and decaying matter. This is their natural role. They return decaying matter into forms that can support plants. So – are the fungi similarly feeding on damaged cells in the mouths, throats and lungs of AIDS victims? Is there a breakdown in the protective systems surrounding these cells? If cells are intact, fungi rarely infect them. But if the cells are already dying, their protective systems will be weak and fungi and bacteria may move in.

The arrival of fungi is not automatically a bad thing. The fungi naturally living in us may help by fighting damaging bacteria with a range of chemicals. Indeed some of the latter have been extracted and proved extremely valuable as medicines, such as penicillin and erythromycin. Thus, by living in us, fungi may serve to protect us

But, despite a rigorous search, I found there is surprisingly little in medical texts on the relationship between cells and fungi. One textbook, currently in use in US universities, reported: 'There is very little information about mechanisms of fungal pathogenicity, in contrast to what is known about molecular mechanisms of bacterial pathogenesis.' [470] I found this surprising, given the fortune invested in researching HIV.

---

[469] After 26 years, how does HIV really cause AIDS? Report on the July 2007 4th International AIDS Society (IAS) Conference on Pathogenesis, Treatment and Prevention. Quotation from Michael Lederman, professor of medicine and pathology at Case Western Reserve University

[470] Medical Microbiology Fourth Edition, University of Texas. Edited By: Samuel Baron, MD. Chapter entitled Disease of Mechanisms of Fungi by George S. Kobayashi

It seems that there has been a neglect of research on the fungal diseases from which many AIDS victims actually die.

But why in AIDS cases are fungi found multiplying out of control in mouths, throats and lungs?    Is anything poisoning, or otherwise damaging, the cells of the respiratory tract, destroying their natural ability to protect themselves, making them decay and thus into food for fungi?

As I delved deeper, I found that toxicologists have long known that certain inhaled drugs damage the cells of the respiratory tract,  making them unable to do their job of absorbing oxygen, thus robbing our entire body of energy while leaving the cells of the respiratory tract vulnerable to fungi. In fact PCP, the fungal infection of the lungs found in AIDS cases, is first diagnosed by detecting a lack of oxygen in the blood. Thus long-term exposure to these drugs eventually produces widespread cellular malnutrition – and body wasting – the signature symptom of AIDS.

Statistics reveal an 80 to 90% correlation between the use of nitrite inhalants in the early AIDS cases in the USA and the UK – and a 60% correlation with crack cocaine. This contrasted to a 10 to 15% exposure to injected drugs. (More on this later)

These inhaled drugs have a cumulative impact on the mitochondria within our cells that must have oxygen to produce the energy our cells need. This in turn weakens T-cells – another symptom of AIDS. It may also make Kaposi sarcoma more likely, as cells turning cancerous stop relying on mitochondria for energy and turn to the less efficient method of raising energy by directly burning sugars. Cancers are thus also associated with body wasting. These drugs also produce NO – and this in turn weakens our cells' defences against damaging free radicals, again possibly leading to increased fungi infestation.

From the AIDS-related fungal diseases of the West, I then turned to the biggest killer in AIDS cases in Africa, TB – another illness mostly of the respiratory tract. It also deprives the blood of oxygen, causing cellular malnutrition.

TB is a frequently linked to poverty. Often environmental factors first damage the lung cells – such as heavy exposure to toxic dust, malnutrition or impure water supplies – although TB also strikes the well nourished and well off, particularly when their work exposes them to the same conditions as the poor.  For example, in 2006 I spent time in southern Africa with diamond mineworkers in townships and with medical professionals. What I learnt was that, although TB bacteria live contentedly in every healthy adult, they multiply when silica dust and asbestos fibres from mines shred lung cells.

I interviewed a woman who worked as a health and safety officer at a De Beers' owned diamond mine, Sandy Murray. Her duties took her underground just twice a week. From her x-ray records, within a year her lungs were seriously damaged, within 4 years she had TB and had lost a major part of her lungs. She could no longer pick up her small daughters.

Silica dust and asbestos fibres I discovered are scandalously uncontrolled in De Beers diamond mines. [471] The company says the dust is safe, so does not spray water to suppress it. Scientists report the dust is often full of asbestos fibres and sharp silica fragments. This cuts their lungs, giving them consumption – the old name for TB, making the product of their hands truly 'blood splattered diamonds'. Asbestos fibres are present because diamonds are often found in asbestos rock (altered serpentine, crystolite) – while rocks containing silica often surround the shafts going into the mines.

In most mines, the normal mandatory safety practice is to drill while spraying the rock with water to suppress rock dust.  However, in De Beers mines in South Africa, the company has obtained legal exemptions from this on the basis that the dust in their mines is uniquely safe! It thus conducts what is called 'dry mining.'

---

[471]  Janine Roberts *Glitter and Greed: The Secret World of the Diamond Cartel*. 2007 edition.  Disinfo Inc. New York. The first chapter of this new edition contains the scientific evidence behind these allegations. The author researched this in South Africa in 2006.

A driller who had lost part of his lungs to surgery, told me he thought the mine owners wanted the mine dusty 'to hide the diamonds from us.' It seemed difficult to think of other reasons, apart from parsimony. From all reports, the company has since blamed the consequent TB on AIDS rather than installing the normal, and usually compulsory, 'wet-drilling' dust-suppression measures. It is always easier to blame germs. If the cause is dust or toxins, someone might be sued.

Wherever there is widespread and long-term malnutrition, whether from lack of food, constant diarrhoea, damaged lungs, or produced by drugs, then our cells can die, fungi flourish, and our bodies waste away. So, what were the social conditions in which the AIDS epidemic was first reported?

The earliest medical case reports were made in the late 1970s. They told of young gay men in London and New York falling desperately ill mostly with fungal diseases as mentioned above. The victims came from a gay partying subculture in which frequent sex was fuelled by an incredible amount of drug taking. These reports were from St. Mary's Hospital near Paddington Station in London, and from Dr. Joseph Sonnabend's clinic in downtown Manhattan.[472]

It soon became evident that these patients were dying of a new deadly 'cocktail' of diseases, including a fungal or protozoa pneumonia (PCP) that kills within a year of diagnosis, a gross Thrush that obstructs the mouth and throat and can thus also kill, and a disfiguring dangerous skin cancer called Kaposi Sarcoma sometimes found near the mouth or even inside it, although often elsewhere. None of these illnesses were new. PCP ravaged severely malnourished European children at the end of the Second World War. Thrush was widespread, but very rarely this extreme. Kaposi Sarcoma is found among the elderly in the West. But never before had these diseases combined to afflict so many young men.

From the lifestyle of the early victims, there seemed to be a hundred reasons why they might be ill. They were having unprotected sex with strangers perhaps a dozen times a night at the bathhouses, fuelling these orgies with cocktails of drugs. They were suffering from multiple sexually transmitted diseases – and for these were being prescribed large doses of steroids and antibiotics, both very immune suppressant.

The government health organisations did little to help at first, perhaps because many doctors were uncomfortable with the amount of promiscuity and the scenes of 'indulgence' in the bathhouses, and had decided the condition was self-inflicted. The disease complex was named GRID, meaning Gay Related Immune Deficiency.

The first official CDC report was issued in 1981 and focussed on 5 young Los Angeles men, hospitalised with fungal PCP and Thrush. As I previously mentioned, this report said the patients 'did not know each other and had no known common contacts or knowledge of sexual partners who had had similar illnesses,' and moreover did not have 'comparable histories of sexually transmitted diseases'.

But the report did note a common factor. 'All five reported using inhalant drugs' – particularly the amyl nitrite inhalant called 'poppers'.[473]

I then found in London, St. Mary's Paddington Hospital had reported the same. They undertook in 1982 ' a survey of male homosexual patients attending' ... 250 men were interviewed...[of which] 215 (86%) had inhaled nitrites within the past five years, a proportion similar to the 86.4% reported for homosexual men then attending sexually transmitted disease clinics in New York, San Francisco, and Atlanta.' [474]

---

[472] . Also http://www.aidsinfobbs.org/articles/quilty/q04/1528 referred to by J Whitehead, BMJ Rapid Responses re AIDS, 2004

[473] M.S. Gottlieb, H.M. Shanker, P.T. Fan, A. Saxon, J. D. Weisman and J. Pozalski. Pneumocystis Pneumonia – Los Angeles, *Morbidity and Mortality Weekly Report*, 30 (1981): 250-252.

[474] McManus TJ et al. Amyl nitrite use by homosexuals. Lancet. 1982 Feb 27.

Among the recreational drugs, poppers are still today uniquely favoured by gay men since they relax the sphincter muscles, making anal sex easier, while giving a pleasurable buzz and more fun.[475] In the early days of the AIDS epidemic, crucially less than 1% of heterosexuals or lesbians took them.

For the toxicologists investigating AIDS, these inhaled drugs were thus an obvious suspect – especially since AIDS was reported as rarely affecting heterosexuals or lesbians. The multiple infections reported for the partying gay community, of cytomegalovirus, herpesvirus, and STDs, were eliminated from the early searches into a cause of AIDS, for, unlike poppers, they were not specific to the gay community.

For toxicologists, it was not the occasional use of poppers that was suspect, but their intensive use many times a night, and for years. All toxins will accumulate in us until they reach dangerous levels – and that is exactly what these drugs did. They came into common use in the gay clubs and bathhouses of major Western cities in the mid-1960s. The first cases of AIDS appeared a decade later among gays using these facilities. This might explain why AIDS seemed to need a long time to develop. Not because the virus was slow, a 'lentivirus,' but because the toxins in the drugs took years to accumulate until reaching a dangerous level.

Poppers were invented back in 1867 as a medical drug for angina pain. They helped by relaxing blood vessels and came in capsules 'popped' to release the acidic fumes of amyl nitrite for inhalation, hence their name. But in the 1960s they started to be widely used among US troops in Vietnam and in the gay community. In 1968 the US government imposed a medical prescription requirement, but this led to them being marketed instead as 'liquid incense' or 'room odorizers' in multi-dose small brown bottles.

Ian Young then reported in *Steam*: 'In the gay ghettos of the Seventies and early Eighties, poppers were always at the center of the action ... On any given night ... a large percentage of the men on the dance floor would have poppers in hand ... Some disco clubs would even add to the general euphoria by ... spraying the dance floor

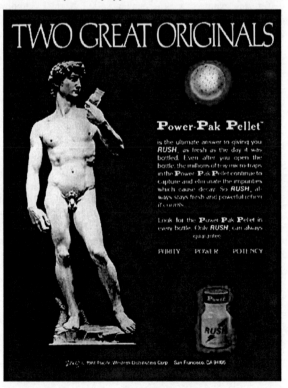

TWO GREAT ORIGINALS

**Power-Pak Pellet⁻**

is the ultimate answer to giving you *RUSH*, as fresh as the day it was bottled. Even after you open the bottle, the millions of tiny micro-traps in the Power-Pak Pellet continue to capture and eliminate the impurities which cause decay. So *RUSH*, always stays fresh and powerful when it counts.

Look for the Power-Pak Pellet in every bottle. Only *RUSH* can always guarantee

PURITY     POWER     POTENCY

───────────────
[475] 'Amyl nitrite is used widely in the male homosexual population and there are even illegal 'pushers' of this drug. It is used by the passive partner in anal intercourse to relax the anal musculature and thereby facilitate the introduction of the penis.' Labataille L. Amyl nitrite employed in homosexual relations. Med Aspects Human Sexuality. 1975;9:122 [DL].

with poppers fumes. Many gay men ... find they're no longer able to enjoy sex without them.' In the bathhouses, 'the musky chemical smell was constantly in your nostrils.' [476] It was the same in London, where John Lauritsen reported; 'Every Saturday night an estimated 2,000 gay men attend a dance club where drug consumption is the main activity ... Poppers are sold legally in London.'

I knew of this scene – it still exists in London today. I have gay friends who boasted of the good times they have had.

When the CDC in 1982 examined a further 170 cases of AIDS, it found 96% were on poppers, with 40 to 60% also taking cocaine, Crystal Metaqualone and LSD – sniffed or swallowed drugs – but not so much the injected. Heroin was around 10%. This was quite a surprise, for today only injected drugs are officially listed as a risk factor for AIDS. [477] I found the original AIDS victims used poppers nine times more than heroin.

A doctor stated in 1981: 'The patients are typically young homosexual men, most of whom live in large cities and many of whom use drugs ...The leading candidates are the nitrites, which are now commonly inhaled to intensify orgasm. Users of amyl nitrite are more likely than nonusers to have had hundreds of sexual partners and to contract venereal diseases. Preliminary data indicate that this 'liberated' subgroup may be at highest risk for immunosuppression.'[478]

The Atlanta study of 1983 confirmed much of this. It reported 96% of AIDS victims were on 'poppers,' and that they mostly also took crack cocaine, LSD and Crystal, while only 10% took heroin.[479] Furthermore, in February 1982 scientists at the US National Institutes of Health (NIH) acknowledged in *Lancet* that poppers might well suppress the victims' immune systems. Nevertheless the advertising continued – as in the example opposite.

The dangers of 'poppers' had been recognised early by many toxicologists. In 1981 Dr. Thomas Haley, a leading toxicologist, surveyed 115 recent studies, finding; 'Accidental prolonged inhalation of amyl nitrite [poppers] has resulted in death from respiratory failure ... 1 to 2 days after cessation of exposure. [It] interferes with oxyhemoglobin, causing anoxia [oxygen starvation] of vital organs' and thus diminishes the number of T-cells in the blood.

His words caught my attention. 'Anoxia of vital organs' meant these drugs would create severe malnourishment in those that over-indulge. Severely malnourished World War 2 children got fungal pneumonia – so malnutrition may lead to conditions in which this illness flourishes – and thus also to body wasting. He also reported that the drugs cut T-Cell numbers –the very thing that HIV is usually given the sole credit for doing. If poppers have the same effect – then surely, they also could cause AIDS?

The reason for the skin cancer, KS, was not so obvious from the early reports. Although it was found in or around the mouth and thus could be related to inhaled drugs, it was also found on legs and other parts of the anatomy. But a study by Michael Marmor et al. published in the Lancet in 1982, reported all the victims of Kaposi Sarcoma they studied were heavily into sniffing poppers. 'Amyl nitrite was the only drug that 100% of patients [with Kaposi's Sarcoma] reported ever having used, although 1 patient reported using it only once in his life...Only amyl nitrite had significantly elevated risk ratios at the [99%] probability level in the time periods 5 to 9 and over 10 years before disease.'[480]

---

[476] From Michael Rumaker's book , *A day and a Night at the Baths*,

[477] Jaffe et al 1983 Table. CDC 1983: Drug use by American male homosexuals with AIDS and at risk for AIDS. (Percentage users among 50 AIDS cases and 120 at risk for AIDS.)

[478] Durack DT. Opportunistic infections and Kaposi's sarcoma in homosexual men. N Engl J Med. 1981 Dec 10

[479] Kaslow et al 1989, , Ostrow et al 1990, Ostrow et al 1993.

[480] Marmor M et al. Risk factors for Kaposi's Sarcoma in homosexual men. Lancet. 1982 May 15.

I knew that chronic diarrhoea also causes severe malnourishment – and has also long been a common AIDS symptom.[481]   Were these the clues I was looking for? Was chronic severe malnourishment, drug-induced or otherwise, a possible cause of AIDS internationally?

I wondered also if crack cocaine, Crystal and LSD might have similar long-term effects? Could these, taken in combination with poppers over a long time, do the damage to the immune system associated with AIDS?

I had to ask, because of this very strong epidemiological evidence (see table towards the end of this chapter), why are inhaled drugs currently omitted from all AIDS surveillance reports and why are the much less associated injected drugs included? From what I can discover, it is solely on the theoretical grounds that a virus cannot be spread by inhaling acidic popper fumes, but can be spread by contaminating a needle. I cannot stress enough the seriousness of this omission. It has been done in the face of epidemiological evidence that there is more than a 500% greater risk of a link between inhaled drugs and AIDS than between injected drugs and AIDS. It means we have been robbed of absolutely vital data.

It is evident from accounts that many scientists by 1982 believed they knew the cause of AIDS. The remedy was obvious to them. These drugs would have to be removed from the scene. A powerful drug education campaign was essential, and possibly legislation. Anti-toxin and anti-fungal medical treatment was clearly required for those affected, as well as nourishment to counter the effects of severe malnutrition.

Nevertheless, a very different view ultimately prevailed. For the dominant school of

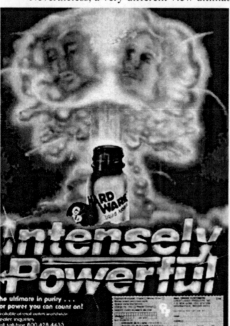

virology, a virus is the first suspect in every epidemic. They thus looked on this outbreak as a major opportunity to virus-hunt. Also many Gays lobbied hard against the illness being linked to homosexual lifestyles – and hoped a virus would be found to be its cause – thus exonerating their lifestyle.

This led in the summer of 1982 to the director of the CDC making perhaps the most important scientific decision of his career. Despite over a hundred toxicology reports on the link to drugs, despite no virus yet being found to cause AIDS, he put the prestige of his institution wholly behind the viral theory of AIDS. According to a memoir by a senior and respected colleague, Dr. William Blattner, CDC researchers were intending that day at an AIDS workshop to blame AIDS on poppers and drug taking. But, when they heard of the Director's decision, he said they immediately revised their presentations to say that these drugs, while being toxically dangerous, were only related to AIDS because they helped an unknown virus spread by

---

[481] Merck Manual, entries on malnutrition and on diarrhoea

encouraging sex! [482] Soon after this the name of the illness lost its gay lifestyle tag –and became officially AIDS.

But, his decision was welcomed by those gays who did not want to change their partying lifestyle. Charges of homophobia were levelled at the toxicologists who still blamed the drugs.

Blattner confessed they initially thought AIDS was caused by poppers because 'people who had the most severe immune deficiency had the strongest history of amyl nitrite [poppers] use,' but they had then realised; 'What this really reflected was the fact that people who had the heaviest nitrite use were the people who had the largest amount of anal receptive sex. As a result they probably got the virus earliest.' The sexual transmission of 'HIV' was thus presumed before it was discovered.

But others in the clubbing gay community were not so convinced. They started a very active campaign against poppers that appears to have been particularly effective in San Francisco. By 1983 the use of poppers had sharply declined in this city – and with it, equally sharply, the incidence of Kaposi Sarcoma and AIDS. A 1987 Public Health Department study of gay men in San Francisco found by 1983 the incidence of AIDS among gays had tumbled down from the 1982 peak height of 21% to just 2% - and had continued downwards since. [483]

Also, many scientists openly disagreed with the CDC declaration in support of the viral theory of AIDS. Dr. Albert Sabin, the inventor of one of the first polio vaccines, said at a 1983 meeting of scientists, 'the CDC and the NCI [where worked Dr. Robert Gallo] were the only people who believed that AIDS was caused by a retrovirus.'[484] Some FDA scientists were so incensed by the CDC's endorsement of a virus that they accused the CDC of inventing a viral epidemic to give jobs to its virologists. They charged the CDC with assembling a collection of disparate diseases and calling it AIDS.

Professor Etienne de Harven has stated: 'I feel the viral theory won primarily because retrovirus pathogenicity in humans had to be saved at all cost, even at the cost of scientific integrity! Too much money and politics had been put, in the 60s-70s, in the theory according to which retroviruses were the cause of human cancer! It was politically impossible to just drop retroviruses in human pathology! To find another role of retrovirus in human pathology was salvation for the respectability of Gallo's lab, and many other US cancer research centres.' [485]

The CDC defended its position so fiercely that a conclusion was added to a CDC 1983 paper that did not match its data. The misfit conclusion was, 'at the levels tested, isobutyl nitrite had no significant detrimental effect on the immune system of mice.' But the text of this paper stated that male mice exposed to poppers for 'up to 18 weeks' had a sharply lowered white blood cell count, down to nearly one third of that of the controls. It added: 'These drugs do have toxic effects. They have been shown to be mutagenic in vitro and are highly flammable. Reported side effects include: dizziness, headache, tachycardia, syncope, hypotension, and increased intraocular pressure; nitrites have also been associated with methemoglobinemia and, rarely, sudden death ... their role as a cofactor in some of the illnesses found in this [AIDS] syndrome has not been ruled out.' [486]

Months later the CDC published a pamphlet entitled, *'What gay and bisexual men should know about AIDS.'* It stated: 'Current research favors the theory that AIDS is

[482] This is recounted by Dr William Blattner, in his page in a section of the current (2004) NIH website dedicated to the pioneers of AIDS research. He was at the NIH's National Cancer Institute at the time. He recalls attending a meeting called to discuss AIDS research when the Director announced he favoured a virus as the cause of AIDS. He recounts how papers prepared for this meeting on other possible causes such as drugs were then hastily changed.

[483] Dr George Rutherford of the San Francisco Public Health Department, at the US 1987 Federal AIDS conference
[484] NIH website 2004 – Interview with James Curran.
[485] Email to author, October 2007.
[486] *Morbidity Mortality Weekly Reports* **September 09, 1983**

caused by an infective agent, possibly a member of the retrovirus group'.[487] The pamphlet then tried to clear poppers from blame by citing the false conclusion to the above paper. The Clinical Director of the NIH National Institute of Drug Abuse, Dr. Harry Haverkos, pointed out in vain that this paper said nothing of the sort.[488]

The CDC leaflet soon was the central feature in a major advertising campaign organised by the largest manufacturer of poppers, Great Lake Products. It announced the CDC had confirmed that poppers were safe. Jim Curran of the CDC swiftly issued a somewhat timid correction, saying poppers might be an AIDS cofactor, but his words were ignored. Sales of poppers soared, much to the bitter frustration of those who had campaigned so effectively against them. The drug now came in many varieties: amyl, butyl and isopropyl nitrites.

While the scientists debated, full-page adverts for poppers appeared in the leading gay magazines, stressing the role poppers could now 'safely' play in the 'gay lifestyle'. The activists who found the scientific evidence against poppers convincing, now found themselves marginalized by many in the gay community. They instead began to form alliances with toxicologists and other 'dissenting' scientists. The continuing bitter debate caused further hardening of the lines as the CDC was forced onto the defensive. It is today still defending its position from such dissenting scientists – and it is still a debate highly charged with anger.

The CDC henceforth would take little note of the toxicology evidence, as witnessed by senior NIH official, Dr. Harry Haverkos. He reported: 'I almost had a question about nitrites put on the CDC surveillance form back in 1984, but they had to weed it, make it a little shorter, and that was one of the questions they took off. [489] Thus the CDC, and its parallel institution, the NIH, ended the investigation of poppers, rejecting even the cures the toxicologists had suggested for AIDS (and had tested to show they would work!) on the theoretical basis that, as anti-toxins, they simply could not work against a virus.

Since then, other evidence has accumulated that implicates poppers and other drugs in producing AIDS-like symptoms. Dr. Sidney Mirvish reported that isobutyl nitrite (the 'mildest' of the popper drugs) causes mutations (as demonstrated with the industry standard Ames Test) that might lead to cancer. [490] In 1988 a government study reported. 'The studies presented here [on mice] show that chronic inhalation of AN [amyl nitrites] can lead to a decrease in helper cells, thus alternating the T-cell H/S [CD4/CD8] ratio, which is the same phenomenon that occurs in AIDS victims. This suggests a link between AN inhalation and cellular immunity depression.' [491]

A 1997 study of 2,822 gay men in San Francisco reported that the use of amyl nitrite for sex was associated with increased risk of being 'HIV positive,' that 'injection drug use was not associated' and 'a history of sexually transmitted disease did not appear to contribute an increased risk of seroconversions [HIV positivity]'. [492] One experiment took '8 HIV-negative male volunteers' and over four days had them take part in 13 sessions in which they inhaled either amyl nitrite or a placebo – without knowing which they were breathing. [493] 'The results showed that exposure to amyl nitrite can induce

---

[487] US Public Health Service, 1983.

[488] This was pointed out by a senior NIH figure who remained highly sceptical of the HIV theory of AIDS, Dr. William Havekos – http://www.posh-uk.org.uk/gmh/poppers_tbethell.html

[489] http://www.duesberg.com/articles/tbpoppers.html

[490] Mirvish et al., 1993

[491] Ortiz JS, Rivera VL. Altered T-Cell Helper/Suppressor Ratio in Mice Chronically Exposed to Amyl Nitrite. NIDA Research Monograph. 1988

[492] McFarland W et al. Estimation of human immunodeficiency virus (HIV) seroincidence among repeat anonymous testers in San Francisco. Am J Epidemiol. 1997 Oct 15.

[493] Dax EM et al. Effects of Nitrites on the Immune System of Humans. NIDA Research Monograph. 1988.

changes in immune function even after short exposure to moderate doses.' The table below lists the results from numerous academic studies in different cities.

## Drug use by homosexuals with AIDS and at risk for AIDS

| Drug | Atlanta 1)1983: 5 AIDS, 120 at risk | San Francisco (2) 1987: 492 at risk | San Francisco (3) 1990: 182 AIDS | Chicago (4) 1993: 5000 at risk | San Francisco (5) 1993: 215 AIDS* | Vancouver (6) 1993: 136 AIDS | USA, Europe, Australia (7) 1994: AIDS | London Manchester (8) 1996: 685 at risk |
|---|---|---|---|---|---|---|---|---|
| Nitrite inhalants | 96% | 82% | 79% | 71-100% | 100% | 98% | 50% ** | 0% [8] |
| Ethylchloride | 35-50 | | | 18 | | | | |
| Cocaine | 50-60 | 84 | 69 | 40-66 | yes | yes | 12-34 | 40 |
| Amphetamines | 50-70 | 64 | 55 | 26-46 | yes | yes | 6-27 | 48 ecstasy 57 speed |
| Phenylcyclidine | 40 | 22 | 23 | yes | | | | |
| LSD | 40-60 | | 49 | yes | | | | 48 |
| Metaqualone | 40-60 | 51 | 44 | | | | | |
| Barbiturates | 25 | 41 | 30 | yes | | | | |
| Marijuma | 90 | | 85 | 88 | | | 41-68 | 76 |
| Heroin | 10 | 20 | 3 | yes | | | | 25 |
| Alcohol | | | 46 | 95 | | | 90 | 95 |
| Tobacco | | | 33 | yes | | | 50 | 58 |
| AZT | | | | | most | most | 15-64 | |
| Drug Free | 0 | 0 | 0 | 0 | 0 | 0 | 0 | 0 |

** 6 month reported use

1) Jaffe, H. W., Choi, K., Thomas, P. A., Haverkos, H. W., Auerbach, D. M., Guinan, M. E., Rogers, M. F., Spira, T. J., Darrow, W. W., Kramer, M. A., Friedman, S. M., Monroe, J. M., Friedman-Kien, A. E., Laubenstein, L. J., Marmor, M., Safai, B., Dritz, S. K., Crispi, S. J., Fannin, S. L., Orkwis, J. P., Kelter, A., Rushing, W. R., Thacker, S. B. and Curran, J. W. (1983) National case-control study of Kaposi's sarcoma and *Pneumocystis carinii* pneumonia in homosexual men: Part 1, Epidemiologic results. *Ann. Intern. Med.* 99: 145-151.

2) Darrow, W. W., Echenberg, D. F., Jaffe, H. W., O'Malley, P. M., Byers, R. H., Getchell, J. P. and Curran, J. W. (1987) Risk factors for human immunodeficiency virus (HIV) infections in homosexual men. *Am. J. Publ. Health* 77: 479-483.

3) Lifson, A. R., Darrow, W. W., Hessol, N. A., O'Malley, P. M., Barnhart, J. L., Jaffe, H. W. and Rutherford, G. W. (1990) Kaposi's sarcoma in a cohort of homosexual and bisexual men: epidemiology and analysis for cofactors. *Am. J. Epidemiol.* 131: 221-231.

4) Kaslow RA, Blackwelder WC, Ostrow DG, Yerg D, Palenicek J, Coulson AH, Valdiserri RO. No evidence for a role of alcohol or other psychoactive drugs in accelerating immunodeficiency in HIV-1-positive individuals. *J Am Med Assoc* 1989; 261: 3424-3429; Ostrow DG, Beltran ED, Joseph JG, DiFranceisco W, Wesch J, Chmiel JS. Recreational drugs and sexual behavior in the Chicago MACS/CCS cohort of homosexually active men. *Journal of Substance Abuse* 1993; 5: 311-325; Ostrow, D. G., Van Raden, M. J., Fox, R., Kingsley, L. A., Dudley, J., Kaslow, R. A. and the Multicenter AIDS Cohort Study (MACS) (1990) Recreational drug use and sexual behavior change in a cohort of homosexual men. *AIDS* 4: 759-765.

5) Ascher, M. S., Sheppard, H. W., Winkelstein Jr, W. and Vittinghoff, E. (1993) Does drug use cause AIDS? *Nature (London)* 362: 103-104. Ellison, B. J., Downey, A. B. and Duesberg, P. H. (1996) HIV as a surrogate marker for drug-use: a re-analysis of the San Francisco Men's Health Study. In: *AIDS: virus- or drug induced?*, pp. 97-104, Duesberg, P. H. (ed.) Kluwer Academic Publishers, Dordrecht, The Netherlands.

6) Schechter, M. T., Craib, K. J. P., Gelmon, K. A., Montaner, J. S. G., Le, T. N. and O'Shaughnessy, M. V. (1993) HIV-1 and the aetiology of AIDS. *Lancet* 341: 658-659. Craddock, M. (1996) A critical appraisal of the Vancouver men's study; does it refute the drugs/AIDS hypothesis? In: *AIDS: virus or drug-induced*, pp. 105-110, Duesberg, P. H. (ed.) Kluwer Academic Publishers, Dordrecht, Netherland.

7) Veugelers PJ, Page KA, Tindall B, Schechter MT, Moss AR, Winkelstein WW, Cooper DA, Craib KJP, Charlebois E, Coutinho RA, Van Griensven GJP. Determinants of HIV disease progression among homsexual men registered in the tricontinental seroconverter study. *American Journal of Epidemiology* 1994; 140: 747-758.

8) Gibbons, J. (1996) Drugs & Us. *Gay Times (London)* September, p17-37.

Poppers and some other recreational drugs, if taken intensely, may chemically change numerous blood cells, making it impossible for them to carry the oxygen the body needs. Thus they are associated with blackouts, cell starvation and worse. It has been known since 1981 that 'Nitrites are powerful oxidizing agents which are recognized to cause haemoglobin [red blood cells] to be oxidized to methaemoglobin.' [494] They thus will particularly damage the highly exposed cells of the respiratory tract – the very place where deadly PC and severe thrush appear in so many AIDS cases.

A typical case report stated: 'A 21-year-old homosexual man presented ...complaining of severe headache, nausea, vomiting, chest pain, and shortness of breath. The patient reported that the onset of symptoms had occurred late in the evening prior to admission. He admitted to the ingestion of methaqualone (Quaalude) plus the inhalation of 'Hardware' [brand name for isobutyl nitrite] every 2-3 minutes for a period of 5-6 hours ending at 11:00 PM the evening before admission. Examination revealed a deeply cyanotic [blue skin due to oxygen deprivation] male ...Arterial blood gas samples ... were extremely dark, ...Methemoglobin [haemoglobin unable to carry oxygen] was 37% of all haemoglobin [normal values are 1-2%].' [495]

Taken much less intensely, over time such poisoning will cause considerable immune system damage – but it should not be forgotten that most taking poppers were also taking other drugs.

Other studies showed that injected cocaine has a 'strong association' with the presence of 'HIV' antibodies, as detected with the HIV blood test – but that 'conversely the frequency of current heroin injection was only weakly associated with HIV infection.' [496] Another study found 'surprisingly a significant relationship between non-intravenous use of cocaine and crack and seropositivity.' [497] These studies significantly contradict the established thesis that only injected drugs are associated with HIV infection. They also suggest that cocaine, and perhaps poppers, may falsely test positive for HIV.

The 'MACS' Multicenter AIDS Cohort Study is a much-cited authority on HIV transmission. The authors admitted: 'We did not attempt to quantify nitrite usage... It is thus possible that we missed or obscured a meaningful association.' [498]

However, important data were collected. At a 1994 workshop on nitrites held at the National Institute on Drug Abuse, Lisa Jacobson of Johns Hopkins University (Baltimore, MD) reported that 60-70 percent of the several thousand gay men at risk for AIDS who participated in the above study had used nitrites. 'Data from the MACS showed that the HIV-negatives surveyed had, on average, 25 months of nitrite use, HIV-positives had 60 months of nitrite use, and AIDS patients had over 65 months of nitrite use.'

We may now know why cocaine may help cause AIDS. 'Cocaine-induced oxidative stress appears to involve decreased glutathione and lipid peroxidation, potentiating [making more powerful] the oxidative stress associated with HIV-1 infection.' [499] It has been found that oxidative stress and decreased glutathione are common to all AIDS cases – but more about this later.

James Curran, who headed the CDC team investigating AIDS, has since owned; 'If it [the cause of AIDS] had been something like isobutyl nitrite, it would not have taken us

---

[494] Romeril KR, Concannon AJ. Heinz body haemolytic anaemia after sniffing volatile nitrites. Med J Aust. 1981 Mar 21.

[495] Guss DA et al. Clinically significant methemoglobinemia from inhalation of isobutyl nitrite. Am J Emerg Med. 1985 Jan

[496] Chaisson RE e a. Cocaine use and HIV infection in intravenous drug users in San Francisco. JAMA.1989 Jan 27.

[497] Sterk C. Cocaine and HIV seropositivity. Lancet. 1988 May 7.

[498] Polk et al. 1987

[499] Shor-Posner G et al. Neuroprotection in HIV-positive drug users: implications for antioxidant therapy. J Acquir Immune Defic Syndr. 2002 Oct 1;31 Suppl 2:S84-8 [DL].

very long to get rid of that as a risk.'[500] But instead they launched a search for a remedy against a then unknown virus that has absorbed over \$180 billion dollars over 23 years of research.

Dr. Harold Jaffe, the director of the division of HIV/AIDS at the Centers for Disease Control and Prevention, explained: 'The difficulty is this. Nitrite use among gay men also tends to be associated with other behaviours. Men with a heavy use of nitrite inhalants often also are highly sexually active, and have other sexually transmitted diseases. So it's very hard in doing studies to be able to separate out all these behaviours that are highly associated'. Nevertheless, he chose to focus on a sexually transmitted virus as the one and only cause of AIDS.

In 1990 the US Congress amended the law to ban 'volatile alkyl nitrites that can be used for inhaling or otherwise introducing volatile alkyl nitrites into the human body for euphoric or physical effects.' But today these inhaled drugs remain readily available, cheap – and highly profitable.

In the UK, in 1996 the Royal Pharmaceutical Society succeeded in the Crown Courts to have amyl nitrite banned – but a subsequent legal action in 2001 failed to have butyl and isobutyl nitrites similarly banned.[501] As in the USA, all these drugs are still widely and cheaply available in the UK – even in many secondary schools.

But why, when the evidence seems so strong, did the theory not carry the day that AIDS was the result of internal starvation caused by poppers, cocaine and prolonged severe malnourishment?

It seems the viral theory won in great measure, not just because of the influence of the 'germ theory' at the CDC and NIH, but because of the 'HIV' test. A significant number of people tested positive who were not taking any recreational drugs at all – particularly among haemophiliacs. Blood supplies also tested positive to an extent that could not possibly be explained by drug addiction. Also, Africans were testing positive who did not take such drugs. These HIV Test results seemed to bury the drugs exposure theory of AIDS in the West, despite all the correlations between inhalant drugs and AIDS cases.

But, as we have seen, testing positive does not mean one must be infected with HIV, for the positive result is for an antibody that is also reported to target fungal and mycobacterial infections and possibly drug-related toxins. This may well be why exposure to poppers statistically correlates with the presence of this antibody. Other toxins may cause similar damage, especially when patient has low levels of selenium and other antioxidants – or is taking certain prescribed drugs. Many factors can be implicated in causing such a broadly defined condition as AIDS.

As for blood supplies – the HIV test originally greatly over-reported positive results. In 1997 it was recognized that 'There is no recognized standard for establishing the presence or absence of HIV-1 antibody in human blood.' (Abbott Labs test kit instructions). It has since been pointed out that HIV would not survive the processes used with stored blood. Also, as we have seen, the diagnostic definition of AIDS has been made so very broad that it now includes many illnesses apart from those caused by recreational drugs.

In 1984 an Australian scientist submitted for publication a paper setting out a non-viral theory of AIDS based on the oxidising damage done by chemicals, including recreational and prescribed drugs, and by malnutrition. Her name was Eleni Papadopulos-Eleopulos – the same woman who would contest with Robert Gallo in an Australian courtroom in 2007.

---

[500] From the interview with Curran on the NIH website giving the memories of those of its staff engaged in the fight against AIDS.
[501] http://www.posh-uk.org.uk/gmh/poppers

Another scientist contested with Robert Gallo in the mid 1980s. His name was Peter Duesberg at Berkeley University, a member of the US National Academy of Science – and perhaps the brightest star in virology of that time. He had made his reputation by analyzing the genome of retroviruses and with work on oncogenes. He won the NIH Outstanding Researcher award – but he simply did not believe that his colleague Robert Gallo had got things right with HIV. It did not fit with what he knew of retroviruses.

Instead he suspected poppers and other recreational drugs were much to blame, as well as malnutrition in Africa – and published a scientific paper followed by a book setting out the evidence for this.[502] The reaction from the establishment was as if their favourite son had betrayed them. He was told that he would lose his research grants unless he retracted this heresy – but he refused.

But as time passes, many other independently minded scientists have joined with them in a scientific dissent that is rarely acknowledged by the media.  Thus in 2007 the biochemist, Professor Jean Umber of Nancy in France published an article entitled: 'What if HIV was simply a natural signal of cellular death (apoptosis)?' [503]

Like many others, he had been intrigued by the work of Benigno Rodriguez et al., published September 2006, the same work that was quoted with approval by the Prosecution's experts in the Australian trial. This revealed the viral load taken to be of HIV, could explain only about 5% of the decline in numbers of the CD4+ immune cells associated with AIDS diagnosis.

This meant something else must be killing these immune cells if AIDS were to develop. He noted that Professor Luc Montagnier now states the major killer of these cells must be oxidative stress, not HIV – and had observed that 'AIDS patients had an enormous deficit in glutathione', the body chemical that naturally defends us from oxidants. This strongly suggests that AIDS is principally not a viral infection, but a bio-chemical reaction.  In so doing, Montagnier had adopted the theory on oxidation and AIDS first put forward in 1988 by Eleni Papadopulos, the same Australian scientist whose testimony on AIDS was characterised as 'non-expert' by the judge in the Australian court case.

Umber pointed out poppers and other drugs produce nitrogen monoxide (NO), a slow destroyer of glutathione: 'This includes recreational drugs: nitrites (known as poppers), tertiary amines such as cocaine and secondary amines such as crystal meth.' Some medically prescribed drugs will also produce NO, he added, including antiretrovirals.[504]  The NO they produce will eventually use up all our cells' natural protector against oxidation, glutathione, leaving the cells very susceptible to oxidative damage.  But why would the doctors of patients on antiretrovirals not see this happening? Because, he said, it takes time for the cell's glutathione to be used up. In the meanwhile, the additional NO may combine with glutathione to prevent normal cell death. 'These donors of nitrogen monoxide have an anti-apoptotic [preventing normal cell death] action as long as the quantity of glutathione (and of glutathione peroxidase) is normal.'

By stopping natural cell death, the viral load will fall sharply – simply because the two metres of genetic code in each cell are not being released into our blood as our cells die. This includes the host of retroviral genetic codes in everyone's DNA. This is why, he explained: 'Nobody, except a person consuming HAART (Highly Active Anti-Retroviral

---

[502] *Inventing the AIDS virus* by Peter Duesberg.

[503] Jean Umber Professeur agrégé de chimie (Chemistry Professor) Nancy, France. What if HIV Alberta Reappraising AIDS Society. 2007 Feb. http://aras.ab.ca/articles/scientific/Umber-apoptosis.html

[504] 'Finally and especially, we find donors of nitrogen monoxide in all the medicines which contain a bond between a nitrogen and an atom (Chlorine, Nitrogen, Oxygen) whose electronegativity is superior to that of carbon. Examples are: bactrim (isoxazole ring); chloramphenicol (now mostly used in developing countries), metronidazole, nitrofurantoin (nitrocompounds); isoniazide against tuberculosis (mainly in Africa) and AZT.'

Therapy) has a zero viral load.' Such a viral load may well be unnatural – if it means that even normal cell death is not happening.

He gave a specific example. The antiretroviral drug Lamivudine (3TC) is oxidised by our defensive chemistry, producing chemicals that prevent cell death. This resulted in ' an important decrease in the apoptosis [deaths] of CD4+ cells in medicated AIDS patients from 1996.' But, he warns, eventually these drugs, whether prescribed or not, will leave our cells much weakened. They may then produce body wasting, an AIDS symptom.

Umber added significantly: 'Another interesting study, that of the Huber et al, published in December [2006], reminds me that the apoptotic immune cells themselves are the source of 'infectious' particles, independently of any infection. [505] He thoughtfully concluded: 'Finally, I wonder if HIV is not simply a natural signal of cellular death, but so weak that it passes unnoticed in a healthy person.'

It would be remiss of me if I did not also point out in this chapter the role played by the terrible life-changing curse of simply being told you are HIV positive, that you have an incurable sexually transmitted disease and will surely die of AIDS.

This is surely enough to make most people highly depressed. In 2007 it was reported by WHO scientists that 'depression significantly worsens the health state of people with chronic diseases.' [506] Long-term chronic depression is widely reported to have a devastating effect on the state of one's immune system. It thus makes one liable to get AIDS – as originally defined, as an acquired immunodeficiency syndrome.

## BUT, WE KNOW HIV IS PRESENT. IT HAS BEEN SEEN?

The evidence from electron micrography is not as clear as once thought. It now appears that the creators of the micrographed images that so far have been labelled as of 'HIV', or even of other viruses, have been optimistic in identifying minute particles as the pathogenic viruses sought. The particles differ in shape and size – as can be seen from the images below.

Recent micrographs reveal cells are normally surrounded by an absolute host of tiny particles – most self-produced as Umber noted above! Our cells naturally release these particles, varyingly labelled as 'microvesicles,' 'exosomes' and retroviruses, for a wide range of purposes. Some go to other cells, enter them, and 'tell' them that it is their natural time to die. This process appears identical in an electron microscope to what is often diagnosed as a 'virus infection.'

The scientists who took the micrographs on the next page, said to be the best available of HIV, explained that it was difficult for them to distinguish microvesicles from HIV. Their concluding words were of a hope for the future: 'The development of various purification strategies to separate microvesicles from HIV-1 particles and the use of cell lines that produce fewer microvesicles will greatly enhance our ability to identify virion [HIV] associated cellular proteins.[507]

---

[505] Apoptosis. 2007 Feb;12(2):363-74. The role of membrane lipids in the induction of macrophage apoptosis by microparticles. Huber LC, Jungel A, Distler JH, Moritz F, Gay RE, Michel BA, Pisetsky DS, Gay S, Distler O.

[506] Depression, chronic diseases, and decrements in health: results from the World Health Surveys Saba Moussavi et al. MPH

[507] Bess, Julian et al. 'Microvesicles are a source of contaminating cellular proteins found in purified HIV-1 preparations.' 1997 Virology 230 134-144.

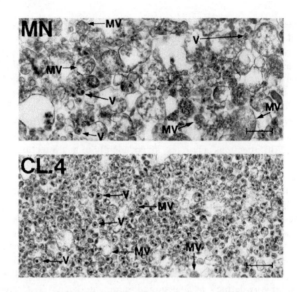

'Micrographs of HIV' 1997.  The authors state these are 'purified preparations of HIV-1' produced after centrifugation, even though clearly many kinds of particles are present. Those that are marked as 'MV' by the authors are said to be normal microvesicles and those marked 'V'' are said to be HIV.  The later were selected apparently because they resembled the particles identified by Robert Gallo.  The scale in lower right is of one micrometer.  Since a retrovirus is typically about one tenth of this, the particles labelled as HIV are apparently about twice the right size for a retrovirus. [508]

What then about the micrographs that Professor Montagnier had published of his virus LAV, the one we now call HIV? He reported it was budded off a lymphocyte cell from an infant's umbilical birth cord. [509] It was, and still is, well known that the human cord and placenta are full of natural 'endogenous' human retroviruses.[510] He also stated, in another paper, that he could not grow these suspect viruses from normal 'peripheral' blood cells from AIDS or 'pre-AIDS' patients, where one would expect HIV to be if it is produced by infection.

And how did Montagnier persuade cells to produce retroviruses? He added 'polybrene' to the cell culture, following which 'a relatively high level of reverse transcriptase activity was observed' which he took to be from the production of retroviruses. However, polybrene is a chemical which comes with this warning; 'May cause irritation of the eyes, skin and mucous membranes. Use in a chemical fume hood. Wear safety goggles and rubber gloves … assume highly toxic if ingested. May cause lesions of the adrenal cortex.'[511]

He had thus exposed the cells in his culture to a dangerous toxin, as did Gallo and Popovic, to make them produce his suspect AIDS virus. No mention of infecting them

---

[508] http://www.sigmaaldrich.com/Brands/Aldrich/Tech_Bulletins/AL_118_Polybrene/Appearance___Handling.html Montagnier's micrograph of LAV is on page 130 above

[509] 'These were detection of: 'umbilical cord lymphocytes showed characteristic immature particles with dense crescent (C- type) budding at the plasma membrane...' Barre-Sinoussai et al. Isolation of T-lymphotropic retrovirus from a patient at risk for acquired immune deficiency syndrome (AIDS). Science 1983;220: 868–71.

[510] Isolation of a T-lymphotropic retrovirus from a patient at risk for acquired immune deficiency syndrome (AIDS) Science 1983 May 20;220(4599):868-71.

first! (How could he, when he had not yet proved any virus to cause AIDS?) What provable relationship had polybrene to AIDS? None I suspect. In other words, his 'possible AIDS viruses' were more likely to be human retroviruses (HERVs) produced by cells to defend themselves from the toxin, or the cells mobilising retrotransposons as a form of immediate defence. In both cases reverse transcriptase activity is caused. I suspect this is exactly what bacterial cells do in hospitals when they are exposed to antibacterial toxins.

What I have learnt about AIDS science has frequently made me despondent. Surely research on toxins – and on their impact on cellular chemistry – should not have been so marginalised by what seems to have been an utterly unscientific discrimination in favour of virology? Surely the AIDS challenge demands all scientists pull together and keep an open mind to alternative theories? Many theories that challenge the orthodoxy are never fully tested. The heretics who dare to challenge conventional science are instead isolated, ignored and not funded – no matter how eminent their previous academic standing. (See below – *The Silenced Voices*)

This clearly has to change – but for this to happen, the amount of pride that will need to be swallowed, the amount of face-saving required, will make it very difficult to achieve – despite the desperate need of hundreds of thousands of suffering people.

But before concluding this book, I must tell of something that does give me hope, that is revolutionising cellular biology and hopefully will eventually do the same to virology. It may even remove the fear many of us have for viruses! It now even seems feasible that advancing scientific knowledge may force the most die-hard establishment scientists to eventually agree with Professor Duesberg and other dissidents in saying that HIV cannot be the cause of AIDS.

# Chapter 20

# Why Cells make Retroviruses

Western medicine has long focussed more on understanding disease rather than health. This is possibly its major handicap. Thus its scientists have tended to examine nature through the prism of illness, looking mainly for the harmful particle, while not being so ready to observe the beneficial. [512]

Before the electron microscope was invented in 1931, scientists searching for the causes of illnesses theorised that germs might exist that could pass through filters fine enough to remove all known bacteria. They threw an enormous amount of effort into this hunt and neglected other avenues of research.

Then, when particles were detected with the electron microscope that were small enough to go through these filters, many thought these might be the enemy, the dangerous 'filterable viruses' they had long sought – in particular the poliovirus they were then hunting. These particles were indeed miniscule – shorter than light waves, under 200 nanometres in diametre – that is, under 200 thousandths of a millionth of a metre. [513] When these were seen entering cells, this was immediately called 'infection.' When they were found in fluid from sick people, they were named as 'viruses,' the Latin for poisons [514] – and so the general public was taught to regard them. When retroviruses were discovered, they too were presumed dangerous and thus also called viruses.

But much more than viruses had passed thorough these fine filters. We now know that tiny infectious mycoplasmas (parasitic bacteria), slipped through, as also did toxins and cellular fragments. Mycoplasmas are true living cells, the smallest but many times bigger than a virus. Soft like a jellyfish, they can readily change their shape and were thus hard to recognize and study. [515]

When the evidence for characterising every virus as dangerous could not be found, the New York Academy of Science held a conference in 1960 entitled: '*Viruses in search of a Disease*,' during which, according to a participant, Etienne de Harven, 'many viruses were described … that could not be associated with any disease.' He argued that therefore 'at that time' these were not thought of as 'poisons.' [516] But they were not renamed – and today most of the public are still misled into seeing all viruses as foes and poisons – as indeed I was once myself. (Also, without an official renaming, it remains difficult for me to call such particles anything different in this book.)

Many virologists still describe many such particles as invasive and cunning foes, as if they posses some kind of intelligence, even while contradictorily saying they must be dead; since unlike mycoplasmas they lack the ability to reproduce and are inert outside cells – and because some have been turned into crystals and then reactivated, something

---

[512] This is even true of some of the laboratory techniques used. The plaque purification method is designed only to detect particles that kill.

[513] Recently giant 'mimiviruses' have been described, with over 1,000 genes. However, the definition of these as viruses may be mistaken. I would argue that a virus is a messenger vesicle and thus normally very small. http://www.giantvirus.org/intro.html

[514] Medical Dictionary 1940

[515] http://lungdiseases.about.com/od/pneumon2/a/mycoplas_pneum.htm

[516] Etienne De Harven: Personal communication by email with the author, January 2008.

surely that cannot be done to a living particle? For example, a recent article in the *Annals of Science* started by saying viruses are 'so rudimentary that many scientists don't even consider them to be alive' and then went on immediately to characterise them as 'parasites' – as something that is alive. [517]

Nobel Laureate biologist Joshua Lederberg is quoted as saying the 'single biggest threat to man's continued dominance on this planet is the virus' – despite us having evolved alongside them and with their help, as we will see. Luis Villarreal is likewise quoted as predicting that nearly the entire population of Africa would perish of HIV without an AIDS vaccine – 'we can expect a few humans to survive' – this despite the population in southern Africa having almost doubled in size according to official US statistics during twenty years of the 'AIDS epidemic.' [518]

They may well believe their predictions – but I must note, even if this is somewhat cynical, that spreading fear is a good way to raise research funds. I have seen this happen far too often. Their predictions, however, enliven science reporting. It makes gripping journalism to depict viruses as engaged in an unending battle against us.

As for retroviruses, they are often spoken of as cunningly evading our immune systems, penetrating, infecting, turning cells cancerous and hijacking – despite them being targeted to little effect in Nixon's War against Cancer and despite most now being seen as harmless. The above-quoted *Annals of Science* article states that retroviruses 'insinuate' themselves into cells. Some scientists even describe retroviruses that do not hurt us as 'defective.' In other words, they presume their nature is to be dangerous. Thus harmless retroviral codes found in our DNA have been described as 'defeated by evolution.' [519]

Peter Duesberg explained in a 1987 paper why we came to fear retroviruses and should not: 'The virus-cancer hypothesis steadily gained support because, in efforts to identify causative agents, retroviruses and DNA viruses were frequently isolated from animal leukemias and other tumours, and occasionally from human leukemias. However … most of these viruses were subsequently found to be widespread in healthy animals and humans.'

I had earlier learnt that viruses invade cells in order to reproduce, and that cells are the victims of this process. I also learnt that HIV was a retrovirus that hijacked' cells. But I now realised there was an entirely different way to see this process. Biology, a science that unlike virology has no focus on illness, has taught me that no virus exists that is not made by a cell, that these are produced by all healthy cells, whether of plants, fungi, birds, fish or animals, and that cells apparently consider retroviruses so harmless that they will trustingly incorporate codes brought by them into their very genomes, into the protected centres of their being. [520]

Why do we presume that viruses take the initiative when they enter a cell, when viruses are universally recognised to be inert? What if it is the other way around? What if cells actively attract the passing retrovirus because they need the information they carry? They reportedly carry markers that enable cells to recognize them. [521]

Viruses are essentially, as we will see, cell-made transport particles, similar to the vesicles cells make to use internally as transports. If cells send out such particles to share

---

[517] Specter, Michael. 'Darwin's Surprise.' Annals of Science, December 3, 2007

[518] Quoted in Specter, Michael. 'Darwin's Surprise.' Annals of Science, December 3, 2007. For population doubling, see US Bureau of the Census, International Database 2001

[519] Ibid.

[520] For plant retroviruses, see Plant retroviruses: structure, evolution and future applications, https://tspace.library.utoronto.ca/handle/1807/1315 For retroviruses from several fish species, see http://www.ncbi.nlm.nih.gov/books/bv.fcgi?rid=rv.section.8063

[521] 'Exosomes express cell recognition molecules on their surface that facilitate their selective targeting and uptake into recipient cells.' From 'Exosomal transfer of proteins and RNAs at synapses in the nervous system.' Neil R Smalheiser. Biol. Direct; published online Nov. 30th. 2007

information between themselves, perhaps this explains why cells evolved viral receptors and can absorb many such particles without ill effect? It would even explain why cells invest a great deal of energy in making them. Since these transport particles seem to be no more living than a text message, this explains also why we cannot kill them with antibiotics.

What then of the viruses said to kill cells, the 'cytolytic'? Cytolysis in biology is defined as the death of a cell due to osmotic imbalance, due to the pressure being too great or low within. Could viruses jointly mount enough pressure to burst a human cell? Today, this is thought very unlikely. The virus is simply too small and the cell's self-protection too able.[522] Currently, medical courses teach instead that viral-infected cells die mostly because of an 'allergic' reaction; or because our immune system will naturally kill a sick cell. [523] We will look more at this in the next chapter.

If 'viruses' are essentially messenger particles, this may explain why the genomes of viruses can vary so much. It might not be always because they are 'unstable', or subject to chance 'mutations'. It could be because they are designed by cells to carry a wide variety of messages. This would explain why the NIH reports that it is hard to classify them into 'species': 'Since viruses can evolve with enormous rapidity under selective pressure, it is difficult to define by sequence precisely what a virus 'species' is;' so it has been decided that they may be identified as of a particular species if less than 20% of their genetic code is different from other members of that species. [524] (Yet the genetic codes of monkeys and humans have only a 2% difference.)

I wondered if the 'selective pressure' the NIH mentioned may be a factor that leads cells to alter the code in a virus? Once it is produced, then its codes are static – so its variability is due to the cell that makes it.

We still know remarkably little about why cells make retroviruses and their possible usefulness. The same applies to other viruses. The cells of our world clearly invest a vast amount of energy in making milliards of them. We live in a sea of them. Every breath we take is full of them; but they rarely hurt us. We evolved among them. But two characteristics they all have by definition: viruses are all produced by cells, whether from animals, fungi, plants or bacteria, and they all contain short segments of genetic code.

Comparing a cell's size with that of a virus is, to put it simplistically, like comparing an elephant to a scrap of paper. A virus is approximately a billion times smaller than a cell. In contrast, each cell of a multicellular organisms, whether animal, plant or fungi, contain nearly two metres of genetic code in its core – with even more in its mitochondria and organelles (small organs). And they are certainly not inert. Today techniques like X ray crystallography reveal that living cells pulsate with energy, colour and movement.[525]

The vast difference between the amount of genetic code in a virus and in a cell reflects the immensely greater capability of the latter. Yet much too often some scientists and journalists have permitted themselves to speak of viruses as if they are as intelligent as cells and have the same survival instincts.

If we want to better understand why cells make retroviruses, and other viruses, it might help to first look at the similar particles cells make to use internally as transports. Our cells are constantly making vast numbers of hollow transport particles ('vesicles') in their 'ribosome' organelles;' sending these out carrying cargo along intricate 'road-

---

[522] Definition of cytolysis from Biology Online. http://www.biology-online.org/dictionary/Cytolysis

[523] For example, see http://www.kcom.edu/faculty/chamberlain/Website/Lects/MECHANIS.HTM and also http://mansfield.osu.edu/~sabedon/biol2065.htm

[524] http://www.ncbi.nlm.nih.gov/books/bv.fcgi?rid=rv.section.285

[525] Mae-Wan Ho Bioenergetics and the Coherence of Organisms  Neuronetwork World 5, 733-750, 1995.

systems' of 'microtubules.' [526] This system is extremely busy – supplying materials for some 100,000 chemical reactions a second[527] including cargoes of protein, enzymes and even DNA: 'The final proof that DNA actually entered the vesicles came from import experiments, in which radiolabeled ssDNA [single stranded DNA] was shown to accumulate inside the vesicles.' [528] Communication systems are thus as vital for our cells as they are for the largest of our hi-tech factories.

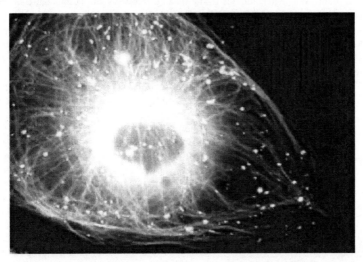

**Cell with its internal microtubule network. The dots are reported to be the vesicle transports that travel or 'walk' along them.**[529] **(This cell is from the kidney of an African Green Monkey – the same cell that is used to make the polio vaccine.)**

The 'Golgi Apparatus' is the cell's 'post office.' It directs these cargoes to where they are most needed. This system also supplies the materials for the assembly of retroviruses on internal membranes.[530] It can transport large mitochondria organelles and is of vital importance to the division of cells into new cells.

Extraordinarily these vesicles, with their cargo inside them, are carried along the 'roads' of microtubules by motors that walk! They 'walk' with 'two legs ... stepping along just like a porter carrying some cellular material as cargo.' 'Kinesin, one of the best-studied molecular motors, walks with precise steps of 8 nanometres.' They can go forwards and backwards. Some molecular stepping motors even have a gear system! [531]

The sketch below, not drawn to scale, illustrates how vesicles are carried along the 25nm-wide microtubules. They move at about 100 steps a second. The Kinesin particle,

---

[526] LabNotes http://www.mbl.edu/publications/pub_archive/labnotes/2.3/Langford.html
In recent video tapes made by Langford and colleagues with high-powered light microscopes, packages could be seen travelling along microtubules.

[527] Eugen A. et al. Puzzles of the living cell... Digest Journal of Nanomaterials and Biostructures Vol. 1, No. 3, September 2006, p. 81 – 92 http://www.chalcogen.infim.ro/Preoteasa.pdf

[528] Fabrice Dumas et al. An Agrobacterium VirE2 channel for transferred-DNA transport into plant cells. *Proceeding of the National Academy of Science*, USA January 2001.

[529] Nature Cell Biology 3, 473 - 483 (2001) Published online: 18 April 2001; | Caveolar endocytosis of simian virus 40 reveals a new two-step vesicular-transport pathway to the ER Lucas Pelkmans, Jürgen Kartenbeck & Ari Helenius

[530] http://www.ncbi.nlm.nih.gov/books/bv.fcgi?highlight=virus,golgi&rid=rv.section.2497

[531] http://www.tifr.res.in/~roop/NaturesNanotech.htm

some 70nm long, has two 'feet' powered by ATP molecules. It also has two 'hands' that grip a cargo that may be far wider than itself, perhaps a vesicle over 500nm wide. The cargoes thus can be far wider than the 'roads.' Several kinesin working together can drag whole strands of DNA. Illustrations of this may be found on a Max-Planck-Institute of Molecular Cell Biology and Genetics website.[532]

The microtubule 'roads' are linked to a finer network of actin threads. A scientist researching them said: 'Microtubules (MT) are like freeways and actin filaments are like local streets.'[533] Both networks constantly carry thousands of moving particles.[534']

Another study reported: 'Eukaryotic cells create internal order by using protein motors to transport molecules and organelles along cytoskeletal tracks. Recent genomic and functional studies suggest that five cargo-carrying motors emerged in primitive eukaryotes and have been widely used throughout evolution.'[535]

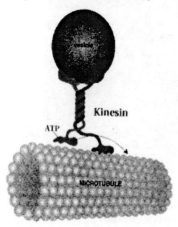

In 2006 Drs. Andrew Z. Fire and Craig C. Mello jointly won their Nobel Prize for Medicine for describing how cells use another extremely important messenger – the 'messenger RNA' (mRNA) particle. It carries information in the form of double-stranded RNA to control the making of proteins 'involved in all processes of life, for instance as enzymes digesting our food, receptors receiving signals in the brain, and as antibodies defending us against bacteria.' The cells also make smaller 'microRNAs' capable of carrying only 20 or so base pairs of code.[536] Our cells thus control and regulate the genes that were previously thought to reign supreme.

In 2006, discoveries in cellular biology won not only the Nobel Prize for Medicine but also the Nobel Prize for Chemistry. The latter went to Roger D. Kornberg: 'for his fundamental studies on how the information stored in the genes is copied and transferred to the parts of the cells that produce proteins.' In his Nobel speech he emphasised that, if this communication 'is interrupted, the organism will soon die, since all protein production in the cells ceases.' He added: 'Many illnesses – like cancer, heart disease, and different kinds of inflammation are linked to disturbances in the transcription process' that is vital to these cellular communications.

Cells also make larger elements known as transposons and retrotransposons. These can travel within their nuclei. They are the tools by which the cells adjust their genetic codes to meet environmental challenges and may contain up to five thousand 'base-pairs'[537] of code. They can carry the code for cellular genes, help regulate our genes – and even re-wire our gene control systems! For example: 'Many retrotransposons carry enhancer sequences responsive to host gene regulatory systems so that they are capable of

---

[532] http://www.emccd.com/downloads/?doc=Watching%20Single%20Motor%20Molecules%20at%20Work.

[533] How Does Intracellular Molecular-Motor-Driven Transport Work?
http://eiffel.ps.uci.edu/cyu/talks/actin04.ppt

[534] LabNotes Fall 1992. http://www.mbl.edu/publications/pub_archive/labnotes/2.3/Langford.html

[535] http://www.ncbi.nlm.nih.gov/pubmed/12600311?dopt=AbstractPlus

[536] Processing of Pre-microRNAs by the Dicer-1–Loquacious Complex in Drosophila Cells. Kuniaki Saito. Akira Ishizuka Haruhiko Siomi Mikiko C. Siomi
1 Institute for Genome Research, University of Tokushima, Kuramoto, Tokushima, Japan. PLOS Biology.

[537] Our double stranded code is made up of nucleotides that pair themselves with nucleotides on the other strand. Each of these couples is called a 'base-pair'.

rewiring the regulation of adjacent genes—perhaps another example of 'genomic altruism.' [538] (A contradiction to the theory of the selfish gene?)

There are also 'plasmids.' These are molecules containing circular DNA.[539] Bacteria cells seemingly make these to facilitate the movement of DNA both within and without themselves. They may carry around 4,000 base pairs of code. Some have been found to confer antibiotic resistance – and it seems plasmid codes are sometimes incorporated into mammalian DNA. (They are now being experimented with as 'vectors' for gene therapy.)

The genomes of plants are mostly made of retrotransposon-transported codes. As for humans, it seems from the evidence left within our genome, that around 42% of it has been moved around by transposons or retrotransposons, and perhaps plasmids, at one stage or another of our evolution.[540]

## THE CREATION OF RETROVIRUSES

Cells do not only make internal transports. We now know that they also make particles that travel through 'extra-cellular space' to other cells, not to 'perniciously infect' them, but to pass information to them. We are multi-cellular organisms and inter-cell communication is absolutely vital to us. An adult human contains approximately 100,000 billion cells and for us to survive, these must 'talk' to one another, learn from each other, share and cooperate.

A cell can transform its retrotransposons, give them the ability to travel between cells with their variable load of genetic codes, make them retroviruses, by simply appending to each an additional piece of code. An 'intracellular, non-infectious retrotransposon' becomes 'a budding, infectious retrovirus merely by appending a retroviral MA domain.' [541] This may well be how retroviruses first evolved.

They leave their home cell by 'budding' from it. On arrival at another cell, the codes they carry are incorporated into that cell's DNA – and with this these retroviruses as such cease to exist. They have served their function. They are strictly one-use vehicles. Our genome has been thus constructed in part from codes created by other cells over a very long period of time. [542] In other words, this system is vital to evolution.

Retroviruses can carry a wide variety of messages. 'Retroviral particles contain a variety of cellular RNA's'. The scientists who noted this, added that these 'are presumed to be packaged fortuitously during virion [virus] assembly.' [543] But this is only a presumption made because the authors did not see a reason for the presence of these codes. I would ask if the 'parent' cell put these RNAs into retroviruses to have them taken as cargo to other cells?[544]

---

[538] White

[539] http://www.life.uiuc.edu/molbio/background/background.html

[540] Lander ES, Linton LM, Birren B, Nusbaum C, et al. Initial sequencing and analysis of the human genome. Nature, 2001; 409(6822): 860-921

541 Higher-Order Oligomerization Targets Plasma Membrane Proteins and HIV Gag to Exosomes Yi Fang, Ning Wu, Xin Gan, Wanhua Yan, James C Morrell, and Stephen J Gould. Department of Biological Chemistry, Johns Hopkins University School of Medicine, full text available at http://www.pubmedcentral.nih.gov/articlerender.fcgi?artid=1885833#pbio-0050158-b058 - also Denzer K, Kleijmeer MJ, Heijnen HF, Stoorvogel W, Geuze HJ. Exosome: from internal vesicle of the multivesicular body to intercellular signaling device. Journal of Cell Science 113, 3365-3374 (2000). The MA domain is added to the 'N-terminus of its Gag-like protein.'

[542] David J Griffiths Endogenous retroviruses in the human genome sequence. Genetic Biol. 2001; 2(6): reviews1017.1–reviews1017.5. Published online 2001 June 5.

[543] http://www.ncbi.nlm.nih.gov/books/bv.fcgi?highlight=ribosomes,cell&rid=rv.section.2542#2547

[544] Similar arguments also apply to the exosomes as noted later.

The vesicles leaving cells do not all swim free. Recent micrographs, such as that reproduced below, reveal slender 'nanotube' bridges slung from cell to cell, carrying proteins, organelles and encoded information.[545] 'Transfer of molecules and organelles can occur directly from the cytoplasm of one cell to that of the other.' Note the particle on the connecting nanotube. From 50 to 200nm wide, these connections might accommodate a retrovirus. We do not yet know if retroviruses do, but vesicles have been observed moving along them from one cell to another. [546] (See image below.)

These nanotube 'highways' are made of actin (once thought to be a constituent of HIV) and can link immune cells together. It is reported: 'We think the cells make these connections so that they can work in a coordinated fashion to collect antigens from pathogens rather than working as individuals. This would seem to make the likelihood of successful delivery of the antigen to a distant lymph node much more likely.'[547]

This nanotube network also extends within the cell to carry the vesicles that move by 'stepping.' 'Mitochondria and intracellular vesicles, including late endosomes and

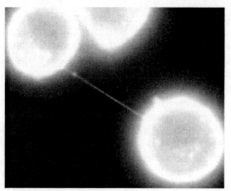

lysosomes, could be detected within thick, but not thin, membrane nanotubes. Analysis from kymographs demonstrated that vesicles moved in a stepwise, bidirectional manner at 1 μm/s, consistent with their traffic being mediated by the microtubules found only in thick nanotubes.'[548]

It seems every year we are learning more about how vital and complex is the cell's transport system. Some of the particles they send out mineralise the spaces between cells to create bone and cartilage.[549] So surely it is not too far fetched to suggest that retroviruses also play a vital role in carrying codes from one cell to another?

The National Institutes of Health (NIH) reported that retroviruses 'are so irregular and so labile that we have been unable to apply the tools of structural analysis to good effect.' It also reported that retroviral DNA 'closely resembles a cellular mRNA' messenger vesicle. Retroviruses are also said to be 'unique among animal viruses in that some groups exhibit considerable polymorphism in receptor usage.' They are thus particularly well suited for carrying messages – as they can deliver 'irregular', or varying, code 'similar to' mRNA to many kinds of cellular receptors.

Today, I am glad to say, many biologists are no longer automatically naming all such travelling elements as 'viruses'. Many of these now called 'exosome vesicles,' a name widely used since 1997. [550] These are generically described as 'cargo-loaded small vesicles released into extra-cellular space,' a description that surely applies to all viruses?

[545] Demontis F (2004) Nanotubes Make Big Science. PLoS Biol  Published: July 13, 2004

[546] Demontis F (2004) Nanotubes Make Big Science. PLoS Biol 2(7): e215 doi:10.1371/journal.pbio.0020215 Image courtesy of Hans-Hermann Gerdes

[547] Nanotubes link immune cells. The Scientist, 20 September 2005.

[548] Björn Önfelt et al 'Structurally Distinct Membrane Nanotubes between Human Macrophages Support Long-Distance Vesicular Traffic or Surfing of Bacteria *The Journal of Immunology*, 2006, 177: 8476-8483

[549] Bonucci, E. (1967), "Fine structure of early cartilage calcification", *Journal Ultrastructure Research*, **20**: 33-50

[550] Exosome 'vesicles' are not be confused with the unrelated 'exosome complex' that helps break down RNA within cells.

Scientists varyingly describe them as particles of a width 'up to 120nm',[551] 'from 40 to 100nm',[552] from '60 to 90nm' [553] or even 'up to 150nm'. They thus include vesicles of the size of the typical retrovirus, from 80 to 120nm wide, as well as sizes pertaining to other viruses.[554]  In 2006-7 several scientists placed the retroviral family itself among the exosomes.

All kinds of cells make exosomes, including T-Cells – and, it seems, often for very good reasons.  In an important experiment, 'exosomes secreted by bone-marrow-derived dendritic cells were challenged with tumour-derived peptides, activated CTLs, causing the eradication of established tumours.'[555]  When near tumour cells, exosomes are reported to sometimes produce very strong anti-tumour reactions.[556]  Radiation-damaged cells also produce exosomes, perhaps as a genetic code repair mechanism.  They are also thought to help against streptococcus pneumonia bacteria and to generally stimulate our immune systems, including T-cells.[557]  They can transport antigens that protect us.

When I read the above reports, it made me wonder if this explains why retroviruses were initially discovered near tumour cells. They could be there to help cells repair themselves. It might also explained why they are found entering and leaving T-cells – a phenomenon long associated with 'HIV infection.' It could be that they are there for a very different reason – to help these cells fight pathogens.

Exosomes are now called 'one of the most important protein complexes' involved in controlling the 'RNA-processing machinery' in mammals.[558]  They vitally help ensure accuracy in the reading of RNA messages and help deactivate old RNA messages that are no longer needed.[559]  Because of their many functions, they are also called 'secreted organelles' – external cellular organs. [560]  (Yet, 'anti-retroviral therapy' is based around the out-of-date notion that all retroviruses are useless or dangerous particles.)

In 2007 it was described how 'cells send RNA messages to each other by packing these into exosomes' and how exosomes can carry a 'large amounts of RNA' from one cell to another – up to 1,300 different mRNAs! Among these are vital messages that

---

[551] Martin P. Bard, Joost P. Hegmans, Annabrita Hemmes, Theo M. Luider, Rob Willemsen, Lies-Anne A. Severijnen, Jan P. van Meerbeeck, Sjaak A. Burgers, Henk C. Hoogsteden and Bart N. Lambrecht; Proteomic Analysis of Exosomes Isolated from Human Malignant Pleural Effusions American Journal of Respiratory Cell and Molecular Biology. Vol. 31, pp. 114-121, 2004

[552] Nicolas Blanchard*, Danielle Lankar*, Florence Faure*, Armelle Regnault, Céline Dumont*, Graça Raposo and Claire Hivroz2,* TCR Activation of Human T Cells Induces the Production of Exosomes Bearing the TCR/CD3/ Complex1 The Journal of Immunology, 2002, 168: 3235-3241.

[553] The Journal of Immunology, 2001, 166: 7309-7318. Proteomic Analysis of Dendritic Cell-Derived Exosomes: A Secreted Subcellular Compartment Distinct from Apoptotic Vesicles Clotilde Théry,, Muriel Boussac,, Philippe Véron*, Paola Ricciardi-Castagnoli, Graça Raposo, Jerôme Garin and Sebastian Amigorena*

[554] http://www.ncbi.nlm.nih.gov/books/bv.fcgi?rid=rv.section.285

[555] Denzer et al. op.cit. – cites this experiment as carried out by Zitvogel et al., 1998.

[556] Banchard et al. 2002. Cited above.

[557] Infection and Immunity, January 2007, p. 220-230, Vol. 75, No. 1 Dendritic Cell-Derived Exosomes Express a Streptococcus pneumoniae Capsular Polysaccharide Type 14 Cross-Reactive Antigen That Induces Protective Immunoglobulin Responses against Pneumococcal Infection in Mice Jesus Colino and Clifford M. Snapper*

[558] Houseley J, LaCava J, Tollervey D. RNA-quality control by the exosome. Nat Rev Mol Cell Biol. 2006 Jul;7(7):529-39. PMID: 16829983

[559] Raijmakers R, Shilders G, Pruijn G. The Exosome: a molecular machine for controlled RNA degradation in both nucleus and cytoplasm. European Journal of Cell Biology, Vol. 83, 5 July 2004. Pp 175-183

[560] Yi Fang, Ning Wu, Xin Gan, Wanhua Yan, James C Morrell, and Stephen J Gould; Higher-Order Oligomerization Targets Plasma Membrane Proteins and HIV Gag to Exosomes. PLoS Biol. 2007 June; 5(6): e158. Published online 2007 June 5

'regulate cellular development and protein synthesis' – in other words regulate some of the most important functions in our bodies and in all multicellular organisms.[561]

Professor Peter Duesberg at Berkeley was the first to describe the genome of retroviruses as I have mentioned. He wrote of how their genetic codes 'are integrated as proviruses [viral DNA] into the germ line of most if not all vertebrates' after being carried from one cell to another. He also described them as totally harmless.[562]

In summary: retroviruses, like retrotransposons and messenger RNA (mRNA), carry information encoded into double-stranded RNA. They are formed inside cells on membranes.[563]  They are then budded out through the cell wall, which, on the way through, donates to them their protective coating of proteins.  On arrival at another cell, their RNA is passed inside, converted and incorporated into that cell's library of DNA.

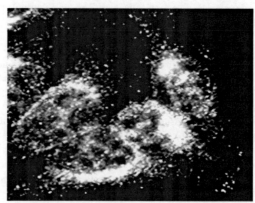

**Cells surrounded by clouds of particles.**

We have many 'endogenous' (self-made) retroviruses. Many evolved earlier than us. For example, ERV-L are in all placental mammals, suggesting they evolved at least 70 million years ago.[564]  The HERV-K retrovirus is said to go back to some 30 million years ago. ERV-3 is described as 'evolutionarily conserved human endogenous retrovirus' with a coding envelope gene 'potentially involved in important placental functions.'[565]

Our cells also send out 'microvesicles' under 1 micron wide that can carry as cargo mitochondria, lysomes and even DNA.[566] They are a 'much overlooked' and 'important' 'cell to cell communication system that appeared very early in evolution.' Cells send out many of these when injured. [567]

---

[561] '*The Exosome Exchange.*' The Journal of Cell Biology. 21 May 2007.  Also, Denzer K et al. *Exosome: from internal vesicle of the multivesicular body to intercellular signaling device'* Journal of Cell Science, Vol 113, Issue 19 3365-3374,

[562] Retroviruses as Carcinogens and Pathogens: Expectations and Reality By Peter H. Duesberg.  Cancer Research, Vol. 47, pp. 1199-1220.(Perspectives in Cancer Research), March 1, 1987.

[563] Graziella Griffith, and Marie-Christine Dokhélar Arielle R. Rosenberg, Lélia Delamarre, Claudine Pique, Isabelle Le Blanc,  Early Assembly Step of a Retroviral Envelope Glycoprotein: Analysis Using a Dominant Negative Assay
Cell Biol., Volume 145, Number 1, April 5, 1999 57-68

[564] ERV-L Elements: a Family of Endogenous Retrovirus-Like Elements Active throughout the Evolution of Mammals. J Virol. 73(4):3301-3308. 1999.

[565] de Parseval, N., and T. Heidmann. 1998. Physiological knockout of the envelope gene of the single-copy ERV-3 human endogenous retrovirus in a fraction of the Caucasian population. J Virol. 72(4):3442-5

[566] Neil R Smalheiser. 'Exosomal transfer of proteins and RNAs at synapses in the nervous system.' Biol. Direct; published online Nov. 30th. 2007

[567] http://bloodjournal.hematologylibrary.org/cgi/content/full/108/9/2885

But how does all this relate to HIV research? Today, in order to maintain the hypothesis that HIV is a retrovirus, researchers strive to show that cells make HIV in the same way as are made other retroviruses – and that HIV is an exosome.

Thus, HIV specialists reported in 2007 that they 'thought' our cells make HIV in the same place where are made all healthy retroviruses. To quote them more fully, they said: 'human immunodeficiency virus type 1 (HIV-1) is generally thought to assemble at the [cellular] plasma membrane' like all retroviruses. [568]

Pelchen-Matthews and others reported: 'Our data indicate that most of the infectious HIV produced by primary macrophages is assembled on late endocytic membranes [where absorbed particles are broken down] and acquires antigens characteristic of this compartment.' HIV is thus made, they say, in great part, from the normal 'antigens' (proteins) used naturally in this compartment. [569]   Others add that HIV's GAG protein, that makes up the shell of the virus, appears to be 'secreted from cells in exosomes.' [570]

HIV specialists have now named HIV as a 'viral exosome.' [571] *The Journal of Cell Biology* reported in 2003: 'Hildreth now proposes that: "the virus is fully an exosome in every sense of the word."' [572] Then, in a 2007 paper, they advanced the 'hypothesis that HIV and other retroviruses are generated by a normal non-viral way of exosome biogenesis' and added; 'We proposed that retroviruses are, at their most fundamental level, exosomes.' [573] '(The result of this has been astonishingly the authorisation of a course of drugs designed to stop our cells making exosomes; no matter how important these might be to us, in fear that the cells might thus also make HIV.)

HIV specialists also suggest that the 'Golgi apparatus' dispatches proteins to help make HIV in the same manner as it does to help make other retroviruses. [574] A recent paper vaguely concluded: 'It is therefore interesting to speculate that HIV, and perhaps other viruses, may benefit from a normal cellular process in order to facilitate exit from the cell.' [575]   Other HIV specialists say that 'viruses' in general have proteins allotted to them by 'the same signals that target proteins to exosomes.'

On arrival at another cell, HIV is again said to behave like a normal retrovirus. A 2002 paper concluded 'we propose that HIV uses the microtubule network to facilitate the delivery of the viral genome to the nucleus of the cell … using the highly ordered … cellular motor pathways.' [576]

---

[568] Infectious HIV-1 assembles in late endosomes in primary macrophages. Annegret Pelchen-Matthews, Beatrice Kramer and Mark Marsh Published online 28 July 2003. The Journal of Cell Biology

[569] Annegret Pelchen-Matthews, Beatrice Kramer and Mark Marsh. Infectious HIV-1 assembles in late endosomes in primary macrophages The Journal of Cell Biology. Published online 28 July 2003.

[570] Amy M. Booth, Exosomes and HIV Gag bud from endosome-like domains of the T cell plasma membrane. J Cell Biol. 2006 March 13; 172(6): 923–935

[571] Gould S.J, Hildreth J.E. 'The Trojan Exosome Hypothesis'. Proc Natl Acad Sci U S A. 2003 Sep 16;100(19):10592-7. Epub 2003 Aug 28: also Pelchen-Mathews A., Raposo G., Marsh M. 'Endosomes, exosomes and Trojan Viruses. Trends Microbiol. 2004 July. 12 (7): 310-6.

[572] The Journal of Cell Biology, Volume 162, Number 6, 960-960 8 September 2003

[573] Yi Fang, Ning Wu, Xin Gan, Wanhua Yan, James C Morrell, and Stephen J Gould; Higher-Order Oligomerization Targets Plasma Membrane Proteins and HIV Gag to Exosomes. PLoS Biol. 2007 June; 5(6): e158. Published online 2007 June 5

[574] Cell Biol., Volume 145, Number 1, April 5, 1999 57-68 Early Assembly Step of a Retroviral Envelope Glycoprotein: Analysis Using a Dominant Negative Assay. Arielle R. Rosenberg, Lélia Delamarre, Claudine Pique, Isabelle Le Blanc, Graziella Griffith, and Marie-Christine Dokhélar

[575] Gluschankof, Pablo et al. 'Cell Membrane Vesicles Are a Major Contaminant of Gradient-Enriched Human Immunodeficiency Virus Type-1 Preparations.' Virology 230, 125–133 (1997)

[576] Visualization of the Intracellular Behavior of HIV in Living Cells David McDonald, Marie A. Vodicka, Ginger Lucero, Tatyana M. Svitkina, Gary G. Borisy, Michael Emerman, Thomas J. Hope; *The Journal of Cell Biology*, Vol. 159, No. 3 (Nov. 11, 2002), pp. 441-452.

But nevertheless, these specialists at the same time insist that HIV is very different from other exosomes or retroviruses. For example, Professor Elizabeth Dax in 2007, in sworn testimony before an Australian court, claimed that HIV deviously coats itself with normal human proteins in order to disguise itself as an endogenous harmless retrovirus, but I wonder? Is HIV really capable of such subterfuge? Is she right in thinking this a super-viral act of deception – or is what she is observing the creation of normal endogenous retroviruses out of normal human proteins?

So I have to ask - how do these specialists claim to know the cells they are studying are making HIV and not normal retroviruses? It surely must be difficult to tell these apart when they have so very many similarities? I went to their experiments to discover how.

I was then astonished to discover that the methods they used were scarcely more advanced than those used in the early 1980s by Popovic and Gallo. In 2003 these modern researchers reported detecting HIV's presence in the cells, 'by measuring levels of p24, or reverse transcriptase activity' – and not by finding HIV itself! When they found more than usual p24 or RT activity, then they concluded that the cell must be making HIV!

But surely every biologist for decades has known that reverse transcriptase activity is common to all cells and not unique to retroviruses, let alone to HIV? So what then of their other way to detect HIV – 'measuring levels of p24'? Again they were relying on an old technique, claimed to work by Robert Gallo back in 1984.

But it has been long known in biology that p24 is a normal constituent of healthy cells and vesicles. For example, Dr. Chris Kaiser recently stated of p24 molecules; 'Because of their abundance, their conservation through evolution, and the fact that they shuttle from the ER [endoplasmic reticulum] to the Golgi compartments in transport vesicles, p24 proteins are thought to be fundamental constituents of vesicles.' [577]

Dr. Kaiser continued: 'The challenge is to explain the following: that p24 proteins are abundant constituents of the vesicle membrane, and their cytosolic tails interact with and powerfully nucleate assembly of both COPI and COPII [from **CO**ating **P**rotein] vesicle coats.' Thus, p24 is an important part both of the vital COPI vesicles that carry proteins to the membranes and of the COPII vesicles that carry proteins from the membranes back to the Golgi. So – in the very sites were HIV assembly was supposed to be detected by finding p24, there are p24s busily at work doing entirely healthy normal things!

HIV specialists recognise this – and now maintain that the p24 they are seeking and detecting is unique. They say it is an `HIV specific p24' called 'p24CA.' [578]

But the 'CA' added to p24 means it is 'of the capsid.' Well, a capsid literally means a 'box'. It is simply the external part of a retrovirus. It is not specific to HIV. Indeed, p24CA is also found in Bovine Leukaemia Viruses. [579]

The idea that there is a different p24 for HIV conflicts with other research. P24 is a major 'conserved' molecule, according to Dr. Kaiser, which suggests that it appeared early in evolution and still plays a vital role, thus ensuring it is protected from variation. The lack of variation of such proteins was endorsed by Nobel Laureate Leland Hartwell who stated in his 2001 Nobel Lecture: 'The genetic control of cell division provided two important lessons that have been repeated over and over in molecular, cellular and developmental biology. The first is the conservation of proteins and their functions

---

[577] Thinking about p24 proteins and how transport vesicles select their cargoChris Kaiser*
http://www.pnas.org/cgi/reprint/97/8/3783.pdf

[578] Bess JW Jr, Gorelick RJ, Bosche WJ, Henderson LE, Arthur LO. Microvesicles are a source of contaminating cellular proteins found in purified HIV-1 preparations. Virology. 1997 Mar 31;230(1):134-44
www.ncbi.nlm.nih.gov/sites/entrez?db=pubmed& uid=9126269&cmd=showdetailview&indexed=google

[579] L. Llames, E. Gomez-Lucia, A. Domenech, A. De Avila, G. Suarez, J. Goyache (2000). Production and Characterization of Monoclonal Antibodies against Bovine Leukaemia Virus using Various Crude Antigen Preparations: a Comparative Study; Journal of Veterinary Medicine Series B  Volume 47 Issue 5 Page 387-397, June 2000

throughout evolution. This was not a surprising conclusion because all living organisms share a common ancestor.' [580]

Another report said that p24 is a normal part of healthy human retroviruses; that it is their structural Gag protein and that: 'The Gag protein is the precursor to the internal structural protein of all retroviruses. …The internal structural proteins of retroviruses are derived from a single polypeptide.' [581]

Gallo and Popovic justified their claim that there was an 'HIV specific' p24 by saying, in a 1985 paper, that they could distinguish the p24 found in HTLVIII from that found in HTLVI and HTLVII with the Western Blot test. But in fact they did not attempt to prove any form of p24 unique to HTLV-III. [582] This paper was written to substantiate Gallo's erroneous claim that he, not the French, found the AIDS virus first, and that HTLV-3 is thus part of his HTLV retroviral family. This is now known to be untrue.

If thus there is no such thing as an HIV-specific p24, this would explain why anti-p24 'responses are minimal or absent in many HIV-infected individuals.' [583] Our bodies simply are not programmed to attack themselves.

These new insights have led to HIV specialists observing: 'An exosomal origin also predicts retroviral antigen vaccines are unlikely to provide prophylactic protection.'[584] If I may put it more simply: this suggests that the putative 'HIV particles' are so much part of ourselves that our immune systems cannot be persuaded to see them otherwise or to remove them, even if helped with a vaccine! Thus it seems there is very little evidence supporting their claim that human cells make a retrovirus that they can reliably identify as HIV during its assembly within the cell.

But now I feel able to set aside their reservations and quibbles as poorly based scientifically. Instead I am now growing more and more fascinated by the incredible world of the cell and the particles it uses to communicate. This clearly reveals the great importance of retroviruses and the other messenger particles. It now is apparent that they are an invaluable part of us – and of every cellular organism.

What I have learnt of cells and retroviruses has now shifted the paradigm with which I started researching this book. I have now learnt that retroviruses are not selfish, devious, or invaders, but primarily inert messages created to travel between cells. This is the task our cells give them. They are thus not individualistic particles with no need for their parents. Instead they serve their parents. Our cells make them because they need them. They are important to our health.

But – what of other viruses? What roles can they play? Why do they differ from retroviruses? Are most pathogenic?

---

[580] Yeast and Cancer Nobel Lecture, December 9, 2001 By Leland H. Hartwell.

[581] Vogt and Eisenman 1973

[582] Gallo and Popovic reported the p24s of HTLVI, HTLVII and HTLVIII could be distinguished from each other by such tests as Western Blot. [582] But the data produced depended on finding unique and specific antibodies and was inconclusive – not surprising as Gallo was then maintaining that his virus, not the French, was the real HIV and related to his other viruses. He hoped this paper would help prove his case. Proc. Natl. Acad. Sci. USA Vol. 82, pp. 3481-3484, May 1985 Immunological properties of the Gag protein p24 of the acquired immunodeficiency syndrome retrovirus (human T-cell leukemiavirus type III)(human T-cell leukemia virus types I and 11/immunological cross reactivity) M. G. SARNGADHARAN, L. BRUCH, M. POPOVIC, AND R. C. GALLO http://www.pnas.org/cgi/reprint/82/10/3481

[583] *The Journal of Immunology*, 2000, 165: 1685-1691. CD40 Ligand Trimer and IL-12 Enhance Peripheral Blood Mononuclear Cells and CD4' T Cell Proliferation and Production of IFN- in Response to p24 Antigen in HIV-Infected Individuals: Potential Contribution of Anergy to HIV-Specific Unresponsiveness Mark Dybul[1,*], George Mercier*, Michael Belson*, Claire W. Hallahan*, Shuying Liu, Cheryl Perry*, Betsey Herpin*, Linda Ehler*, Richard T. Davey*, Julie A. Metcalf, JoAnn M. Mican, Robert A. Seder and Anthony S. Fauci*

[584] Gould SJ, Booth AM, Hildreth JE. The Trojan exosome hypothesis. Proc Natl Acad Sci U S A. 2003 Sep 16;

# Chapter 21

# The Cell and the Virus.

The more I have learnt about the cells that make us, and all the life on our planet, the more I have been amazed by the skills they display. It has transformed my understanding of biology and entranced me. I now cannot learn enough about cells and their creations.

The works of some great women of biology have inspired me, particularly Barbara McClintock. She was one of the first to describe the intelligence of the cell, a concept she developed after studying plant cells! Her view was at first highly disputed among scientists. But, after being practically ignored and belittled most of her life, she was in her old age awarded a Nobel Prize in 1983 for discovering the transposon – from which the retrovirus may have evolved. It was her work that made me ask: if she is right in saying cells make carefully considered responses to their environment, then what are cells doing when they make the viruses that we link to diseases?

In her Nobel Lecture of 8th December 1983 she boldly spoke of cells as intelligent, as sophisticated in their responses to the environment and as making 'wise decisions.' She explained 'a genome may reorganize itself when faced with a difficulty for which it is unprepared.' She gave an example: 'cells are able to sense the presence in their nuclei of ruptured ends of chromosomes, and then activate a mechanism that will bring together and then unite these ends, one with another, a particularly revealing example of the sensitivity of cells to all that is going on within them. They make wise decisions and act upon them.'

McClintock continued: 'Cells must be prepared to respond to many sources of stress. Mishaps that affect the operation of a cell must be occurring continuously. Sensing these and instigating repair systems are essential. ... It is becoming increasingly apparent that we know little of the potentials of a genome. Nevertheless, much evidence tells us that it must be vast.'

She predicted: 'In the future attention undoubtedly will be centred on the genome, and with greater appreciation of its significance as a highly sensitive organ of the cell, monitoring genomic activities and correcting common errors, sensing the unusual and unexpected events, and responding to them, often by restructuring the genome. We know about the components of genomes ... [but] we know nothing, about how the cell senses danger and instigates responses to it that often are truly remarkable.'

This was far from the mechanistic view found in many virological studies in which the cell is described as the passive invaded victim of the cunning hijacking germ. It made me think – might the production of viruses sometimes not be due to 'infections?' Could virus production be sometimes a natural part of a cell's 'wise' response to the environment?

Could viruses have been damned too often? I had found that this happening with polio and perhaps the 1918 flu epidemic? Could it be also true of other 'viral' diseases? If virus production can be a positive intelligently chosen option for a cell, then surely a far more radical rethinking might be called for?

But to return to McClintock, she also observed: 'The establishment of a successful tissue culture from animal cells, such as those of rat or mouse, is accompanied by readily observed genomic restructuring' – adding that cells effect such changes with 'transposons.' A scientist thus cannot presume when making a vaccine that cell and viral genomes stay the same. The very fact of our intervention may mean that the particles present are not the same. This is a challenge that I suspect vaccine manufacturers have mostly ignored.

I wondered if the cell's ability to manipulate genomes might explain why virus genomes are frequently described as 'mutated' (changed)? I had thought that the virus mutated itself, but on reflection this could not be. They are inert, so cannot change their genomes. In contrast, cells modify their DNA. When confronted by a toxin, such as from petrochemical fumes, cells work assiduously to protect themselves by adjusting their DNA. They thus help us survive the many toxins we encounter in modern life.

Transposons are our cells' 'molecular-sized engineers,' that experiment, so-to-speak, with our DNA by swapping fragments of it around as if trying to resolve problems. To date this process has reshaped at least 30% of our genome.[585] It is incidentally the very same process that is used by the 'hospital super-bug' to ensure its survival. These modify their DNA to protect themselves from antiseptics or antibiotics in the same way that our cells seek protection from toxins. Our cells are constantly adjusting to protect us.

When RNA, a more flexible form of genetic code, is manipulated by the cell, we call the 'engineer' employed a 'retrotransposon' – and, as we have seen, these are easily transformed into retroviruses that can pass from cell to cell, thus sharing the results of the retrotransposons' work. Recent studies show that plant retroviruses work similarly to help plants rapidly adapt to new environments.

Retroviruses have a unique role among viruses. They carry genetic codes that are spliced into the DNA in the nucleus of the receiving cell. This process is a vital part of the evolution of all cellular organisms. Although the genetic codes of other viruses are likewise taken into cells, their codes reportedly are not spliced into the cells' genomes but taken into other areas of the cell, such as into the cytoplasm in which the organelles are found.

Another great woman of science, Dr. Lynn Margulis, was, like McClintock, at first marginalised because her theories challenged the orthodoxy, but she also is now recognised as one of the great scientists of our age because of her radical insights into the evolution of cells. She theorized that cells evolved through symbiosis, by working together, by cells coming to live within other cells as organs ('organelles'). Her theory was proved when organelles were found to have their own DNA. Other scientists have similarly theorised that viruses contribute to cellular evolution by symbiosis. Perhaps this is how those viruses whose nucleic acid is absorbed into the cell's cytoplasm contribute to the cells' welfare? The theory of 'Cytoplasmic Evolution' states that genetic codes found elsewhere than in the cell's nucleus also contribute to cellular evolution.[586]

'Cross-species' help between cells is vital and common. In 2007 the cells of invertebrates were found to accept genes from bacterial cells when repairing 'damaged genes.' Dr. Werren and colleagues reported in *Science* there was 'widespread transfer of bacterial genes into the genome of numerous invertebrates.' [587] As most cells within us are bacterial, this points to considerable cooperation happening within us. No talk here of a race between selfish cells or germs as fiercely independent individuals – or of a need to

---

[585] Clustering of human endogenous retrovirus sequences with median self-organizing map. Merja Oja, Panu Somervuo, Samuel Kaski, and Teuvo Kohonen Neural Networks Research Centre, Helsinki University of Technology

[586] Sapp, Jan. *Beyond the Gene: Cytoplasmic Inheritance and the Struggle for Authority in Genetics.* Oxford University Press. 1987. Pp 117 -122

[587] http://www.nytimes.com/2007/09/04/science/04obgeno.html?ex=1346558400&en=7c1ad56945d50a73&ei=512 4&partner=permalink&exprod=permalink

kill this bacteria. Rather the more female vision of cellular survival, evolution and growth, through compromise, symbiosis and cooperation. [588]

Another biologist who inspired me is Dr. Mae-Wan Ho, the founder of the Institute of Science in Society (ISIS), at the UK's Open University. She took the ideas of Barbara McClintock and ran with them. What emerges from her work is a picture of cells as centres of dynamic fields of energy, as fluid crystals, electric, magnetic, coherent and quantum. In one of her papers she shares the vision that drives her. 'I see all nature developing and evolving, with every organism participating, constantly creating and recreating itself anew.' From her I learnt that cells have many ways of communicating, that little is static in nature and that life itself is woven into the fabric of the universe.

Then there is the work of a man – of Professor James A. Shapiro, who teaches in the States but was formerly at the Institut Pasteur. His work reveals our cells use massive amounts of information with seemingly great computational skills, having in their DNA a massive 'read-write' memory. His ideas helped me to better understand the role 'viruses' might play in the cellular world. To continue his metaphor, I now see viruses, exosomes, retroviruses, functioning as the natural flash memory sticks used by cells to share encoded information with each other.

Shapiro wrote: 'The expectation of its pioneers was that molecular biology would confirm the reductionist, mechanical view of life. However, the actual result of molecular studies of heredity, cell biology and multicellular development has been to reveal a realm of sensitivity, communication, computation and indescribable complexity.' He also said: 'The conceptual changes in biology (since the work of McClintock was recognized) are comparable in magnitude to the transition from classical physics to relativistic and quantum physics.' [589]

An editorial in the Journal of Cell Science similarly said of cells: 'their behaviour such as solid-state channelling of substrates, error-checking, proof-reading, regulation and adaptiveness ... imply an 'intelligence.' [590]

Shapiro stated that cells are capable of 'Boolean calculations' during a 2007 lecture in the UK. The intelligence we often credit solely to our brains exists at the cellular level in all parts of our bodies. He said of bacterial cells; 'they display astonishing versatility in managing the biosphere's geochemical and thermodynamic transformations: processes more complex than the largest human-engineered systems. This mastery over the biosphere indicates that we have a great deal to learn about chemistry, physics and evolution from our small, but very intelligent, prokaryotic relatives.' [591] He added: **'there can be no doubt that bacteria received evolutionary benefits by having mobile DNA in their genomes and systems for transferring DNA from cell to cell.'**

Cells carry out this transfer by making the particles that we have called viruses. By using a base of four (the four nucleotides) to encode information into the RNA and DNA of viruses, rather than the base of two used by computers, our cells have achieved the ability to process and pack an incredible amount of information into extremely small spaces – making it possible 'viruses' that can economically transport much information between cells. It has been pointed out that: 'the bases are spaced every 0.35 nm [billionths of a metre] along the DNA molecule, giving DNA a data density of over one-half million gigabits per square centimetre.' [592] However, the transported information is not just stored in the genetic acid. It is also encoded into proteins of viruses, as we will see.

---

[588] Lynn Margulus in 2007 stated she did not agree with the theory that HIV caused AIDS. March 12, 2007 10:21AM http://scienceblogs.com/pharyngula

[589] Boston Review: Is Darwin in the Details? A Debate http://www.bostonreview.net/br22.1/shapiro.html

[590] G. Borisy; 'Beyond cell toons.' Editorial. Journal of Cell Science, Vol. 113, Issue 5.

[591] J. A. Shapiro; Stud. Hist. Phil. Biol. & Biomed. Sci. 38 (2007) 807–819

[592] http://www.etcgroup.org/upload/publication/602/01/synbioreportweb.pdf

Cells do not only communicate by means of exosomes or viruses; they also do so by movement, electric currents, chemical emissions (smells), photons and magnetic fields. They can send light signals to each other to make near instantaneous communications. The water within the cell is also used. Rich in salts, it preserves information, and, as it flows within the cell, it generates the electric current needed for the signals sent through the nerves.

Protein molecules take on specialised functions through the information that cells encode into their folds. For example, cells can produce the specialist p53 protein when exposed to radiation or to other causes of DNA damage. In 2007 this protein was found to vibrate when it detects DNA damage. Other molecules apparently vibrate to help regulate genes, almost as if they are talking.[593] P53 molecules play an important role in regulating the production of exosomes and retroviruses – and thus also help to move information between cells. [594]

I mentioned how McClintock discovered that 'cells are able to sense the presence in their nuclei of ruptured ends of chromosomes' and repair these. Is this why some retroviruses reportedly have powerful anti-tumor effects, as mentioned in the last chapter? Likewise it is reported of the particles called 'retroelements' (including the retrotransposon) that: 'Unusually high activity or unexpected appearance of retroelements within cells is often found in connection with stress events.' It seems these particles are also produced when the cellular DNA is inadequately 'methylated' and thus not properly protected from toxins.[595]

Professor James A. Shapiro noted; 'molecular analysis has confirmed the generality of Barbara McClintock's revolutionary discoveries of internal systems for genome repair and genome restructuring.'[8] I would add that such repair systems do not stop at the borders of a cell in multicellular organisms – they extend to the whole of the organism. Cells produce clouds of 'hundreds of' defensive vesicles whenever they are challenged, 'in response to danger signals.' [596] It is further reported that these viruses or particles help activate our T-cells by merging with them – and this of course could be easily mistaken for HIV infection.

We need an information genetic highway that weaves our cells together, and we have it – the world of retroviruses, viruses, exosomes, microvesicles, mRNA, microRNAs – all carrying information encoded by our cells.

But – I must not leave out the bacteria. These are cells, thus entirely unlike viruses. The use of the term 'germ' for both has confused things. A bacterium is a cell with a more independent style of life that nevertheless lives communally with and communicates with other cells. It can make toxins to kill pathogens, change its DNA, and make viruses that travel to other bacteria. It can use the enzyme RT to change the proteins making up its 'skin' to make it harder for it to be recognised by enemies. It can take on specialisations to serve the collective good of its colony. Shapiro has produced excellent pictures of beautifully constructed bacterial colonies.

There are extremely small bacteria called 'mycoplasmas,' that are true parasites capable of living inside cells without harming them.[597] Like jellyfish each is covered in a

---

[593] Tiana G et al. 'Oscillations and temporal signalling in cells' Phys Biol 4 (2007) R1-R17

[594] The Regulation of Exosome Secretion: a Novel Function of the p53 Protein
Xin Yu1, Sandra L. Harris1 and Arnold J. Levine Cancer Research 66, 4795-4801, May 1, 2006.

[595] Hansen and Heslop-Harrison. 2004. Adv.Bot.Res. 41: 165-193. Page 14 of 34.
(Dahal et al., 2000; Lockhart et al., 2000; Mhiri et al., 1997

[596] Carolina Obregon et al. Exovesicles from Human Activated Dendritic Cells Fuse with Resting Dendritic Cells, Allowing Them to Present Alloantigens 2006 American Society for Investigative Pathology DOI: 10.2353/ajpath.2006.060453

[597] Mycoplasmas: Sophisticated, Reemerging, and Burdened by Their Notoriety by Joel Baseman and Joseph Tully http://www.cdc.gov/ncidod/eid/vol3no1/baseman.htm

thin pliable membrane. Thus they can change shapes dramatically and be hard to recognize in the microscope. They are our smallest life form but still have a genome over 50 times bigger than the typical virus at half a million to 1.2 million base pairs. They are nevertheless so small that they have contaminated many a scientific experiment and been mistaken for viruses, although unlike viruses they are truly alive and can reproduce. Montagnier in 1990 suggested that they might be a co-factor in causing AIDS since he found them in one third of blood samples from AIDS patients. A sneeze can spread them and they are suspected to cause a mild pneumonia.

Surprisingly it is said that there are in us some ten times more bacterial cells than there are of 'human cells'. Thus there must be a great deal of inter-species communication if we are to smoothly function.

Bacteria sometimes take on the role of scavengers. They may multiply within us when cells die during a severe illness. As soon as they have completed this scavenging work, the bacterial numbers will naturally decline.

However, when human cells are severely diseased, bacterial cells may multiply out of control and produce toxic by-products, as in severe TB.  Bacteria are intelligent cells that might well prefer to cooperate, but they might put their own survival first when necessary. They also will bond with other bacterial cells to form self-protective 'biofilms' that are often hazardous to us. The NIH states that '80% of chronic infections are biofilm related' (and thus not viral).[598]

## THE VIRUS

There are estimated to be some $10^{31}$ viruses on Earth,[599] but how this estimate was arrived at was not explained. All I can say is that, as viruses do not usually survive longer than a few days and cannot reproduce themselves, cells must be constantly making and sending out an enormous number of them.

The International Committee on Viral Taxonomy describes a virus as *'an elementary biosystem that possesses some of the properties of living systems such as having a genome and being able to adapt to changing environments. However, viruses cannot capture and store free energy and they are not functionally active outside their host cells.'*

This, however, fails to explain why a cell would make them. It omits entirely their ability to move genetic codes from cell to cell. It also contradictory maintains that viruses are both 'able to adapt' and 'not functionally active.'

But, there is something else interesting about this definition.  It does not differentiate the virus from the vesicles our healthy cells make and it does not define viruses as pathogenic. In fact there is nothing strikingly different in definition, appearance, creation and structure between the 'pathogenic' virus and inter-cellular vesicles.

Our cells invest much energy in sending out transport vehicles. This may be why they locate mitochondria 'power stations' alongside the Golgi apparatus.[600] Sometimes this process may go wrong – but I would argue that our cells would not invest so much energy if this process did not normally serve them well.  As we have seen, some retroviruses are thought to repair DNA – thus doing very much the same as transposons were reported by Barbara McClintock to do within cells.

Cells, whether healthy or sick, are constantly making vesicles or viruses, but virology textbooks normally start their description of virus production from when a virus

[598] Monroe D (2007) Looking for Chinks in the Armor of Bacterial Biofilms. PLoS Biol 5(11): e307 doi:10.1371/journal.pbio.0050307  Published: November 13, 2007

[599] Trends in Microbiology Volume 13, Issue 6, June 2005, Pages 278-284

[600] Rojo et al.1998 Migration of Mitochondria to Viral Assembly Sites in African Swine Fever Virus-Infected Cells. Journal of Virology, September 1998, p. 7583-7588, Vol. 72, No. 9

is about to infect a cell. But, I must ask, is this the best way to depict this process? I would suggest that it presumes too much – particularly that a virus is an independent entity, that it initiates this action and the cell is its victim.

It is universally accepted that cells make every virus that exists, so why not start from where this process starts, from when a living cell creates messenger RNA with instructions to encode and make a virus – for after all that is when all inter-cellular vesicles are created? After all, the first viruses made could not have been the result of a viral infection.

In the first stage the cell encodes information in the form of a strand or double strand of DNA or RNA. It then surrounds this with a protective capsid of proteins, plus sometimes a membrane envelope as well, before sending it out from the cell. On arrival at another cell, its genetic strands and proteins are brought inside that cell and absorbed. After this, the virus no longer exists. Any new virus or vesicle is made afresh.

The codes thus transported include many mRNAs (messenger RNAs). These in turn may contain many 'Open Reading Frames' used to make proteins. The cytomegalovirus carries up to 200 of these. This is an impressive cargo, but it should be remembered that a virus is utterly unable to do anything with these codes. It is only the receiving cell that can use them. Viruses simply do not have the tools or the knowledge to use what they carry. They are messages in bottles, to put it metaphorically.

Viruses have no metabolism so they cannot produce energy or eat. They have no nervous system, no sensory system, no intelligence that can facilitate any kind of invasion or the hi-jacking of a cell a billion times larger.

The conventional theory of viral hijacking is that, after the short genetic code of a virus has been absorbed by a cell, the 'viral genes' absorbed start to 'direct the production of proteins by the host cellular machinery.' It is assumed they are able to force the host cell to do this, It is said they force the cell to assemble proteins into a shell or 'capsid,' to insert into this a clone of the original viral genetic code and then to launch it out of the cell by using the same machinery that the cell uses to harmlessly produce its own exosomes and other extra-cellular particles or vesicles.

But I had to ask, would cells give such minute and 'dead' messenger vesicles the extraordinary ability to pirate cells of the same organism? This is the quandary we are left with if we agree that viruses are not alive and thus incapable of having a survival instinct.

But what if cells create viruses as weapons against other cells? If they do, then this would be remarkably suicidal as viruses usually pass from cell to cell within the same organism.

Such thoughts have left me deeply puzzled about the many pathogenic viruses reported to exist. I have severe doubts about some of these, particularly the poliovirus and HIV. I would have to look again at the evidence on other viruses.

### VIRAL ILLNESSES

Viruses are commonly blamed for illnesses that seem easily passed from one person to another. Bacteria may cause many of these – but viruses are often blamed. Our only medical weapons against them are said to be vaccination and powerful chemotherapy-type antiviral medicines that are designed to stop cells from making viruses, rather than to attack the virus itself, for apparently it is too elusive a target.

But, why do cells make pathogenic viruses? Surely the reason for this has been established in numerous laboratory experiments? It is a doctrine in virology that cells make malignant viruses only after a disease virus arrives and infects them.

I had long presumed this must be so, but when I tried to analyse it, I had problems. I found myself asking, since a virus cannot make a virus, surely the first viruses to cause an illness must have been made by an uninfected cell?

I had earlier learnt how viruses did their damage. I had been told that they burst forth from infected cells, 'exploding' them. I was now surprised to discover that this is not so; that viruses are far too small, at one-billionth of the mass of a cell, to have this effect.

Current courses on Medical Microbiology now teach, as mentioned briefly above, that viruses kill or damage cells indirectly, by triggering cellular processes that do this damage. Professor Tritz blames allergic reactions. 'With animal viruses, cell lyses [death] is usually the result of one of four types of allergic reactions' and 'allergy to viruses usually results in a very localized anaphylactic reaction.' Alternatively, he suggests that the immune system sees the virus-producing cell as foreign and kills it.

Tritz suggests that some illnesses are due to 'toxic substances' produced by cells because they are infected. 'Virus-infected cells, at times, will produce compounds coded for by the host DNA, but which are not normally produced by the host. These are often cytotoxic at relatively high concentrations.' Finally, some viruses might cause 'structural alterations in the host cell', affecting the chromosomes, moving the nucleus or creating bubble-like spaces.[601] Another university course teaches, 'virus infected cells may be recognized by the immune system, which leads to the destruction of the virus infected cells.' [602]

But the above are only said to be suggestions; I have been unable to find experiments that prove viruses acting alone cause such effects. But their theories perhaps make sense. The virus is so minute compared to the cell – and our protective systems will destroy a very sick cell that does not self-destruct. Our cells often seem altruistically to decide to die when not needed, poisoned or otherwise diseased.

But, on further thought, how can we prove cell's illness is caused by the small viral genetic code it's absorbed? How can we be sure that a damaged cell is so solely because it is infected? It may be naturally dying or poisoned. It may even produce viral-like particles for waste disposal, or to attempt a cure or help other cells similarly afflicted.

Also, if cell deaths in viral illnesses are mostly caused by our immune system as Tritz suggested, why do we have such deaths when the immune system is down, as surely it often is in such circumstances?

But nevertheless, viruses are encoded information, and since cells can make errors, I must conclude that they may sometimes wrongly encode the viruses they send out. These in theory could misinform other cells, perhaps sometimes encouraging them to take courses of action that they would not take otherwise. But as to how often the codes thus transported could lead to such effects, I had no idea.

I went to consult a standard textbook, '*Introduction to Modern Virology*' by N. Dimmock and S. Primrose, published by Blackwell Scientific Publications.

On page 230 I found it surprisingly reported that, although people have presumed that flu is spread by coughing, 'transmission experiments from people infected with a rhinovirus to susceptibles sitting opposite at a table proved singularly unsuccessful. Equally unsuccessful was the transmission of influenza from a naturally infected husband/wife to his/her spouse.'

Also on the same page it reported: 'it has been shown that recently bereaved people are susceptible to infectious diseases. Thus one's resistance is influenced by one's state of mind.' It then went on to discuss winter life styles; such as living crowded in unventilated and over-heated rooms, all things it says might make us produce the symptoms of illness – and all things that make cells ill without any need of help from viruses. It then concluded on page 212: 'Evidently viruses do not kill cells by any one simple

[601] Medical Microbiology Fall 2000. Tritz Professor/Chairman Department Microbiology & Immunology
http://www.kcom.edu/faculty/chamberlain/Website/Lects/MECHANIS.HTM
602 http://mansfield.osu.edu/~sabedon/biol2065.htm

process and we are far from understanding the complex mechanisms involved …[it does] seem more akin to death by slow starvation than acute poisoning. Lastly it is by no means clear what advantage accrues to the virus in killing its host cell. This situation may represent a poorly evolved virus–cell relationship or virus in the 'wrong' host cell.'

It thus seems that cells may be sick, poisoned, stressed or malnourished in some way before they show the symptoms of 'viral infection.' There is a considerable body of research that indicates cellular illness or malnourishment often precedes the production of viruses, rather than the converse. For example: it is reported that deficiency in selenium, a metal our cells use as an antioxidant, can precede the symptoms of colds, flu and even AIDS. (There is also a strong correlation between selenium levels in soils in African countries and the prevalence of AIDS symptoms. [603])

Dr. Melinda Beck reported that selenium-deficient mouse cells show symptoms of illness and emit viruses. She and her co-authors deduced from this that a lack of selenium made viruses dangerous – and consequently that these viruses made the cells ill. [604] But was this deduction soundly based? Selenium is a component of glutathione peroxidase (GPX), an enzyme that protects cells from oxidative stress. Selenium-deficiency thus makes cells ill with oxidative stress without any need for a viral illness. They consequently could produce viral-like particles as waste or for repair purposes.

Another research paper reported that, when cells are suffering from 'oxidative DNA damage' (such as from chemotherapy), then they are more likely to get hepatitis due to HCV viral infections. Again, what comes first? The authors presume the virus must cause the illness – but surely the illness started with the earlier oxidative stress.[605]

The first observation of retroviruses is credited to Peyton Rous. 'It is generally accepted that Peyton Rous discovered retroviruses in 1911 when he induced malignancy in chickens by injections of cell-free filtrates obtained from a muscle tumour.' [606] But, when I went back to his records, I found that he also suggested that the cause of his chickens' illness might be a chemical toxin in his filtrate! If retroviruses were indeed also present, might they have appeared as a defence against this toxin?

In earlier chapters we found that toxins, rather than viruses, are likely to be the primary causes of polio and AIDS – but what then about measles, mumps, flu and colds?

I had long presumed the evidence for these illnesses being due solely to viral infection must be overwhelming – but I have found to my surprise that scientists have long known that the guaranteed way to make cells produce viruses in the laboratory, including flu and measles virus, is not primarily by getting them infected, but by exposing them to stress and toxins!

In 1928 the President of the Royal Society of Medicine's Pathology Section, A. E. Boycott, in a report on the 'nature of filterable viruses,' stated that with toxins 'we can with a considerable degree of certainty stimulate normal tissues to produce viruses.' [607]

Then in 1963 the famous Sloan-Kettering Institute for Cancer Research reported that viruses multiplied after cells were exposed to 'x-ray, ultraviolet light or certain

[603] Burcher, Sam. *Selenium conquers AIDS?* Institute of Science in Society. http://www.i-sis.org.uk/AidsandSelenium.php

[604] Melinda A. Beck *Antioxidants and Viral Infections: Host Immune Response and Viral Pathogenicity.* Departments of Pediatrics and Nutrition, University of North Carolina at Chapel Hill, Chapel Hill, North Carolina. April 27 2000 or 1999 issue of the FASEB Journal, a scientific journal published by the Federation of American Societies for Experimental Biology.

[605] Fabio Farinati et al. Oxidative DNA damage in circulating leukocytes occurse as an early event in chronic HCV infection. Free Radical Biology and Medicine, December 1999. Pages 1284-1291.

[606] J. Exp. Med. vol. 13, no. 4, pp. 397-411 (April, 1911). httm://www.jem.org/cgi/reprint/13/4/397

[607] Boycott AE. The transition form life to death; the nature of filterable viruses. Proc. Royal Soc. Med. 1928;22:55-69.

mutagenic chemicals' and that this exposure seemed to 'alter the benign relationship' that otherwise existed between cells and bacteria.[608]

Then in the 1980s Robert Gallo reported that after he added a certain substance (interleuken 2) to cell cultures, these cells both reproduced and made retroviruses. Gallo thus named this his 'T-cell growth factor' – and Montagnier at the Institut Pasteur used the same. If retroviruses were indeed thus produced, what if this were a natural reaction to such chemicals?

In 2007 Dr. Dominic Dwyer, a Senior Medical Virologist, formerly of the Institut Pasteur in Paris, testified that to persuade blood cells to produced HIV retroviruses, 'we stimulate them with compounds such as PHA.' [609] He added; if we want to persuade cells to produce the flu virus 'we use other things like tryspin.' – thus that they expose cells to different chemicals to make them produce different viruses! (Tryspin is destructive to proteins, and Phytohemagglutinin (PHA) is mitogenic. [610]) This surely suggests that virus production can be a cell's response to being exposed to certain substances and perhaps stressed,  - and that there might thus be no need for it to be infected beforehand?

Dr. David Gordon, the Chair of the Clinical Drug Trials Committee at Flinders University in Australia, testified, at the 2007 Parenzee trial, that there is no need to 'purify a virus in order to identify it'. He repeated emphatically: 'No need to purify' then questioned: 'Has any virus ever been purified?' He explained: 'The issues are exactly the same with any virus.' He doubted if any virus was ever isolated from sick cells. It seemed that a cellular illness is all the proof he needed to conclude that unseen viruses were present – no matter how artificial the laboratory circumstances or what chemicals were added.

Gordon concluded: 'acceptance of the Defence Experts arguments [that HIV had not been isolated from AIDS patients and thus not proved to cause AIDS] would lead to the conclusion that no viruses or virus diseases (such as measles, mumps, polio, hepatitis B and C, smallpox and many others) exist at all. ... All the issues, such as antibody testing and virus isolation, these would apply to every single virus. That is impossible.' Yes indeed, demanding the suspected virus is proved present would apparently undermine the validity of many experiments now said to 'prove' that viruses cause illnesses.

The British virologist Robin Weiss confirmed much the same in a 1999 email exchange with the Perth Group. He wrote: 'If we are to doubt HIV as a cause of AIDS, we must cast even more doubt on variola as a cause of smallpox, and the existence of measles, mumps, influenza and respiratory syncytial virus. None of these would pass your definition of purification. None of these has been 'purified' even by culture propagation (my sense) to the extent that has been achieved for poliovirus and for HIV.' He added: 'It is precisely because Val Turner and his colleagues in Perth have not queried the existence of other viruses that I find it difficult to take their ideas on HIV seriously. All the 'failings' they attribute to HIV could equally well, according to their own stringent criteria, be levelled against any virus with a lipid envelope, e.g. small pox, influenza, measles, mumps or yellow fever.'[611]

He also stated in the same email exchange: 'When you have evidence of infection in culture, purification is not particularly important.' Symptoms of cellular illness are frequently allotted to particular viruses without the presence of these viruses having been proved.

Extraordinarily, these orthodox scientists were giving strength to what Dr. Steven Lanka, a virologist, had controversially reported in the 1990s. He stated he could find no

---

[608] Sloane-Kettering Institute for Cancer Research, Progress Report XV, Viruses and Cancer. January 1963

[609] Nucleic Acids Res. 1977 August; 4(8): 2713–2723.

[610] Nucleic Acids Res. 1977 August; 4(8): 2713–2723.

[611] This correspondence is available at http://www.theperthgroup.com/emailcorres.html

evidence for the complete isolation of any pathogenic virus. He then went one step further. He interpreted the electron micrographs published of 'viruses' as solely showing parts of the 'intra- and intercellular transport' system – such as the vesicles. He said viruses were thus 'cell components' [612] I must admit that he stimulated me into asking the same questions and thus I am thankful to him.

The scientists who question if HIV causes AIDS (see some of their names and academic positions in the epilogue to this book) have frequently arrived at their positions by discovering that HIV has never been isolated from an AIDS patient – and thus not proved to cause their illness. But, if the testimonies of Weiss, Gordon and other scientists cited are to be believed, other viruses are likewise not isolated from cellular cultures or from patients before being blamed for an illness.

Confirmation that a virus is responsible for an illness is now usually sought through experiments in which cells are exposed to 2-3 milligrams of fluid from a sick patient. If these cells then fall ill, it is often simply assumed this is caused by a virus in the fluid, while other elements that may cause this are not tested for, such as free DNA, proteins, cellular debris, other viruses, mycoplasmas, possibly prions and of course toxins.

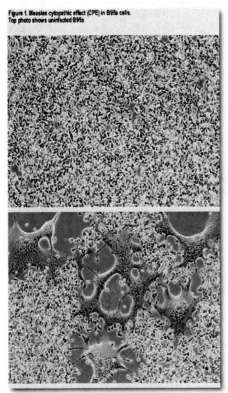

Figure 1. Measles cytopathic effect (CPE) in B95a cells. Top photo shows uninfected B95a

So what has made virologists and doctors so sure that a malignant unseen virus is at work? Dwyer replied, when this was put to him: 'We look to see what the cell lines are looking like. ... The virus will often cause cytopathic effects. In other words, because their cells are infected they look as although they're going to die, and they are dying... in fact sometimes they all clump together and take on a very bizarre shape.' (See images on left of cells before and after, not just infection as the text suggests, but the addition of toxins etc.) [613]

Gordon said much the same when asked the same question. If cells fall ill, the suspect virus must be present and guilty. 'This is a principle for all the viruses we culture.' 'That is the same principle that we use right now for other things – like influenza cultures or measles cultures. You look what the cells look like. If they have a cytopathic effect [if the cells get ill or die] then you have the various measures of the viruses in them.' If there is RT activity, cell disease or death, all these are interpreted as proof of the presence of a deadly virus. In the case of HIV, they even make the cells in the culture turn cancerous before they look among them for signs of damage they may use as signs of retrovirus production!

---

612  http://www.neue-medizin.com/lanka2.htm

613  Images from CDC Measles Lab. Manual.
http://www.cdc.gov/ncidod/dvrd/revb/measles/isol_man_immuno/measles_cytopathic_effect.htm

I cited earlier the currently online CDC paper entitled '*Isolation and Identification of Measles Virus in Cell Culture.*' [614] It is a truly staggering paper for it could not make it more evident that cell sickness is still being taken as 'virus isolation.'

The paper bears summarizing. Take from the person thought to have measles a small fluid sample from mouth, nose or urine .Put this aside. Now prepare a cell culture. Take cells from a marmoset monkey, immortalize these possibly by exposing to radiation (meaning make them cancerous) then give them Epson Barre Syndrome. They are not yet sick enough so expose them to trypsin, taking care to protect yourself from this toxin by wearing gloves and goggles. The cells may now start to 'float free' because they are ill – so the CDC says give them 2 or 3 days to rest up and give them nutrients. There is so far no mention of any need to examine them with a microscope.

After this the cells are to be exposed to the fluid sample from the patient. Add this and an hour later examine the cells with a microscope. If more than half are distorted, floating fee or rounded, the CDC instructs put the cell culture in the fridge and label it as a 'isolated measles virus stock.' No need to see the virus, or to 'isolate' it from the rest of the poisoned cell culture.

If less than 50% are ill at this stage, then the CDC instructs add two antibiotics, Penicillin and Streptomycin. A day later, it says inspect them again with the microscope. If small holes have appeared in the cell layer in the dish, indicating either that the cells have died or floated free, then the CDC says you have your 'isolated measles-virus stock.' No need to actually see the virus, or to find out what other viruses are present. Your 'isolate' is ready to be processed into such products as vaccines. No need for this to remove the toxin added or the parts of monkey cells.

Let us think what this. Injecting such a vaccine into a child would certainly produce antibodies – but we would have no idea if any of these were against measles virus.

This is the whole process as recommended by the CDC. There is no mention of the need to have a control culture, no electron microscopy and no mention of any need to isolate the measles virus from particles or toxins produced by the poisoned marmoset cells. How can they say these cells now have 'measles?'

There is also no consideration of how viruses can cause such deformation – or of the role played by toxin added, or by the artificial circumstances. I wonder to what extent the CDC took into consideration Nobel-Laureate McClintock's observation that cells placed in stress readily mutate?

After learning how the original measles vaccine was similarly developed, I had doubts that they had proved that a virus uniquely caused the cellular distortions that are said to prove its presence, or proved that such distortions are related to measles. How then can the measles virus sometimes cause serious illness? Measles in humans normally does little harm. However some cases are very serious. What happens in such cases? I found that measles is said to kill in the manner of HIV – by damaging the immune system, sometimes over a long period, so that other diseases linked to bacteria, particularly pneumonia and diarrhoea, make the child seriously ill. [615]

Then take the cold viruses. The symptoms of a cold are associated with at least 200 different types of virus and a number of different environmental factors. Any one of these may be present, or even a combination. Rhinovirus is found in about half of colds, but this comes in over 100 serotypes – meaning over a hundred antibodies attach to different types of them. Thus this virus cannot be tested for easily with an antibody test.

---

[614] Enders j et al- Measles Virus: A Summary of Experiments Concerned with Isolation, Properties, and Behavior Am J Public Health Nations Health. 1957 March; 47(3): 275–282. http://www.pubmedcentral.nih.gov/articlerender.fcgi?artid=1551024. Whole text.
[615] The immuno-suppression 'molecular' theory is set forth by the Medical Research Council on http://www.mrc.ac.uk/OurResearch/Impact/Infections/Measles/index.htm#P40_6040

Rhinovirus is preferentially produced in the lab by using human cervical cancer cells (HeLa) – something inexplicable. How can they say the virus is present and 'isolated' when such cells show extra symptoms of illness? How can they deduce the cells have a cold? All that can be said for certain is that during colds we produce a multitude of different viruses along with the many other elements that travel in the fluids spread by sneezes.

In order to explain failures in finding viruses in studies of illnesses blamed on them, many virologists have been driven to speak of viruses as if they possess the cleverness of the cell (and thus as if they are bacteria). Professor Elizabeth Dax spoke of HIV as 'very clever at mutating.' At that time, January 2007, she was the Director of the Australian National Serology Laboratory, with responsibility for 'the quality of HIV, hepatitis and blood-borne viral testing in Australia.'

Virologists frequently similarly describe viruses. But, if viruses are dead, as is also widely held, then surely finding a virus that is cleverly pathogenic must be as unlikely as finding a page in a book that physically attacks its reader!

This seeing viruses as clever perhaps harks back to the earliest days of virology, when scientists theoretically posited the existence of 'viruses' while conceiving of them as mini-bacteria and thus as cells. It seems this early conceptual error has not been entirely eradicated. But modern virology is built upon the idea that viruses invade and destroy. So, could viruses be alive and dangerous when inside cells, and inert outside cells?

They are alive within the cell in the sense that they share the life of the cell that creates them. But can they act independently of it? The virus absorbed on arrival at a cell is nothing much more than food and information for the cell. The idea that this tiny amount of disassembled material is able to force the cell to serve its needs seems to me somewhat questionable. It is rather like saying the pea I ate last night was able to hijack my stomach to force it to make more peas, or that a text message I received made me pregnant! If a virus can thus hijack a cell, it needs to be rigorously established, but I cannot find any experiments establishing this. All I find are suppositions.

I appreciate that such thoughts may be received as rank heresy by many virologists, so I would like to stress that I am open to amending this if anyone is kind enough to send me convincing evidence that a virus once ingested remains independently alive and is more the parent of viruses produced by the cell than is the cell itself. This is simply now a major problem for me. There may be evidence out there of which I am unaware, despite my diligent search for it.

I am not arguing that viral infection never precedes illness in cells. A virus or messenger vesicle might be misinterpreted by a cell – or be dangerously encoded by a sick cell. Dimmock and Primrose suggested an illness could result from a virus going into the wrong cell, although this might be difficult to establish. Can the virus ingested be toxic to some cells? As I said above, its codes may misinform. It is unlikely to be toxic, as it is mostly made of proteins common to the cell itself.

In the laboratory, scientists try to separate viruses from other particles by putting suspensions of likely particles into cell cultures in the expectation that only the true viruses will be 'replicated.' But the viruses, or vesicles, produced by cells in such circumstances cannot be presumed to be the same as those added. They may be quite different, changed or mutated. Some may be exosomes and parts of the cells' defensive system – or even cellular waste products.

Scientists also have to take into account any 'microparticles' present. These are defined as particles somewhat larger than viruses with sizes from 0.1 to 100 μm. These are encountered every day, and include pollen, very fine sand and dust. Some are toxins, metals and cellular waste products. 'Microparticles in air pollution are well known toxicants, contributing to asthma, cardiovascular disease and overall mortality ... more than $10^{12}$ particles per day are ingested (on average).' It is suggested that they play a significant role in Inflammatory Bowel Disease. [616] If cellular waste products, it seems they may also play a significant role in thrombosis. [617]

Dr. L. C. Huber and others suggested that some AIDS symptoms might be caused by our cells producing 'microparticles' when ill from severe stress, for in 'clinical situations with excessive cell death due to malignancies, autoimmune diseases and following chemotherapy, high levels of circulating microparticles' could be produced that suppress 'the immune response due to loss of macrophages.'[618]   Professor James Umber said the impact of microparticles might easily be mistaken for an effect of HIV. He explained; although AIDS-related illnesses do not always correlate with low numbers of CD4 immune cells, such low numbers may be caused by the normal process of programmed cell death going askew under cellular stress, perhaps because of drug intake, perhaps through severe malnutrition or similar factors.

These theories reminded me of the 19th century theory of microparticles expounded by a great rival of Pasteur, Professor Antoine Béchamp. However, he was suggesting something apparently quite different – living elements that are akin in size to what we now call mycoplasmas. He described these as 'a scavenging form of the microzymas (minute fermenting living particles), developed when death, decay, or disease causes an extraordinary amount of cell life either to need repair or be broken up.' They might even be found within bacteria. For him their presence was not the reason for a disease but the consequence of disease.[619]

On reflection, much of what I wrote in my earlier chapters on viruses could have been expressed differently. The vaccine industry tells of how viruses 'grow' in its incubators, but in truth, a virus once created does not grow. It is inert. What seems to happen in these incubators is that cells are so stressed and poisoned that they produce debris, protective vesicles and perhaps poorly made vesicles – and attempt to change their DNA to protect themselves. Lynn Margulis has stated: 'Viruses today spread genes among bacteria and humans and other cells, as they always have...'[620] We then inject into our children these stress products – in the hope that their cells will efficiently deal with the intrusion.

For me the jury is now out on the vesicles long identified as pathogenic viruses. I was severely shaken by discovering the evidence for the poliovirus being possibly harmless, then by discovering the fraud involved in the discovery of HIV. Now there are for me many questions concerning measles and other viruses that also need answers. These too have to be taken seriously. It was after all questions about measles, mumps and rubella that first started me on this investigation. What if the evidence is severely flawed for saying that many illnesses are viral-caused? The viruses blamed are dead, and therefore not susceptible to antibiotics. Instead we are relying on vaccines, despite our health historians telling us that most epidemics were ended by the provision of good hygiene, pure water and adequate food before these vaccines were invented.

---

[616] Schneider Jordan C. Can Microparticles Contribute to Inflammatory Bowel Disease: Innocuous or Inflammatory? Experimental Biology and Medicine 232:1-2 (2007)

[617] Detection and characterization of (circulating) microparticles. Working Group on Vascular Biology. June 18, 2004. http://www.med.unc.edu/isth/ssc/04sscminutes/04wg_vascular_biology.html

[618] Apoptosis. 2007 Feb;12(2):363-74. The role of membrane lipids in the induction of macrophage apoptosis by microparticles.   Huber LC, Jungel A, Distler JH, Moritz F, Gay RE, Michel BA, Pisetsky DS, Gay S, Distler O.

[619] Bechamp wrote thus in 1869 of their role in disease: 'In typhoid fever, gangrene and anthrax, the existence has been found of bacteria in the tissues and blood, and one was very much disposed to take them for granted as cases of ordinary parasitism. It is evident, after what we have said, that instead of maintaining that the affection has had as its origin and cause the introduction into the organism of foreign germs with their consequent action, one should affirm that one only has to deal with an alteration of the function of microzymas.'

[620] Lynn Margulis, Symbiotic Planet: A New Look at Evolution, Basic Books, 1998. p 64.

What else might cause measles? The account of how the measles and 'flu viruses are produced in cell cultures intrigues me. It seems that cells in laboratory cultures produce specific viruses in response to exposure to specific toxins. Is this what happens in measles outbreaks? Could the virus be an exosome produced en masse as a defence? Could these particles be a natural part of the cells' stress reactions?

Poor diet is now recognized as playing a major role in measles. The New York Times reported on July 22nd, 1990 that: 'Vitamin A supplements can significantly reduce the risk of death and serious complications in children with severe measles. The study, conducted in South Africa, found that the vitamin reduced the death rate by more than half and the duration of pneumonia, diarrhoea and hospitalisation by about a third. The researchers reported that the results 'indicate a remarkable protective effect of vitamin A in severe measles.' WHO now gives out vitamin A alongside vaccines in countries where vitamin A deficiencies are common. Recent studies have found that 72% of hospitalized measles cases in America are vitamin A deficient, and the worse the deficiency the worse the complications and higher the death rate. [621]

There is also a surprising lack of a clear causal link between these serious cases and the measles virus. It is instead suggested that measles virus is like HIV in harming the immune system and thus helping opportunistic diseases to occur like diarrhoea and pneumonia – and like HIV a slow virus as well, with cases of SSPE said to happen up to a nearly unbelievable 40 years after measles virus infection.

Could the cases of 'severe measles' that parents are warned about be caused by a vitamin A deficiency rather than a virus that damages the immune system. The eminent journal *Nature* reported in 2008: 'Vitamins A and D have received particular attention in recent years as these vitamins have been shown to have an unexpected and crucial effect on the immune response.' [622] If so, children are exposed to this vaccine quite unnecessarily.

What then of "measles parties" in which parents bring together their children to deliberately expose them to a sick child in order to give them life-long immunities? Might the immune system of one child produce "viral" particles to protectively trigger the immune systems of others?

**We are social animals and it might be entirely natural for us to mount a form of communal self-defence. Could viruses sometimes be messengers alerting both our own immune systems and the immune systems of neighbours? Are similar viruses found in similar diseases because cells respond with a very similar message in response to the same challenge? Many times the only link found between a virus and a disease is that they are present in the same place.**

Of course, it is probable that a sick cell might sometimes send a distorted message. We have evolved defences against unhelpful, dangerous or strange messages, which suggests that they do exist. For example, when viruses arrive at the cell, the code they contribute is immediately assessed, and may then be silenced by mRNAs in a process known as 'RNA interference.' [623] If this process can be overwhelmed, this might help explain why American Indians died of diseases in such numbers when Europeans arrived with many pathogens that their cells had not come across before.

Millions of our cells naturally die every day and, as Dr. L. Huber reported, their natural deaths are sometimes preceded by the arrival of messenger particles and their

---

[621] *Pediatric Nursing*, Sept/Oct 1996 Cod liver oil is an excellent source of vitamin A.

[622] Moro et al. Nature Reviews Immunology 8, 685-698 (September 2008).
http://www.nature.com/nri/journal/v8/n9/abs/nri2378.html

[623] Fire and Mello published their findings in the journal Nature on February 19, 1998. For a simple account, see the press release issued in 2006 by the Nobel Committee.
http://nobelprize.org/nobel_prizes/medicine/laureates/2006/press.html

absorption.[624] Such phenomena would once have been interpreted as death due to infection but now it is thought these particles are simply passing information to the cell. But, what if this entirely natural process goes wrong? Could a poorly coded messenger particle, or virus, disrupt the very complex and brilliantly organised informational process inside the cell? Could it, say, do the damage that a computer virus can do? This perhaps depends on just what is the nature of the relationship between cell and the virus.

## THE EVOLUTION OF THE VIRUS

Is evolution through random choice, as Darwin suggested? Shapiro stated that the work of McClintock and others means that our current notions of evolution 'require a profound re-evaluation. All aspects of cellular biology are subject to computational regulation. So we can no longer make the simplifying assumption of randomness.' An example of such non-randomness, he says, is how the caterpillar transforms into the butterfly. This involves it fragmenting its genome 'into hundreds of thousands of segments which are then processed and correctly reassembled.'[625] This makes me ask, where does the control over this process reside while such genomic reconstruction is in progress? It seems it is not in the nucleus but in the cell as a whole.

James Lovelock described how the world of cells and viruses is united. 'Living organisms and their natural environment are tightly coupled. The coupled system is a superorganism'[626] that can adjust its environment to suit itself.[627] Lynn Margulis preferred to say the earth was 'one continuous enormous ecosystem,'[628] but nevertheless, we now know, thanks to her and others, that our cells evolved out of cells that learnt to live together.

We now know that retroviruses have transported a large part of our DNA from one cell to another in a process that has lasted hundreds of millions of years. Scientists who did not understand why these codes were present once rejected them as 'Junk DNA'. But it is now known that this 'junk' regulates our genes and guides our evolution. This 'junk,' not our genes, is the main DNA difference between chimps and us.

Forget the theory of the competitive selfish gene. This was based on the assumption that our genes are independent entities. We now know that they do not rule, but accept regulation by, and cooperate with, this 'junk DNA.'

Our genomes are a vast library assembled over eons by our cells, using the tools of retroviruses and retrotransposons to adapt and to share. 'The genome-integrated retrotransposons have been recognized as a major evolutionary force' and may have started to evolve some 3.5 billion years ago – at the same time that DNA first appeared. Today, evolutionary biologists are constructing a map of evolution going back over vast periods of time by tracing this assembly.'[629] Viruses seemingly have played a major role in our evolution. 'It is probable that the cross-species transfer [by viruses] of sequences, either as DNA or RNA' has played a major role in evolution.[630]

---

[624] Apoptosis. 2007 Feb;12(2):363-74. The role of membrane lipids in the induction of macrophage apoptosis by microparticles.  Huber LC, Jungel A, Distler JH, Moritz F, Gay RE, Michel BA, Pisetsky DS, Gay S, Distler O.

[625] James A. Shapiro[a]  Genome Organization and Reorganizmation in Evolution: Formatting for Computation and Function. jsha@midway.uchicago.edu

[626] James Lovelock *The Ages of Gaia. A Biography of our Living Earth*, first edition 1988, second edition 1995, 2000. Oxford University Press,

[627] Chapter by Lynn Margulis in which she discusses Lovelock http://www.edge.org/documents/ThirdCulture/n-Ch.7.html

[628] http://www.edge.org/documents/ThirdCulture/n-Ch.7.html

[629] International Human Genome Consortium, 2001

[630] Celia Hansen and JS Heslop-Harrison. Sequences and Phylogenies of Plant Pararetroviruses, Viruses and Transposable Elements. *Advances in Botanical Research* **41** : 165-193.

McClintock bluntly put it: 'Darwin has muddied our thinking about evolution.' [631] Her discovery that cells intelligently respond to the environment contradicts the Darwinian theory of evolution, for the latter is based on the concept that cells make random decisions. Shapiro expanded on this. 'The possibility of a non-Darwinian, scientific theory of evolution is virtually never considered.' '[Yet] our current knowledge of genetic change is fundamentally at variance with neo-Darwinist postulates. We have progressed from the Constant Genome, subject only to random, localized changes at a more or less constant mutation rate, to the Fluid Genome, subject to episodic, massive and non-random reorganizations capable of producing new functional architectures.'

He noted that Charles Darwin had finally modified his theory, by saying he had not previously sufficiently appreciated other modes of evolution: 'It appears that I formerly underrated the frequency and value of these latter forms of variation as leading to permanent modifications of structure independently of natural selection.' [632]

As for the origin of viruses, virologists used to guess they were either degenerate parts of cells or vagrant genes. [633] They more recently suggested that viruses are 'selfish' cellular products produced first in the 'primeval tumultuous soup' of life. [634] In a 2006 paper, Eugene Koonin and colleagues argued that viruses evolved alongside early forms of cells – and after this the typical modern cell evolved. They stated: 'selfish genetic elements ancestral to viruses evolved prior to typical cells, to become intracellular parasites' and that 'viral evolution is inextricably linked to the evolution of the hosts.'

They thus acknowledge that cells are the parents of all viruses – but then assume that viruses must be selfish parasites, despite parasites normally being defined as alive, despite viruses normally being defined as dead, for without such assumptions, how could they explain the fear of these particles that dominates virology? They had to adjust their theory to explain why their viruses specialize in attacking their own parents. If they were right, then cells are poor at the evolutionary game – with viruses their terrifying 'living dead' or 'Zombie' offspring.

But others did not see viruses so negatively. Jean Claverie of the Structural & Genomic Information Laboratory stated: 'Viruses have come a long way from being unbecoming to the *Tree of Life*, to be given a central role in all major evolutionary transitions' in 'a spectacular renaissance in the field of viral evolution.' He further stated 'viruses are the dominant life form on earth' – but I would give this credit to cells. Viruses cannot be understood apart from the cells that create them all. [635]

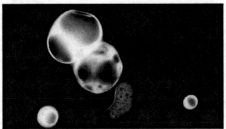

**Images of self-organized water 'molecules' – NASA**

[631] McClintock, 1982.

[632] C. Darwin, Origin of Species, 6th edition, Chapter XV, p. 395

[633] Dimrock and Primrose. *Introduction to Modern Virology. 3rd Edition*. Blackwell Scientific Publications. 1987.

[634] Eugene V Koonin, Tatiana G Senkevich and Valerian V Dolja: *The Ancient Virus World and evolution of cells*. Biology Direct 2006, 1:29doi:10.1186/1745-6150-1-29

635 Virus evolution : from neglect to center stage, amidst some confusion Jean-Michel Claverie. Structural & Genomic Information Laboratory CNRS-UPR2589, IBSM

Recent research on the origin of cells has focused on the water with which cells are filled, and in which they exist. In research funded by NASA, when water was exposed to the conditions of a young Solar system, afterwards they found 'in the water self-organizing structures with dimensions of 10 μm were found ... resembling cells.' 636 ` It seems almost impossible, but does water itself retains the information needed to help create life?

These researchers said their 'studies in molecular self-organization focused on two types of amphiphilic molecules, which are molecules that possess both hydrophobic and hydrophilic regions [water rejecting and attracting]. These molecules tend to self-organize spontaneously in an aqueous environment.' [637] Could such cells have provided an environment in which simple bacteria could evolve, in which they could produce an ocean of viral genetic codes – thus creating the conditions for symbiosis, for sharing information - and hence for multicellular organisms? Is water a universe-wide womb of life?

Life may not be always based on the same chemicals. It seems that non-organic particles in plasmas naturally self-organise into helixes and spirals that, DNA-like, carry out some of the key processes of life.[638] Ultimately we may have to ask if the principles of life, and of self-consciousness, are woven into the very fabric of our universe as the palaeontologist and evolutionary theorist, Teilhard de Chardin, predicted many decades ago, when he wrote of how 'space-time' 'contains and engenders consciousness? '[639]

## CONCLUSION

On this journey I have thus found I was wrong in thinking of viruses as alien foreign creatures that are rivals in the battle of life; and learnt we should not be so scared of them, for we make them, shape them and live within a sea of them. Yes, they can presumably be malformed – but then the fault will lie with the vastly more powerful cells that make them.

The mythology surrounding viruses is deeply misleading. They are frequently targeted and described as intelligent enemies that deserve to have a multi-billion dollar 'war on terror' waged against them – to the great benefit of the pharmaceutical industry.

This table uses official statistics to show how the total US mortality from certain infectious diseases decreased from 1920 to

---

[636] http://www.medicalbiophysics.dir.bg/en/water

[637] Prebiotic Molecular Selection and Organization - Project Investigators: David Deamer, Robert Hazen, Andrew Steele. http://nai.arc.nasa.gov/team/customtags/projectreports.cfm?teamID=14&year=7&projectID=1080

[638] Research by V. Tsytovich et al at the Russian General Physics and the Max-Planck Institutes, published in *The New Journal of Physics*, reported in *Exolife* on 17th August 2007

[639] Teilhard de Chardin *The Phenomenon of Man*. This was written in 1939 but not published until after his death in 1955 due to opposition from the Catholic Church to his work.

being too small to show on this scale after 1950 (on a scale of deaths per 100,000 per year, marked in decades from 1920 to 1960). [640] (Diphtheria is the highest line, pertussis the next down, then measles and the lowest polio.) Yet, as we have reported, most of the great epidemics of the past were successfully fought with clean water, improved nutrition and sanitation before most of the common vaccines were invented. Measles vaccine was released in 1964, mumps in 1967 and rubella in 1967.

The authors of the table below observed that 'from 1900 to 1937, the crude infectious disease mortality rate (bacterial and viral) in the USA decreased by about 2.8% per year from 797 deaths per 100,000 persons in 1900 to 283 in 1937. This was followed by a 15-year period during which the rate fell by 8.2% per year to 75 deaths per 100,000 in 1952 Improvements in living conditions, sanitation, and medical care probably accounted for this trend.

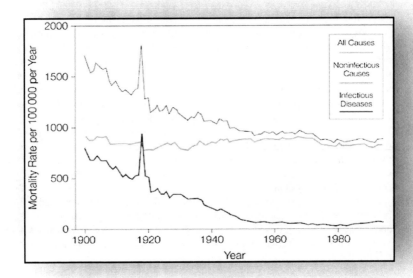

This report came to the conclusion that Westerners have now moved to an "age of degenerative and man-made diseases" and away from infectious. 'In countries like the United States, with established market economies, chronic and neoplastic [cancerous] diseases account for 81.0%' of years lost to disease.' Infectious diseases, including HIV, were of far less importance.

This reinforces everything I have discovered about illness while writing this book. Again and again, it is proving to be toxins and stress that are the major causes of serious illness in the West. We have removed other causes with clean water, good nourishment and public hygiene.

We once thought cancers caused by viruses. We now know they are mostly caused by toxins. It now seems to be toxins that cause the brain diseases of childhood and old

---

[640] Armstrong, Gregory et al. Trends in Infectious Disease Mortality in the United States During the 20th Century. JAMA. 1999; 281:61-66. http://jama.ama-assn.org/cgi/content/full/281/1/61#ACK

age. It was toxins that caused the great polio epidemics – and it is toxins that cause the damage in many AIDS cases.

Our weapons against these are mostly our own cells, with their defense systems, including their ability to change our DNA to give us resistance or immunity to one toxin after another. Nothing else can be so effective. However they need time to do this. We need to nourish our cells, keep our internal balance. Today our hospitals are infested with bacteria that developed resistance to antibiotics by doing what every cell of our bodies does – evolve protection against toxic dangers.

Nevertheless it is 'viral dangers' that still hog our medical research funds. Today TV advertisements stress with apparent horror that a milliard bacteria and viruses inhabit our skin – and that we must destroy them by buying one or another disinfectant. But this is the natural state of our skin. We have been the home to bacteria since we evolved out of them, although this does not mean that we do not need to take precautions. Sick bacterial cells can produce toxins that make other cells ill. But using toxic chemicals to rid our skin of all bacteria is extremely hazardous. We are mostly made up of healthy bacterial cells that live in harmony with us, and even process our food for us.

We need to give priority to nurturing and caring for sick cells, not to going on a virus hunt! The greatest hope we have in medicine right now lies in harnessing the extra-ordinary power of the cell, rather than in poisoning it to stop it from making viral particles. In the month that preceded this book going to the printers, it was reported that an amputated fingertip was restored without scarring by enhancing the power cells have of repair – and a dolphin's fin [641] – and that a skin cancer was removed by growing in the laboratory more of the patient's own CD4 blood cells and using these.[642]

A consequence of the focus on viruses rather than on toxins, as it was with the poliovirus, as it was with the birth of the AIDS epidemic, is that we are distracted away from the far greater tasks of dealing with environmental toxins, lifestyle issues, clean water supplies, sanitation and severe malnourishment; all factors that gravely weaken our cells and immune systems.

In fact, it is far worse. Not only are we distracted from these tasks, but also the priority given to the fight against viruses has resulted in far greater pollution. Our cities and farmers spray organochlorine and other toxins to kill the insects whose cells make viruses and we administer to ourselves powerful toxic drugs to dissuade our cells from making them.

Pesticides, drugs and pollutants all accumulate and weaken, especially when there is a lack of vital nutrients. Over time they can wreck our cells' protective abilities – creating a chaos in which our minute inhabitants may hurt us  - and this is really what AIDS is; a condition that occurs when our cells are stressed, malnourished and crippled.

Is it surprising that birds in China started to fall ill with 'Bird Flu' while flying through the ever-increasing clouds of pollution now enshrouding China? Their cells must have found it incredibly hard to cope. No wonder many died. Why spend billions on chasing tiny bits of genetic code in dead migrant birds, looking for an unidentifiable part of a not-yet-found mutant flu virus, when we put scarcely anything into stopping this mutant-causing pollution?

The fight against HIV has also been disastrously misconceived, creating the black hole of medical research, drawing vast amounts of vital resources away from clean water supplies, sanitation and good nourishment. This causes further poisoning, destroying the immune systems of hundreds of thousands of people.

---

[641] http://www.acell.com/vetfaq.php http://www.youtube.com/watch?v=H73dfmFhMNM

[642] http://news.bbc.co.uk/1/hi/health/7460743.stm
http://www.fhcrc.org/about/ne/news/2008/06/18/T_cells.html

Look again at the 'Great Flu Epidemic of 1918.' Was it surprising that it first broke out on the Western Front of the Great War, after five years of carnage and chemical warfare? We would need another war like this to reproduce those horrific cell-damaging circumstances. Why have we ignored the earlier research that found bacteria to play a far greater role in this than viruses? Why do virologists now scare us with predictions that a similar epidemic is certain to strike hard very soon, not on the Iraqi battlefront but in the comfortable West?

Fear, stress and chemotherapy drugs are the products of the war waged by our virologists on the messages sent by cells. The result is not a happier world but a frightened nervous human population blighted by cancers and stress illnesses.

We must learn to look at health in entirely another way. Ultimately we are the Gaia of our internal world. We rule over bodies that are the natural home for vast herds of bacteria and of a milliard flights of viruses. As long as the whole exists in harmony, we basically stay healthy. They will serve us and not hurt us. Nearly all the so-called dangerous germs, such as TB bacteria, are our inseparable and normally harmless companions that are only dangerous when other factors seriously weaken our cells.

In September 2008 Dr Lynn Margulis gave a lecture to which students flocked in such numbers that screens were erected outside the lecture hall. They heard her speak with passion and enthusiasm about the marvels of the free-living cells, the ones we know of as 'bacteria'. It turns out that nine out of every ten cells in our body are bacteria.[643] In other words, we are made from cells capable of independent life that co-ordinate activity between themselves to sustain us! We are multi-species cities in which communications between inhabitants are absolutely vital to our continued communal health. We truly could not exist if our cells had not evolved ways to communicate.

Surely it is time to leave behind this ugly obsession with unseen dangers – particularly from what are nothing more or less than cellular messengers – and to turn our attention to caring for the utterly marvellous cells of which we are made; that protect us well, that will make healthy viruses or exosomes when they are well nourished and not poisoned. Then we could appreciate the wonder we all are. We synthesize the intelligence of our cells. We are the natural masters of the life enjoyed by billions of cells and part of the greater dance that weaves our universe together.

Health of planet and body are preserved in the same way. Keep both unpolluted and unstressed. Enjoy having such inner and outer worlds to explore – and to nurture.

And don't let anyone use fear to manipulate you.

Janine Roberts

"The majority of viral infections are either entirely asymptomatic or so mildly symptomatic as to go completely unrecognized ... even infection with virulent viruses most often results in subclinical or unapparent infections." [644]

---

[643] The CDC currently state on their website that over 90% of the cells in a human are bacterial.

[644] Mckendall and Stroop. 'Handbook of Neurovirology.' Informa Health Care. 1994. Page 28.

# Epilogue

# Silenced Voices and the Ongoing Debate

The following is a list of just a few of the senior scientists who have long maintained that AIDS cannot be caused by HIV, but can be caused by long-term exposure to certain toxins, to severe malnutrition and other non-viral factors, or who believe that suppression of this debate about the cause of AIDS is wrong.

If you have not heard of their work, this is not a surprise. Ten years ago I had not heard of them either – yet I then regarded myself as a well-informed journalist. It seems their work has mostly been ignored, or presumed to be that of cranks. Do these scientists deserve this? Look at what they have written, the positions they hold, and judge. Many of their papers are freely available on websites. This list is in no particular order.

**Dr. Kary Mullis - Nobel Prize Laureate, won for inventing the Polymerase Chain Reaction (PCR), a vital tool used in the study of genetic code fragments and used for the Viral Load test. http://www.karymullis.com**
He stated: 'Years from now, people will find our acceptance of the HIV theory of AIDS as silly as we find those who excommunicated Galileo.'

**Dr. Lynn Margulis. Discoverer of the symbiotic origins of the cell**
She wrote in 2007: 'From my readings, discussions with knowledgeable scientists close to the story, I simply conclude, as does Kerry Mullis, the Nobel Laureate who wrote a foreword to Duesberg's classical work, that there is no evidence that "HIV causes AIDS."'[645]

**Professor Serge Lang. At the time of his death in 2005, professor emeritus of mathematics at Yale and member of the National Academy of Science.**
'The hypotheses that HIV is a harmless virus and that drugs cause AIDS defining diseases are compatible with all the evidence I know.' 'I regard as scandalous the continued ostracism of people and points of view which go against the orthodoxy on HIV.' See his article published in *Yale Scientific, Spring 1999; The Case of HIV: We Have Been Misled*

**Dr. Peter Duesberg - Professor of Molecular and Cell Biology at the University of California, Berkeley. Member of the US National Academy of Science; first to map the genetic structure of retroviruses; recipient of the NIH's Outstanding Investigator Grant.** His books include '*Infectious AIDS: Have We Been Misled?*' and '*Inventing the AIDS Virus*'. He edited '*AIDS; Virus or Drug Induced*? and in 2003 co-authored a study entitled *The Chemical Basis of the Various AIDS Epidemics;*

---

[645] Posted by: Margulis | March 12, 2007 10:21AM http://scienceblogs.com/pharyngula

*Recreational Drugs, Anti-Viral Chemotherapy and Malnutrition.* This is available on his website; www.duesberg.com

He said of HIV; 'I'm not afraid that HIV exists, because I think retroviruses are not much to be afraid of ... HIV is just a latent, and perfectly harmless, retrovirus'.

**The Perth Group. An international group of academics headed by biophysicist Eleni Papadopulos-Eleopulos at the Royal Perth Hospital, Australia. Other notable members of this group are Dr. Valendar Turner and Professor of Pathology John Papadimitriou. Their many deeply researched articles are available on their website. www.theperthgroup.com**

Eleni Papadopulos-Eleopulos wrote: 'HIV had not been isolated from either fresh tissues or culture, which means that its existence had not been proven and this situation has not changed up to the present day...I am saddened that there are forces at work that have consistently prevented purposeful but friendly debate. To me and my group the problematic nature of the HIV theory was apparent from the very beginning.' She was the first to publicly question if HIV had been provably isolated.

**Dr. Etienne de Harven** - **Emeritus Professor of Pathology, University of Toronto. Former president of the Rethinking AIDS Group and a leading expert on electron microscopy.** http://rethinkingaids.com

'Dominated by the media, by pressure groups and by the interests of pharmaceutical companies, the AIDS establishment lost contact with open-minded, peer-reviewed science ... the unproven HIV/AIDS hypothesis received 100% of the research funds while all other hypotheses were ignored. '

**Dr. Charles L. Geshekter, Ph.D., Three-time Fulbright scholar. Professor of African History, California State University, Chico. Served as an adviser to the U.S. State Department and to several African governments.**

'The scientific data do not support the view that what is being called AIDS in Africa has a viral cause.' 'The scandal is that long-standing ailments that are largely the product of poverty are being blamed on a sexually transmitted virus. With missionary-like zeal, but without evidence, condom manufacturers and AIDS fund-raisers attribute those symptoms to an "African" sexual culture.' 'Traditional public-health approaches, clean water and improved sanitation above all can tackle the underlying health problems in Africa. They may not be sexy, but they will save lives. And they will surely stop terrorizing an entire continent.' 'You're looking at what I think is going to turn out to be one of the great frauds of the late 20th century.'

**Dr. Rosalind Harrison, Fellow of the Royal College of Surgeons, consultant ophthalmic surgeon for the National Health Service, UK**

'Virus isolation is necessary to prove virus infection. Retrovirologists have laid down a set of criteria to distinguish spurious from genuine retroviruses. HIV does not fulfil these criteria.'

**Dr. Heinz Ludwig Sänger, Ph.D., Emeritus Professor of Molecular Biology and Virology, Max Planck Institute for Biochemistry, Germany**

'HIV cannot be responsible for AIDS. After three years of intensive critical studies of the relevant scientific literature, as an experienced virologist and molecular biologist I came to the following surprising conclusion - there is actually no single scientifically really convincing evidence for the existence of HIV. Not even once has such a retrovirus been isolated and purified by the methods of classical virology.'

**Dr. Gordon Stewart, - Emeritus Professor of Public Health, Glasgow University Former WHO Advisor on AIDS.**

'AIDS is a behavioural disease. It is multifactorial.' 'It is a scandal that the major medical journals have maintained a conspiracy of silence over any dissent from the orthodox views and official handouts.'

**Dr. Phillip Johnson, Senior Professor of Law, University of California at Berkeley**

'One does not need to be a scientific specialist to recognise a botched research job and a scientific establishment that is distorting the facts to maximise its funding.'

**Dr. Richard Strohman, Emeritus Professor in Molecular and Cell Biology, University of California, Berkeley.**

'We need research into possible [AIDS] causes such as drug use and behaviour, not a bankrupt hypothesis.' 'My colleagues in molecular biology by and large do not read the AIDS literature. They're just like everybody else who has to believe what they read in the newspapers. We all have to put our faith somewhere, otherwise we don't have time.'

**Dr. Harry Rubin, Professor of Molecular and Cell Biology, Berkeley**

'Who were these people who are so much wiser, so much smarter than Luc Montagnier [the discoverer of what is now known as HIV]? He became an outlaw as soon as he started saying that HIV might not be the only cause of AIDS.'

**Dr. Heinrich Broder; Medical director of the Federal Clinics for Juvenile and Young Adult Drug Offenders for five German counties, including Berlin, Bremen, and Hamburg.**

'The collective virus obsession enables "HIV"AIDS medicine to operate in a lawless sphere without responsibility for the often fatal consequences. It is high time to discuss the ethical consequences of the "virtual medicine" currently practiced, which under the pretence of an imagined global epidemic, force-feeds highly toxic drug cocktails to patients.'

**Dr. Bernard Forscher; former editor of the *US Proceedings of the National Academy of Sciences***

'The HIV hypothesis ranks with the "bad air" theory for malaria and the "bacterial infection"' theory of beriberi and pellagra [caused by nutritional deficiencies]. It is a hoax that became a scam.'

**Dr. Arthur Gottlieb, MD, Chairperson of the Department of Microbiology and Immunology, Tulane University School of Medicine** -the first to report the Los Angeles AIDS epidemic in 1981

'The viewpoint has been so firm that HIV is the only cause and will result in disease in every patient, that anyone who challenges that is regarded as "politically incorrect." I don't think - as a matter of public policy - we gain by that, because it limits debate and discussion and focuses drug development on attacking the virus rather than attempting to correct the disorder of the immune system, which is central to the disease.'

**Dr. Joseph Sonnabend, MD, New York Physician, founder of the American Foundation for AIDS Research (AmFAR); one of the first to report the AIDS epidemic in New York.**

'The marketing of HIV as a killer virus causing AIDS without the need for any other factors has so distorted research and treatment that it may have caused thousands of people to suffer and die.'

'Gallo was certainly committing open and blatant scientific fraud. But the point is not to focus on Gallo. It's us - all of us in the scientific community, we let him get away with it.' 'The notion of "eradication" [of HIV] is just total science fiction. Every retrovirologist knows this. The RNA of retroviruses turns into DNA and becomes part of us. It's part of our being. You can't ever get rid of it.'

**Harvey Bialy, PhD, author of *Oncogenes, Aneuploidy and Aids: A Scientific Life and Times of Peter H. Duesberg*, resident scholar at the Institute of Biotechnology, National University of Mexico and founding scientific editor of Nature Biotechnology.**

'HIV/AIDS [is] the biggest medical mistake and fraud of the past 500 years.'

**Dr. Rodney Richards, Ph.D., Biochemist, Founding scientist for the biotech company Amgen. Collaborated with Abbott Laboratories in developing HIV tests.**

'To date, no researcher has demonstrated how HIV kills T-cells. It's just a theory that keeps money flowing into the pharmaceutical approach to treating AIDS.'

**Dr. Robert Root-Bernstein - Associate Professor of Physiology, Michigan State University. Author *'Rethinking AIDS; The tragic cost of premature consensus'*.**

'No evidence of female prostitutes transmitting HIV or AIDS into the heterosexual community exists for any Western nation. Acquisition of HIV by men from female prostitutes is almost always drug related.'

**Dr. Donald W. Miller, Jr., MD, Professor of Surgery, University of Washington School of Medicine**

'The HIV-AIDS model is untenable. The twenty-plus diseases the government defines as "AIDS" are caused, instead, by immunosuppressive heavy-duty recreational drug use, antiretroviral drugs, and receptive anal intercourse. The elusive HIV, when present, simply goes along for the ride, lodged in a small minority of the body's T cells. It is a passenger on the AIDS airplane, not its pilot.'

**Professor Daniel J. Ncayiyana, the editor of The South African Medical Journal;**

'I am quite confident in my own mind that many cases identified as AIDS (according to their symptoms) are not AIDS. The numbers given must, of necessity, include people who possibly have other conditions.' [646.]

**Professor P.A.K. Addy, Head of Clinical Microbiology at the University of Science and Technology in Kumasi, Ghana:**

'Europeans and Americans came to Africa with prejudiced minds, so they are seeing what they wanted to see...I've known for a long time that Aids is not a crisis in Africa as the world is being made to understand. But in Africa it is very difficult to stick your neck out and say certain things. The West came out with those frightening statistics on Aids in Africa because it was unaware of certain social and clinical conditions.'

---

[646][77] *Now* Magazine, 9-15 March 2000

**Dr. Henry Bauer, Ph.D., Professor Emeritus of Chemistry & Science Studies and Dean Emeritus of Arts & Sciences at Virginia Polytechnic Institute & State University; Author, *The Origin, Persistence and Failings of HIV/AIDS Theory***
'One result of commerce-driven science is the growing number of scandals, especially in biomedical research, where nasty side-effects or lack of efficacy of new drugs seem increasingly to be hidden from public view until significant damage has been done. Nowadays there's the tragedy of AIDS, where the mainstream dogma that HIV is the cause may be subjecting tens or hundreds of thousands to inappropriate, indeed deadly so-called 'treatment' that has brought several drug companies unprecedented profits.' [647]

**Dr. Roberto Giraldo M.D. Author of '*AIDS and Stressors.*'**
'AIDS is neither an infectious disease, nor sexually transmitted. It is a toxic-nutritional syndrome caused by the alarming worldwide increment of immunological stressor agents.'

**Dr. Andrew Herxheimer, MD, Emeritus Professor of Pharmacology, UK Cochrane Centre, Oxford; edited Drug & Therapeutics Bulletin in the UK for 30 years and also helped to found the International Society of Drug Bulletins.**
'I think zidovudine [AZT] was never really evaluated properly; its efficacy has never been proved, but its toxicity certainly is important. I think it has killed a lot of people, especially at the high doses. I personally think it not worth using alone or in combination at all.'

**Lynn Fall (nee Gannett), former data manager, phase III clinical trials AZT (1987-1990)**
'AZT is a poison. AZT commonly causes miscarriages and severe birth defects. AZT is a highly toxic chemotherapy that interrupts DNA synthesis and destroys the immune system. In fact, AZT is a tragedy which I believe has led to tens of thousands of unnecessary deaths, primarily in wealthier countries.'

**Dr. Rudolf Werner, Ph.D., Professor of Biochemistry, University of Miami School of Medicine**
'The HIV-AIDS hypothesis remains just that - a hypothesis. Many experts' predictions turned out to be false. For example, contrary to the prediction that AIDS would rapidly spread into the heterosexual population, the disease in the United States is still restricted to 85 percent males. Yet HIV positives are found with equal frequency in healthy male and female Army recruits. This discrepancy doesn't support the hypothesis that AIDS is caused by HIV.'
'AIDS drugs have been credited for the reduction in AIDS deaths. But there is no scientific evidence that these toxic drugs prolong life. A study in Uganda shows that the time between becoming HIV-positive and the time of death is identical to that in the United States. The Uganda group received no AIDS drugs, while the U.S. group did. Since most people in the Uganda study were malnourished and multiply infected, doesn't that suggest that antiretroviral drugs reduce life expectancy? Malnutrition is the most common cause of immune deficiency.'

**Dr. Manu Kothari, MD, Professor of Anatomy, former Head of Department of Anatomy, Seth Gordhandas Sunderdas Medical College, King Edward Memorial Hospital, Mumbai, India**

---

[647][78] Journal of Scientific Exploration, Winter 2001

'For all we know, it is not HIV that causes AIDS, but the so-called co-factors such as indiscriminate antibiotic use, recreational drugs, poverty, malnutrition, polluted water and pesticised food. AZT and the like (so-called triple therapy) are rank cytotoxic poisons. To give AZT to pregnant women is a crime against the mother and the baby she is making.'

### Dr. Juan Jose Flores, MD, Ph.D., Professor of Medicine, La Universidad Veracruzana, Mexico

'The causes of AIDS are not viral. I have witnessed the fatal effects that the anti-viral drugs have on the immune system. I treated patients diagnosed with HIV who were very poor. Their inability to afford the drugs precluded me from giving them AZT, which is very expensive. As time went by, I began to see that the rich HIV positive patients died, while the poor ones lived and continue to do so.'

### Dr. David Rasnick, Ph.D., Biochemist, Protease Inhibitor Developer. Cancer researcher.

'The National Institutes of Health, the Centers for Disease Control, the Medical Research Council, and the World Health Organization are terrorizing hundreds of millions of people around the world. It would be intolerably embarrassing for them to admit at this late date that they are wrong, that AIDS is not sexually transmitted. Such an admission could very well destroy these organizations, or, at the very least, put their future credibility in jeopardy. Self preservation compels these institutions to not only maintain but to actually compound their errors, which adds to the fear, suffering, and misery of the world - the antithesis of their reason for being.'

### Dr. Joseph Mercola, former Chairman of the Family Medicine department at St. Alexius Medical Center, Illinois; served as editor of HIV Monograph by Abbott Laboratories

'What is not mentioned in any textbook is that AZT has been found in five studies performed after its rushed FDA approval to be equally toxic to T-cells, the very cells whose absence is blamed on HIV. This is not surprising since T-cells are produced in the bone marrow, and AZT depletes all the cells produced there. These studies are but a sample of the evidence that suggest that AZT and other 'antiretrovirals' are causing a variety of AIDS-like symptoms which are being blamed on HIV,' The only studies published that claim positive outcome were short-term and did not have statistically significant results.'

### Anthony Brink, Advocate and Magistrate.

A powerful voice in South Africa, a lawyer who campaigns against the use of antiretroviral drugs in treating AIDS patients because of research evidence documenting their grave defects. His detailed documentation on these drugs is available online at www.tig.org.za

### Dr. Steven Lanka, Virologist and Molecular Biologist.

He holds that there is no evidence for the complete isolation of any pathogenic virus, saying the viruses so far detected are 'cell components,' part of the 'intra- and intercellular transport' system. [648] 'Not only I am maintaining that the so-called AIDS virus "HIV" has never been scientifically demonstrated to exist, but it is only being maintained to exist because of a purported consensus.' 'If I expose cells in a test-tube to a quantity of artificially produced gene substance and albumins, they die faster than under

---

648   http://www.neue-medizin.com/lanka2.htm

the standard conditions for cells dying in a test-tube. This is being presented as proof of the existence, as proof of the isolation and as proof of the multiplication of the purported virus – this is now "normal science.'[649]

### Dr. B.L. Meel MD, Head, Department of Forensic Medicine, University of Transkei, South Africa

'There are several risks associated with HIV/AIDS, but the most important immediate risk, soon after an individual becomes aware of his/her HIV status, is committing suicide. This is as a result of sudden unexpected, unprepared disclosure of HIV test result, leading to mental breakdown, i.e., severe acute depression... A study carried out in New York City (1997) found that 9% of suicide victims were HIV positive.'

This is not all. There are over 2,000 doctors and medical researchers who have taken the bold, and professionally risky, stand of making public their disagreement with the HIV theory of AIDS. They have signed a list maintained on the web at http://www.rethinkingaids.com/quotes/rethinkers.htm, but for this list I will make the final entry not on AIDS, but on modern medicine.

### Ivan Illich, Author of *Medical Nemesis*.

'Modern medicine is a negation of health. It isn't organised to serve human health, but only to serve itself as an institution. It makes more people sick than it heals.'

---

[649]   http://www.gnn.tv/A02138

# THE ONGOING DEBATE

Back in 1991, as the official investigation of Robert Gallo for fraud got under way, other scientists boldly began moves to get the HIV theory of AIDS reassessed, They formed 'The Group for the Scientific Reappraisal of the HIV/AIDS Hypothesis.'[650] But their letters calling for an independent reassessment were refused initially by the major scientific journals. In 1994 the establishment tried to try to remove from dissident ranks Professor Duesberg, a Member of the National Academy of Science, by suggesting that he would be fully restored to favour if he signed a paper already accepted for publication entitled: *HIV Causes AIDS: Koch's Postulates Fulfilled.*[651] He refused, and instead he with some 2000 others from 68 countries signed a letter published in *Science* in 1995 calling for a 'thorough reappraisal' by 'a suitable independent group.'[652] As a result he was denied research grants and post-graduate students.

Their call went mostly unheeded until 2000 when President Mbeki of South Africa decided to set up a 'Presidential AIDS Advisory Panel' of scientists for and against the HIV hypothesis. As I have mentioned, to this he invited Gallo and Montagnier – and Duesberg along with other scientists. Its purpose was to seek agreement on experiments that would settle once and for all this grave dispute.[653]

But this open dissent and calls for reassessment greatly disturbed the virology establishment. Robin Weiss, the professor I met at the SV40 Conference, who had earlier had to apologize like Gallo for using the French virus in patenting an HIV test, now helped to circulate an email calling for signatures to a counter statement. This email stated: 'Peter Duesberg is back in the columns of *Nature* and *Science.* ... The situation has taken a serious turn in that President Mbeki of South Africa is consulting him. The consequences are being felt in Africa and Asia. An international group of scientists and doctors has come up with something called the Durban Declaration to be published in Nature on July 6. You will find it at the bottom of this message. As a scientific statement in plain language, it attempts to set the record straight by stating the facts.'[654]

Some 5000 signatures were thus gathered in support of the HIV theory, and the statement they signed was published in Nature as the *Durban Declaration*. It bluntly asserted: 'The evidence that AIDS is caused by HIV-1 or HIV-2 is clear-cut, exhaustive and unambiguous, meeting the highest standards of science. The data fulfils [*sic*] exactly the same criteria as for other viral diseases, such as polio, measles and smallpox. ... To tackle the disease, everyone must first understand that HIV is the enemy.'[655]

In response to this, a *'Rebuttal to the Durban declaration'* was published on July 26th 2000.[656] This stated that the evidence given for HIV causing AIDS violated the Koch Postulates that are the guiding principles of virology. The UK and USA health authorities state AIDS can occur in the HIV negative, in the apparent absence of the virus. In

---

[650] A group that is still going strong, see its website http://rethinkingaids.com
[651] http://www.duesberg.com/about/bribepd.html also
http://www.reviewingaids.org/awiki/index.php/Document:Alpha_and_Omega
[652] http://www.reviewingaids.org/awiki/index.php/Group_for_the_Scientific_Reappraisal_of_the_HIV
[653] This Panel's Report is available at www.visusmyth.com/aids/panel/
[654] http://www.healtoronto.com/durban/wain-hobson.html
[655] http://www.nature.com/nature/journal/v406/n6791/full/406015a0.html
[656] http://www.healtoronto.com/durban/

September 21$^{st}$ 2000 a reply dissenting from the Durban Declaration also appeared in *Nature.* [657]

In turn, an unsigned response to this appeared on the National Institutes of Health website in November 2000.  It indignantly insisted that the 'HIV theory of AIDS does satisfy the Koch Postulates.'  This response was further updated in 2003.  It now stated; 'With regard to [Koch] postulate #1, numerous studies from around the world show that virtually all AIDS patients are HIV-seropositive; that is they carry antibodies that indicate HIV infection. With regard to postulate #2, modern culture techniques have allowed the isolation of HIV in virtually all AIDS patients ... Postulate #3 has been fulfilled in tragic incidents involving three laboratory workers with no other risk factors who have developed AIDS or severe immunosuppression after accidental exposure to concentrated, cloned [artificial] HIV in the laboratory.' [658]

Yet this too met with an immediate rejection – not just from scientists but from organizations of the 'HIV positive' who have refused antiretrovirals and remained healthy. [659]  Scientific studies were cited of Africans diagnosed with AIDS that showed well over half were not infected with HIV. Thousands of similar cases in America were cited – as well as studies demonstrating that the antibody test is not specific to HIV.

The argument today remains fierce, but continues to be one-sided in terms of publicity.  When do you remember the BBC acknowledging in its reports on AIDS the existence of scientific dissent to the HIV theory? Its extensive website on AIDS ignores this dissent entirely, reporting the establishment view as if undisputed.

I have to say that this is, in my opinion, a violation of the code of journalistic ethics mandatory at the BBC. I know because I have worked as a producer and journalist on projects with the BBC. They must be balanced in their reporting, and thus must ensure that all sides are included whenever there is serious scientific dissent. (These guidelines are of course the same for journalists elsewhere.)

This imbalance is most regrettable, given that even the *British Medical Journal* has recently hosted a major debate for and against the HIV theory.  This raged fiercely for over a year in their online "Rapid Responses" site. *De Spiegel*, the leading German news magazine, and *Harpers*, a major New York publication, have also recently ran controversial major articles covering the debate over the HIV theory. The Internet also is full of this debate. It is thus hard to see why this lively debate on an issue of great public concern has been so shamefully neglected by the popular media.  I fear it is because our medical authorities advise all journalists, as they did me, that we should not to mention the flaws in current theories as this 'may dissuade patients from taking their medicines'!

The scientists who come out against the HIV theory risk much.  They are setting themselves against the medical establishment that awards research grants.  Many will also find themselves labeled as "Denialists' on AIDS websites to deliberately and nastily link them with those who deny the existence of the Holocaust.

They are accused of putting thousands of lives at risk simply by questioning the sexual transmission of AIDS (as also I was when I started my research into HIV and AIDS). No notice is taken of the alternative remedies they discover. Many are instead punished by the loss of research funds, as happened to Professor Peter Duesberg of Berkeley.

It thus takes a great deal of bravery for a working scientist to publicly object to the HIV theory, and even this author, a writer and television producer on medical issues, feels somewhat nervous at taking on the AIDS establishment by writing this book. It is most intimidating. The white coats seem to have become the priests of this age, revered even by

---

[657] http://www.reviewingaids.org/awiki/index.php/Document:Durban_Declaration_Stewart_Response

[658] www.niaid.nih.gov/factsheets/evidhiv.htm

[659] www.healtoronto.com - also see their page www.healtoronto.com/nih/main.html

liberal journalists who do not respect the establishment when it comes to decisions over wars.

I hope that this book helps in some way to remedy this gross imbalance. Given that the world has now spent over 180 billion US dollars on AIDS research without finding a cure, it is surely time to broaden our vision, to seriously look at all alternatives and consider what else than HIV might cause AIDS?

## PRESIDENT MBEKI OF SOUTH AFRICA ON AIDS.

The only international politician to take note of the serious implications of the research work of the above-mentioned scientists has been President Mbeki of South Africa. For this, he has been internationally maligned, forcing him to issue the following letter.

'Our search for these specific and targeted responses is being stridently condemned by some in our country and the rest of the world as constituting a criminal abandonment of the fight against HIV-AIDS. Some elements of this orchestrated campaign of condemnation worry me very deeply.'

'It is suggested, for instance, that there are some scientists who are "dangerous and discredited" with whom nobody, including us, should communicate or interact. In an earlier period in human history, these would be heretics that would be burnt at the stake!'

'Not long ago, in our own country, people were killed, tortured, imprisoned and prohibited from being quoted in private and in public because the established authority believed that their views were dangerous and discredited. We are now being asked to do precisely the same thing that the racist apartheid tyranny we opposed did, because, it is said, there exists a scientific view that is supported by the majority, against which dissent is prohibited. The scientists we are supposed to put into scientific quarantine include Nobel Prize Winners, Members of Academies of Science and Emeritus Professors of various disciplines of medicine!'

'Scientists, in the name of science, are demanding that we should cooperate with them to freeze scientific discourse on HIV-AIDS at the specific point this discourse had reached in the West in 1984. People who otherwise would fight very hard to defend the critically important rights of freedom of thought and speech occupy, with regard to the HIV-AIDS issue, the frontline in the campaign of intellectual intimidation and terrorism which argues that the only freedom we have is to agree with what they decree to be established scientific truths.'

'Some agitate for these extraordinary propositions with a religious fervour born by a degree of fanaticism, which is truly frightening. The day may not be far off when we will, once again, see books burnt and their authors immolated by fire by those who believe that they have a duty to conduct a holy crusade against the infidels.'

Signed **THABO MBEKI**

# Appendix

## Some Scientific Enigmas explained

If the dissident professors who say AIDS is caused by other factors are right, then many enigmas faced by AIDS science today might be explained.

It would explain why WHO today recommends that doctors do not try to find HIV in AIDS patients. The 1994 edition of 'AIDS Testing,' a 400-page text edited by CDC experts, stated that that 'the virus cannot be detected directly by conventional molecular biology techniques'. The work adds that detection is particularly difficult because HIV is 'highly inactive' – that surely means that it is not out doing great damage.

It would explain the difficulties found by AIDS scientists when they do look for the AIDS virus in blood taken from AIDS victims. They can only find fragments of genetic codes that have no consistency; leading some to conclude of HIV 'no two of its genomes are the same, even from the same person.'[660] Others have said, in despair, that in samples taken from any one patient, they can find more than 100 million genetically distinct variants [of the virus].[661] They even give different numbers of genes to the virus. All this they put down to the devilish ability of the virus to protect itself by constantly mutating in their laboratory vessels. Yet this phenomenon could be explained by cellular breakdown within a very ill person, or by accepting that retroviruses as basically messenger RNA vesicles that can carry different codes.

It explains why we still do not know how HIV destroys T-Cells – despite Gallo saying this is how it gives us AIDS. Joseph McCune reported in Nature in 2001: 'We still do not know how, in vivo [in the patient], the virus destroys CD4+ T cells... Several hypotheses have been proposed to explain the loss of CD4+ T cells, some of which seem to be diametrically opposed.'[662]

It would also explain why the HIV test does not look for HIV itself, but for an antibody. The antibody selected has been shown by leading 'orthodox' AIDS researchers, such as Myron Essex of Harvard, a member with Gallo of the US Task Force on AIDS, to react to fungal and yeast infections and to TB bacteria as if all of these are HIV, leading Essex to recommend that AIDS tests not be relied on in Africa.

It helps explain why the 'Viral Load' test used to determine the intensity of HIV infection, does not actually count HIV but incomplete fragments of genetic codes in the blood, which might also be produced by cellular breakdown due to long term drug abuse or by severe malnutrition – or by a cellular need to send out messengers.

It explains why the UK and other national Health Authorities have to tell doctors they may readily diagnose AIDS in patients that have no HIV –despite contradictorily insisting that HIV is the cause of AIDS. They list some 18 diseases that can be diagnosed as AIDS in the absence of HIV. This is a direct violation of the Koch Postulates said to govern virology. The Postulates state the agent of a disease must be present in every case.

---

[660] Eigen, M. and Biebricher, C.K. (1988). Quoted in Emerging Viruses, ed. S.S. Morse, Oxford University Press, New York, 1993, pp.219-225.

[661] Wain-Hobson, S. (1995). Virological Mayhem, Nature, January 12, 1995: p.102. Also According to researchers from the Pasteur Institute, 'an asymptomatic patient can harbour at least 106 genetically distinct variants of HIV, and for an AIDS patient the figure is more than 108. Vartian JP, Meyerhans A, Henry M, Wain-Hobson W. High-resolution structure of an HIV-1 quasispecies: Identification of novel coding sequences. AIDS 1992

[662] 'The Dynamics of CD4+ T-cell Depletion in HIV Disease' by Joseph McCune in *Nature*, April 19, 2001

It explains why the World Health Organization has likewise defined AIDS in Africa as not needing HIV. In Africa, under its official Bangui definition of AIDS, it can be diagnosed if a person has persistent diarrhoea, a persistent cough and persistent itching. With half the population south of the Sahara not having access to clean water, and one third suffering from 'chronic hunger,' such symptoms of illness are surely not surprising?[663]

It explains why the drugs provided to fight HIV, antiretrovirals, are not designed to specifically target HIV but instead to destroy the whole class of 'retroviruses', most of which are native to us.

It would explain that while anti-retroviral drugs initially lower viral load, the underlying illness is not removed. The subsequent failure of the drugs to arrest AIDS is inevitably blamed on HIV surviving and acquiring resistance, but it could also be that the disease is not caused by a retrovirus.

It explains why no cure for HIV infection or of AIDS has been discovered, despite the spending of some $180 billion dollars over some 21 years.

It explains why it has likewise proved impossible so far to market a vaccine against HIV. These commonly use whole weakened or dead viruses and are relatively simple to make. If AIDS researchers had isolated such a virus, they would have used it. If they had part of a virus, then they would have used that. There is also another problem. Vaccines work by stimulating the production of antibodies — but HIV antibodies, ever since Gallo's *Science* papers were published, are uniquely said to be an indication of illness, not of health.

It explains why the largest study ever done on the heterosexual transmission of HIV, the Padian study, found no case of transmission over several years of monitoring a large number of couples, of which one partner was HIV positive at the start of the study and despite one third not using condoms.

It explains why Gallo and other scientists have only been able to strongly link passive anal sex with AIDS – as on this route natural protective chemicals in spermal fluid may get into the blood and suppress the immune system. If it were a viral infection, it would be in both partners.

It helps to explain the strong correlation between suffering from AIDS and possessing a gravely damaged 'redox' system that starves our cells of energy. This can be created by poisoning and produces both body-wasting and severe liver damage. Such damage is associated less with viral infections than to exposure to certain prescribed or recreational drugs – or to severe malnutrition as in Africa. Among recreational drugs, nitrite inhalant Poppers, Crack Cocaine and Crystal, have all been strongly linked to redox damage. Corticosteroids also can produce similar symptoms.

And it helps to explain the puzzling scientific finding that when mice are subjected to the same levels of nitrite inhalants that are commonly used in the gay clubbing scene, they acquire major symptoms of AIDS; then, when they are given anti-toxins, the same mice become healthy. The only explanation seems to be that drugs can cause AIDS – and amazingly and wonderfully, that AIDS is curable – with antitoxins, something that is so scientifically heretical that it is not checked.

---

[663] UNDP Human Development Report 2006 and FAO Sofi Report 2006.

# A selection of HIV documents

## Unearthed by US Governmental Investigations into the scientific work of Dr. Robert Gallo.

A. In this Gallo explains why HIV (here called HTLV) is 'extremely rare' in the AIDS patients. This is dated 1 day before he sent his papers claiming HIV causes AIDS for publication in *Science*.

Building 37, Room 6A0S
(301) 496-6007

March 29, 1984

Jun Minowada, M.D.
Staff Physician
Edward J. Hines, Jr. Veterans
Administration Hospital, and
Professor of Pathology and Surgery
Loyola Univ. Stritch School of Med.
Hines, Illinois 60141

Dear Jun,

In answer to your letter of March 9, I would like to address some of the points you made. First, there is no evidence that the situation with HTLV is similar to EBV. On the contrary, the epidemiological evidence shows a close association between disease and HTLV infection. EBV is ubiquitous. Second, I don't understand why there is a problem with one virus causing "clonal inducer T-cell malignancies" and immunosuppressive disorders. In the cat system it's been accepted for years (at least 10) that FeLV more often induces an immunosuppressive state than leukemia. The age of initial infection, route of exposure and whether there is repeat exposure are all apparent factors in the disease outcome of FeLV infection. If the T4 cells are the target of HTLV and this infection abrogates their function (as shown by M. Popovic, B. Dupont, A. Fauci and myself), then I can easily see that infection could lead to immunosuppression. Third, I'm not surprised that you have not found p19 expression on fresh cells of "AIDS" patients. It's extremely rare to find fresh cells expressing the virus. As in the bovine system, cell culture seems to be necessary to induce virus. This is probably due to removal of inhibiting factors present in the patient. The antigens p24 and p19 are almost always detected simultaneously. Finally, we know now there are many variants of HTLV-I. We believe the cause of AIDS is a more highly cytopathic variant.

Sincerely yours,

Robert C. Gallo, M.D.

AHS:tas

B. Letter from Dr. Gonda, the Head of Electron Microscopy at the NIH, to Popovic, copied to Gallo. He reports that images wanted for the *Science* papers, do not contain HIV (HTLVIII) as Gallo had claimed, but only cellular rubbish. This was received only 3 days before Gallo sent in the Science papers for publication, When the papers appeared in print, they still contained photos credited to Gonda, with Gallo saying they contain HIV.

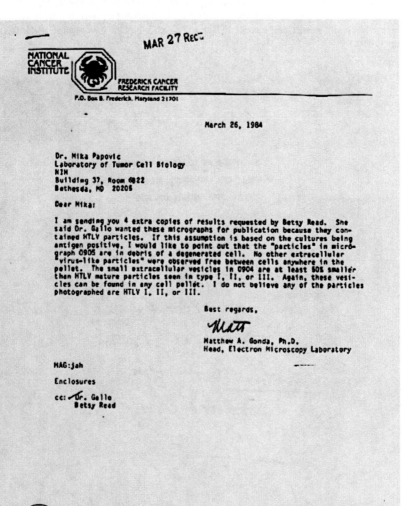

MAR 27 REC'

NATIONAL CANCER INSTITUTE

FREDERICK CANCER
RESEARCH FACILITY

P.O. Box B. Frederick, Maryland 21701

March 26, 1984

Dr. Mika Papovic
Laboratory of Tumor Cell Biology
NIH
Building 37, Room 6B22
Bethesda, MD 20205

Dear Mika:

I am sending you 4 extra copies of results requested by Betsy Read. She said Dr. Gallo wanted these micrographs for publication because they contained HTLV particles. If this assumption is based on the cultures being antigen positive, I would like to point out that the "particles" in micrograph 0905 are in debris of a degenerated cell. No other extracellular "virus-like particles" were observed free between cells anywhere in the pellet. The small extracellular vesicles in 0904 are at least 50% smaller than HTLV mature particles seen in type I, II, or III. Again, these vesicles can be found in any cell pellet. I do not believe any of the particles photographed are HTLV I, II, or III.

Best regards,

Matthew A. Gonda, Ph.D.
Head, Electron Microscopy Laboratory

MAG:jah

Enclosures

cc: Dr. Gallo
    Betsy Read

PRI  PROGRAM RESOURCES, INC. • Operations and Technical Support

   C. The first and the most important of the four *Science* Papers said to prove
HIV the cause of AIDS.  This is the typed draft produced by the Lead Author M.
Popovic, with all the handwritten editing and comments made by R. Gallo just 7
days before the manuscript went in for publication. (The cover page unfortunately
has faded.)

Science — First draft

*Popovic*

RESCUE AND CONTINUOUS PRODUCTION
OF HUMAN T-CELL LYMPHOTROPIC RETROVIRUS (HTLV-III)
FROM PATIENTS WITH AIDS

— WAY TO deal c̄ this
LAV - originally
① Lack of cross before c̄ I, II
② "    "  Ag₁ "  'action
③ Relationship to CIA
④ im published series,

When the
hell are the

## ABSTRACT

A [handwritten edits] permissive human neoplastic T-cell population is described for [routine isolation of] cytopathic variants of human T-cell lymphotropic retroviruses (HTLV-III) [handwritten edits] from pre-AIDS or AIDS patients. The infected T-cell population preserves its capacity for permanent in vitro growth [and] exhibits continuous virus expression [handwritten edits] for isolation of cytopathic variants of HTLV from patients with lymphadenopathy (pre-AIDS) and AIDS. [handwritten] virus production in high amounts. [Therefore,] enables us to prepare specific viral probes for immunological and nucleic acid studies. [can be prepared. One] The cytopathic effect of HTLV-III [on the infection is the induction] [handwritten] of multi-nucleated giant cells which [can] be used as an indicator for the detection of [this] virus.

*This abstract is rather trivial for [too] a [handwritten] putative breakthrough paper for Science.*

A family of human T-cell lymphotropic retroviruses (HTLV) comprises
two major and well characterized subgroups of human retroviruses, called
HTLV-I (      ) and HTLV-II (      ). Recently a new variant of HTLV
has been isolated from a patient with lymphadenopathy named also as lymphadenopathy associated virus (LAV) (      ) which is described here as
HTLV-III. The most common isolate obtained from patients with mature T-
cell malignancies is HTLV-I (      ). Seroepidemiological and nucleic acid
hybridization data indicate that HTLV-I, including the new subtype, is
etiologically associated with T-cell leukemia/lymphoma of adults (      ).
The disease clusters in the south of Japan (      ), the Caribbean (      ),
Africa (      ) and can be found in other parts of the world. HTLV of subgroup II (HTLV-II) was first isolated from a patient with a benign form of
T-cell variant of hairy cell leukemia (      ). To date, this virus represents the only isolate obtained from a patient with neoplastic disease.
However, isolation of retroviruses and seroepidemiological data suggest
that HTLV of both subgroups, including new variants from subgroup III, may
be involved in the pathogenesis of the acquired immune deficiency syndrome
(AIDS) (      ). Here we report
Epidemiologic data strongly suggest that AIDS is caused by an infectious agent which is transmitted by intimate contacts or blood products (      ).
To date, over 3000 cases of AIDS have been reported in the U.S. (      ).
Patients with the disease include mainly homosexuals (      ), intravenous
drug users (      ), Haitian immigrants to the U.S. (      ), and hemophiliacs (      ). Recently, an increased number of AIDS cases have been
reported in children whose parents have AIDS or intimate contact(s) with
a person having the disease (      ). Although the disease in patients is

manifested by opportunistic infections, predominantly Pneumocystis carinii
pneumonia and Kaposi's sarcoma, the underlying disorder affects the
patient's cell-mediated immunity (    ). ~~The T-cell dysfunction is often
marked by an absence of delayed hypersensitivity~~ with absolute lymphopenia and
reduced helper T-lymphocyte (OKT4+) subpopulation(s). ~~This~~ is
reverse ratios of helper-to-suppressor T-lymphocyte subpopulation, poor
lymphocyte responsiveness to mitogens (    ). In some cases, a decreased
~~natural killer cell activity~~

~~Despite intensive research efforts, the causative agent of AIDS has
not yet been identified.~~ Although patients with AIDS are often chronically
infected with cytomegalovirus (    ), or hepatitis B virus (    ), we
have proposed that a    causing AIDS to a    from a family
of HTLV. This assumption, besides being a well known precedence of causing
immune deficiency in cats by feline leukemia virus (    )    
the facts that retroviruses of the HTLV family are characterized by T-cell
tropism    preferentially infect "helper" T-cells (OKT4+),
cytopathic effects on various human and mammalian cells as demonstrated by
syncytia induction (    ); and the
even    of a specific T-cell function    in some
cases may result in a selective    cell killing (    )    
demiological    showed that the presence of antibodies directed to cell
membrane antigens of HTLV infected cells is from 30-40% of patients with
AIDS (    ). In addition, over 20 HTLV isolates of both subgroups and
new variants were obtained from patients with AIDS (    ). The successful detection and isolation of HTLV was made possible by    discovery of
TCGF which enabled selectively to grow different subsets of normal and

*and by the development of* [handwritten annotations]

neoplastic mature T-cells ( ). The viral rescue and transmission of

HTLV into permissive cells followed a well established procedure

worked out in the system of avian sarcoma virus transformed mammalian cells

( ). The cocultivation procedure using cord blood T-cells from new-

borns as recipient cells for enabled preferential

with immortalizing (transforming) capability ( ). HTLV

variants which possess "weak" or lack immortalizing properties for

normal T-cells from peripheral and exhibit

mainly cytopathic effect on the can only be transiently using

cells as target in cocultivation or cell-free transmission experiments.

This main obstacle for more frequent isolation and

particularly for detailed biological, immunological and nucleic acid char-

acterization of cytopathic variants of HTLV. To overcome these obstacles,

we have performed an extensive survey for a cell population which

highly susceptible to and permissive for cytopathic variants of HTLV and

preserve capacity for permanent growth after infection with the

virus. We report here the establishment and characterization of an immort-

alized T-cell population which is susceptible to and permissive for HTLV

cytopathic variants and can be used for the rescue and continuous pro-

duction of these from patients

Several in vitro established permanent cell lines originated from

human malignancies were assayed for susceptibility to infection with

of HTLV a reference virus (HTLV from Dr.

Montagnier) used in the first series of experiments. Two cell

lines with characteristics of mature T-cells susceptibility to

infection as determined by reverse transcriptase (RT) assays,

[handwritten margin note:] MIXa
You or
CRAZY

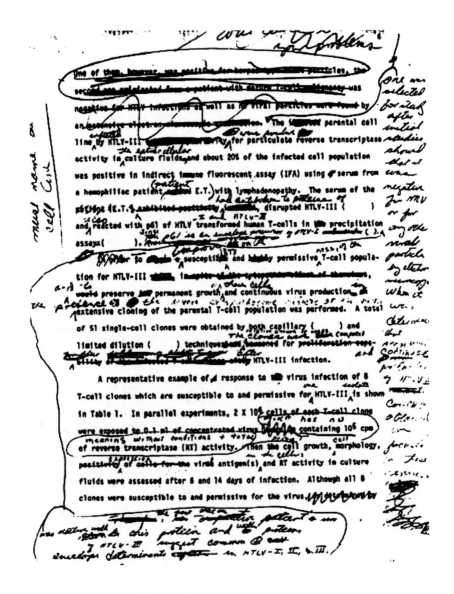

One of them, however, was positive for herpes-like particles, the second one originated from a patient with Burkitt lymphoma was negative for HTLV infections as well as no viral particles were found by an extensive electron microscopic examination. The parental cell line by HTLV-III for particulate reverse transcriptase activity in culture fluids and about 20% of the infected cell population was positive in indirect immune fluorescent assay (IFA) using serum from a hemophiliac patient E.T. with lymphadenopathy. The serum of the patient (E.T.) inhibited positivity, disrupted HTLV-III ( ) and reacted with p61 of HTLV transformed human T-cells in the precipitation assays( ).

susceptible and highly permissive T-cell population for HTLV-III, in-spite-of-the-cytopathic-effect-of-the-virus, would preserve permanent growth and continuous virus production, extensive cloning of the parental T-cell population was performed. A total of 51 single-cell clones were obtained by both capillary ( ) and limited dilution ( ) techniques and assessed for proliferation HTLV-III infection.

A representative example of response to virus infection of 8 T-cell clones which are susceptible to and permissive for HTLV-III is shown in Table 1. In parallel experiments, 2 X 10⁵ cells of each T-cell clone were exposed to 0.1 ml of concentrated virus containing 10⁶ cpm of reverse transcriptase (RT) activity. Then the cell growth, morphology, positivity of cells for the virus antigen(s) and RT activity in culture fluids were assessed after 6 and 14 days of infection. Although all 8 clones were susceptible to and permissive for the virus.

*Redundant*

ed for the presence of viral antigen(s) and RT activity in culture fluids. there were considerable differences between infected clones in capability to proliferate after infection. In early days of infection a cytopathic effect was manifested by 10-90% of the initial cell number and, a high proportion of multinucleated (giant) cells were consistently found in all 8 infected clones. The percentage of T-cells positive for viral antigen(s) in IFA with the patient's serum, and hyperimmune rabbit serum raised against the whole disrupted virus in the range from 10% to over 80%. After 14 days of infection, total cell number increased in all 8 clones. The highest proliferation was found in clone H/4, H/6; and lowest was in clone H/3. The virus positive cultures exhibited consistently round giant cells which in Wright-Giemsa staining revealed nuclei (Fig. 1a). Electron microscopic examinations of the infected cultures showed abundant number of viral particles (Fig. 1b).

To determine whether HTLV-III is continuously produced by the infected T-cells in long term cultures, both virus production and cell viability of the infected clone H4, were followed for several months. As shown in Figure 2a, there was a fluctuation in the amount of virus production, however, culture fluids harvested from the H4/HTLV-III cell cultures at approximately 14 day intervals consistently exhibited particulate RT activity which been followed for several months. The viability of the cells range from 65-85% and the doubling time of the H4/HTLV-III cell culture was approximately 36-48 hours (data not shown) infection. Thus, the data clearly indicate

8

~~can continuously produce~~ *that this* ~~produce~~ permanently growing T-cell population *NTLV-III* in ~~in~~ long term culture.

*assays* ~~Further.~~ The yield of ~~the~~ virus produced by H4/HTLV-III cells was assessed by purification of concentrated culture fluids through a sucrose density gradient and particulate RT *activity* ~~assay was performed~~ in each fraction collected from the gradient. As shown in Figure 2b, similar to other retroviruses, the highest RT activity was found at density 1.16g/ml. Electron microscopic (EM) examinations of ~~the~~ aliquots from the fractions with highest RT activity revealed that the banded virus particles ~~were~~ ~~st~~ ~~LAs~~ were highly purified. An approximate estimation (      ) ~~of~~ the number of viral particles determined by EM and RT activity suggests that the ~~final yield from~~ *amo* ~~culture ( )~~ is about $10^{11}$ particles, ~~Thus, the data clearly indicate that~~ the established T-cell clones are susceptible to and highly permissive for cytopathic variants of HTLV; ~~and~~ all of them preserve proliferation capacity after infection; *and* ~~In~~ addition, as demonstrated in the case of H4/HTLV-III ~~cell lines.~~ ~~that~~ some ~~of them~~ can proliferate and continuously produce large amounts of HTLV-III in long term culture.

We have used two clones, H/4 and H/9, for the rescue of cytopathic variants of HTLV from patients with lymphadenopathy (pre-AIDS) or AIDS.

~~As shown in Table   , both approaches, cocultivation and cell-free virus infection, were effective for virus rescue.~~ HTLV-III isolates have been successfully obtained ~~by~~ cocultivation ~~from~~ (4 patients) and ~~by~~ cell-free infection of T-cell clones ~~H4/H9~~ ~~as target cells~~ ~~(1 patient)~~ In all five cases, the virus released into culture ~~fluids~~ was found ~~by~~ RT assay and extracellular virus particles ~~were~~

~~More than~~ ~~additional~~ *resolate or detection* of *HTLV-III* *have been* obtained *in our laboratory* all those detected by other techniques will now be adopted ... T. cell clones for ... position ... detail ...

... with sera reacted with acetone fixed cells and.

and the positivity was ... by Tween ... 2005. ... the data indicate that the T-cell clones are suitable for HTLV-III rescue either by cocultivation or by cell-free infection. The transient expression of cytopathic variants of HTLV in cells from AIDS patients and ... proliferative cell system which would be susceptible to and permissive for the virus represented a major obstacle in detection, isolation, and elucidation of the ... agent of this disease. The establishment of a T-cell population, which, after virus infection can continuously grow and produce the virus, ...

the possibility for ... biological, immunological ...

studies of any agent. ...

(CONCLUSION NOT COMPLETED)   cytopathic ... variants of HTLV in ... A IDS

and provides the first opportunity for detailed ... molecular immunological analyses ...

REFERENCES NOT DONE

(per Mika)

insert — here at end

**End of Popovic's Draft.**

D. The Office of Research Integrity, US Department of Health,| produced in 1993 a detailed report indicting Robert Gallo for medical fraud. These charges are extraordinarily important as they were drawn up by a panel of scientists appointed by America's most prestigious scientific institutions, the Academy of Science and the Institute of Medicine, in 1992. They had spent months investigating the veracity and integrity of the research into the cause of AIDS carried out by Laboratory Chief Robert Gallo and Senior Investigative Scientist Mikulas Popovic. I include the opening pages – and then one of the key conclusions concerning the above Popovic paper, but as finally edited by Gallo and published in *Science*.

5

BEFORE THE UNITED STATES
DEPARTMENT OF HEALTH AND HUMAN SERVICES
DEPARTMENTAL APPEALS BOARD

RESEARCH INTEGRITY ADJUDICATIONS PANEL

In the matter of:     )     Board Docket No. A-93-91

Robert C. Gallo, M.D.     )

OFFER OF PROOF
OF THE
OFFICE OF RESEARCH INTEGRITY

COMES NOW the Office of Research Integrity ("ORI") and files this Offer of Proof in compliance with the Board's Preliminary Determination of Respondent's Motion (July 6, 1993) and Clarification of Panel's Order and Ruling on Request for Extension of Time (July 21, 1993). In support of its Offer of Proof,¹ ORI would respectfully show as follows:

I.   INTRODUCTION

---

¹    In addition to the Offer submitted by ORI, the Witness and Exhibit Lists will be finalized with additional information concerning the areas noted by the Board, including designations as expert/fact witness, area(s) of testimony, and academic and other relevant credentials. Copies of supplemental exhibits will be provided with the revised exhibit list. Witnesses and exhibits listed in the Offer are identified to satisfy the purposes of the Offer rather than to preclude presentation of additional or different testimonial or documentary evidence at the hearing which may be necessary for logistical reasons.

In its Final Report on the allegations of scientific
misconduct against Dr. Robert C. Gallo, the ORI concluded that
Dr. Gallo committed scientific misconduct with respect to his
following statement published in his article in Science:[1]

> These findings suggest that HTLV-III and LAV may be
> different.  However, it is possible that this is due to
> insufficient characterization of LAV because the virus
> has not been transmitted to a permanently growing cell
> line for true isolation and therefore has been
> difficult to grow in quantity.

ORI Report at 28, 52.

This finding of scientific misconduct was made by ORI after an
extensive investigation, including the efforts of its predecessor
the Office of Scientific Integrity ("OSI"), the NIH, the Richards
Panel (a panel of ten preeminent extramural scientists/scholars
nominated by the National Academy of Science and appointed by the
Acting Director of the NIH), and an Expert Scientific Panel
(three extramural experts appointed by the OSI and ORI to provide
advice on the conduct of the investigation and evaluation of the
evidence).  See Exhibits H-184, H-185, H-186, H-188, H-199, H-
200, H-224.

---

[1]     "Detection, Isolation, and Continuous Production of
Cytopathic Retroviruses (HTLV-III) from patients with AIDS and
Pre-AIDS," Popovic, M; Sarngadharan, M.G.; Read E., and Gallo,
R.C.: Science 224: 497-500 (May 4, 1984).  This publication is
referred as the "Popovic Paper" or the "Science paper."

- 2 -

In its Final Report, ORI also specifically identified four
findings of inappropriate conduct Dr. Gallo which had provided
the essential context for its evaluation of the allegations
against Dr. Gallo.[3]  These are summarized below:

Allegation A1.[4]  In April - May 1983, Dr. Gallo
inappropriately inserted changes into a paper written by
scientists at the Pasteur Institute (the "Barré-Sinoussi
paper.").[5]  The paper had been forwarded to Dr. Gallo for his
assistance in having it accepted for publication by Science.
Exhibit H-6.  In the process of shepherding the paper, and
eventually serving as its peer reviewer, Dr. Gallo both authored
an Abstract and made significant substantive modifications which
advanced his own hypotheses rather than those of the Pasteur
scientists.  Exhibits H-11 through H-13.  These representations
were not identified as comments by Dr. Gallo but rather added as
gratuitous and self-serving changes purportedly representing the
views and findings of the French authors.  Exhibit H-13.

Allegation A2.  Dr. Gallo was Senior Author on the Popovic
paper.  Exhibit H-81.  ORI has found that Dr. Popovic committed
scientific misconduct based on four groupings of nine separate

---

[3]    These allegations were raised publicly in an article in
the Chicago Tribune by John Crewdson, "The Great AIDS Quest- A
Special Report" (November 19, 1989  (Exhibit H-177).

[4]    These findings are identified with the number and
letter assigned by the Board in its Preliminary Determination.

[5]    F. Barré-Sinoussi, et al., Science 220: 868 (May 20,
1983).  (Exhibit H-13).  This publication will be referred to as
the "Barre-Sinoussi paper."

- 3 -

falsifications in that paper. However, the 3-1/2 page paper
contains 13 additional erroneous statements, as well as the false
statements concealing the use and significance of LAV (Allegation
8, *infra*) and the identity and origin of the cell line
(Allegation A4, *infra*). Thus, the paper was replete with at
least 22 incorrect statements concerning LTCB research, at least
11 of which were falsifications amounting to serious deviations
from accepted standards for conducting and reporting research.
*See also* Allegation A3.

*Allegation A3.* Dr. Gallo was the Laboratory Chief at the
Laboratory of Tumor Cell Biology during the relevant period. As
Laboratory Chief, Dr. Gallo was responsible for ensuring the
research in his laboratory was conducted and reported in a manner
consistent with the applicable standards. The fulfillment of
this responsibility included the institution and management of
recordkeeping and data retrieval systems sufficient to support
the methodologies and reports of research in the laboratory. His
responsibilities also included supervision of laboratory
activities concerning the appropriate use and release of
reagents. *See* Allegation A4, *infra*. As Laboratory Chief, Dr.
Gallo was responsible for ensuring the accuracy, integrity, and
safety of the conduct of scientific research in the LTCB as well
as the reporting of that research.

ORI found that Dr. Gallo's failure or refusal to meet his
obligations as Laboratory Chief created an atmosphere which
interfered with, rather than ensured, the accurate and

- 4 -

appropriate conduct and reporting of scientific research. See
Allegations 8, A2, A4.

Allegation A4. ORI determined that Dr. Gallo failed to
determine the source of "H9" in a timely manner and placed
inappropriate restrictive conditions on access of other
scientists to LTCB reagents. See also Allegations A2, A3 supra.
Dr. Gallo knew or should have known that the cell line termed
"H9" in the Popovic paper was merely a clone of a widely-known
and readily available T-cell line, HUT-78. Dr. Gallo's obscuring
the identity and origin of this cell line, especially when
coupled with his selective and restrictive release of this and
other reagents, constitutes a serious deviation from accepted
standards for the conduct and reporting of scientific research.

ORI noted the perhaps singular importance of the research
reported by LTCB scientists in their four Science papers in May
1984. The failures and deficiencies noted above have marred
these advances because of the unacceptable circumstances of the
research, the interwoven inaccuracies and falsifications in its
manipulated reporting, and the monopolistic hoarding of its
reported reagents. These activities have permanently clouded any
legitimate discoveries made by the LTCB, inviting and culturing
indefensible allegations ranging from fraud to misappropriation.

ORI determined that the preferable course of reporting its
findings was to announce its finding of scientific misconduct
that Dr. Gallo misrepresented the use and significance of LAV in
the Popovic paper in light of the inseparable context of its four

- 5 -

other findings. Thus, in its Final Report, ORI not only explained its finding of scientific misconduct in Dr. Gallo's false reporting of the use and significance of LAV but also explained the context in which that finding was made and should be evaluated, i.e. the pattern of inappropriate conduct and scientific misconduct articulated in Allegations A1 through A4.

The inclusion of these four areas of deficiencies is particularly important in light of the recommended sanctions of placing the ORI Report in Dr. Gallo's personnel file and supervision for a period of three years. The Report should be as complete as possible both to relay the appropriate information to the limited number of officials with access to the personnel file and to inform those charged with the laboratory supervision of the appropriate areas for special scrutiny during the period of supervision.

The Board, however, has now ordered ORI to parse its findings to identify which of these areas of censurable conduct, either separately or in the aggregate, constitute scientific misconduct and, for each instance of scientific misconduct, to identify sufficient documentary and testimonial evidence to support a finding of scientific misconduct. In response to this directive, ORI submits this Offer of Proof.

II.  ALLEGATIONS OF SCIENTIFIC MISCONDUCT
ORI alleges the following findings of scientific misconduct:

- 6 -

(The pencil lines above are on the copy released.)

I jump forward to page 18 of the conclusion to the report... please note that the ORI stated that Gallo has 'seriously undermined the ability of the scientific community to reproduce and/or verify the efforts of the LTCB (Gallo's Lab) in isolating and growing the AIDS virus'... making retracing the steps extremely problematic and, in some aspects, impossible.' This greatly damages the credibility of his team's work, as it is normal for scientists to have their work so verified.

knew or should have known of the laboratory's deficiencies. He had an affirmative obligation to take steps to ensure that the LTCB operated in a responsible and appropriate manner. Nonetheless, Dr. Gallo took no such steps. Indeed, his failings as a Lab Chief are evidenced in the Popovic *Science* paper, a paper conspicuously lacking in significant primary data and fraught with false and erroneous statements.[M] ORI will prove that each of Dr. Gallo's deficiencies as a Lab Chief is significant and each can be clearly seen to manifest itself in concrete ways that, at worst, put the public health at risk and, at a minimum, severely undermined the ability of the scientific community to reproduce and/or verify the efforts of the LTCB in isolating and growing the AIDS virus.

Thus, ORI will demonstrate that it was the manner in which Dr. Gallo operated his lab that cultivated an environment which made retracing the steps of the LTCB's AIDS research extremely problematic and, in some respects, impossible. ORI will show that Dr. Gallo has demonstrated a pattern of behavior which effectively disregards and violates the acceptable standards of conduct at NIH and the scientific community at large. He has demonstrated a pattern of conduct that repeatedly misrepresents, distorts and suppresses data in such a way as to enhance his own claim to priority and primacy in AIDS research. Exhibit H-224.

---

[M] Despite the numerous inaccuracies and problematic contentions in the paper, Dr. Gallo has filed no retraction or correction to the paper.

- 45 -

This is a pattern that can be clearly seen in Dr. Gallo's
statement in the Science paper that LAV had not been fully
characterized or transmitted to a permanent cell line. See
Allegation 8.

In short, ORI will demonstrate through testimony and
documentary evidence that there was a standard of conduct in 1983
and 1984 for Laboratory Chiefs at NIH, including Dr. Gallo,
requiring them to, among other things, ensure that the scientists
within the lab adequately document their experiments, share cell
lines and reagents with other scientists and abide by commonly
accepted practices within the NIH for the conduct and reporting
of research.

    4.   ORI Witnesses

ORI will present the following witnesses to establish the
duties of a Lab Chief at NIH and elsewhere and how Dr. Gallo's
conduct seriously deviated from the commonly accepted practice in
the scientific community and NIH in 1983-1984:  Dr. Richard
Adamson; Dr. Edward Brandt; Dr. Walter Dowdle; Dr. Alfred Gilman;
Dr. Robert Goldberger; Dr. Suzanne Hadley;  Dr. Arthur Levine;
Dr. Malcolm A. Martin;  Dr. James O. Mason; Dr. J. Michael
McGinnis;  Dr. Howard E. Morgan; Dr. Mary Jane Osborn; Dr. Joseph
E. Rall; Dr. William H. Raub; Dr. Frederic Richards; Dr. Joseph
Sambrook; Dr. Priscilla Schaffer; Dr. John Stobo; Dr. Robert R.
Wagner.

- 46 -

Ultimately, since this case was dropped and none of these witnesses were
summoned, this Popovic/Gallo scientific paper was allowed to remain available
uncorrected, despite being found seriously flawed and deceptive. It is thus still
scandalously undermining the work of the many AIDS scientists who rely on its veracity.
It is unfortunately and incredibly today one of the most scientifically referenced scientific
papers every printed.

# Glossary

**ACTIN** A protein that is part of the cell's cytoskeletal and transport system. Its weight is approx. 42 kiloDaltons.

**ADULT T-CELL LEUKAEMIA** A rare blood-cell cancer.

**ANTIBODY** A protein made by a B white blood cell that fits onto a surface feature of mostly foreign molecules.

**ANTIGEN** A molecule that stimulates the production of an antibody.

**ANTISERUM** Blood serum known to contain antibodies to a particular antigen

**AUTOIMMUNE** Disease caused by the immune system attacking the cells of its own organism.

**BACTERIUM** A single-celled organism. There are typically a million of these in a millilitre of fresh water and 40 billion in a gram of soil. Their genome is half the base-pair length of a human cell; their size typically 10 times smaller than a human cell at 0.5 to 5 micrometres width.

**B CELL** A white blood cell that produces antibodies

**BASE PAIRS** Opposing nucleotides on double-stranded DNA or RNA

**BIOFILM** A thin layer of microorganisms adhering to each other.

**CAPSID** The protein shell of a virus.

**CD4** A protein found on the surface of Helper T cells, macrophages and nerve cells.

**cDNA** A double stranded DNA copy of an RNA molecule

**CELL** The basic unit of life with its own metabolism and ability to reproduce.

**CELL CULTURE** Cells kept alive in the laboratory away from their host organism.

**CELL LINE** A culture of the same class of cells.

**CHEMOTHERAPY** Commonly refers to treatment of cancer with chemicals that target our most rapidly dividing cells, preventing them from so reproducing. This affects not just cancer cells but at the same time healthy immune system cells that also rapidly divide. Similar drugs are used against AIDS where they are intended to prevent cells from making vesicles or viruses.

**CHROMOSOME** A strand of DNA with codes for genes

**CLONE** An identical copy

**CLONING** The process of making copies of nucleic acid fragments by PCR or by inserting them into bacteria where they will be multiplied as the bacteria reproduces.

**CONTINUOUS CELL LINE** Cells made cancerous and grown in the laboratory.

**CTL** Cytotoxic T Lymphocyte cells ('Killer' T-Cells)

**CYTOPATHIC** Causing disease symptoms in cells

**DALTON** A unit of mass equal to the weight of a hydrogen atom

**DNA** Double-stranded molecule made up of encoded information – as found in the nucleus of cells and in cellular organelles. The information is encoded in the sequences of four nucleotides on the strands – the four being adenine, guanine, cytosine and thymine.

**DOUBLE HELIX** Shape taken by the two strands of DNA when they are bonded in a nucleus.

**ELISA** Enzyme-Linked Immunoabsorbent Assay. A serologic test used for the detection of antibodies in, say, a blood sample.

**ENDOSOMES** A membrane-bound compartment within cells.

**ENVELOPE, Viral** A lipid membrane that covers the capsid shell of some viruses.

**ENZYME** Protein molecule that accelerates ('catalyses') chemical reactions.

**EPIDEMIOLOGY** A statistical study of a population to find causal relationships – for example between living conditions and disease occurrence.

**EUKARYOTES** The organisms whose cells are organised into complex structures by internal membranes – including animals, plants and fungi.

**EXOSOME** A cellular vesicle containing nucleic acid that is capable of being absorbed by cells other than its parent.

**GAG PROTEIN** The proteins encoded by the GAG gene that make up the structural elements of a retrovirus. These include P24 and other proteins. These make up the capsid or shell. GAG is short for Group Antigen.

**GENE** DNA encoding the production of a protein

**GENETIC CODE** Information encoded in nucleic acid (DNA or RNA)

**GENOME**         The total information encoded in DNA within a cell's nucleus including hereditary information and newly acquired genetic codes. The mitochondria organelles within a cell have their own genomes.

**GLUTATHIONE**    A molecule synthesised by cells that serves as an antioxidant to remove unstable and damaging free radicals.

**GLYCOPROTEIN**   A protein with an attached carbohydrate molecule. E.g. gp120

**GP120**          A glycoprotein of 120 kiloDaltons mass

**HAEMOPHILIACS**       People suffering from a hereditary genetic disease that impedes blood clotting and thus can produce excessive bleeding.

**HELPER CELLS**   CD4 T-Cells said to help in the recognition of foreign particles

**HERV**           **Human** endogenous retrovirus

**HIV**            Human Immunodeficiency Virus

**HTLV**      Human T-Cell Leukaemia Virus originally – but in 1983 the 'L' in it was changed to stand for Lymphadenopathy (Swollen Lymph Glands) to make it applicable to AIDS.

**HTLV-III**          Robert Gallo's AIDS virus

**HYDROPHOBIC and HYDROPHILIC**   Hydrophobic molecules like oils and fats are expelled from water, while hydrophilic molecules dissolve in water by forming a hydrogen bond with water molecules. Soap has both properties, allowing it to dissolve in both water and oils. Cell membranes have both hydrophilic and hydrophobic properties, allowing them to selectively admit fluids.

**HYPERIMMUNE ANTISERUM**          Blood serum obtained usually by inoculating a rabbit with the appropriate antigens to caused the production of specified antibodies. Used to test for antigens from a virus.

**IMMORTALIZED**   Made cancerous

**IMMUNE SYSTEM** System by which an organism detects within it a foreign body, or other hazard, and removes it

**INTERLEUKIN-2**   A cellular signalling molecule produced during a cell's immune response to foreign particles that encourages the production of Killer and Regulatory T-Cells.

**ISOLATE** Varying definitions in virology. Logically a biological element removed from all others – but in practice this is rarely if ever done. Often now means little more than the detection of symptoms of cellular distress that have been associated with the presence of a virus;

**IN VITRO**          Biological material experimented on in the laboratory. Literally means 'in glass' as in a test tube.

**IN VIVO**  Biological material in its natural living state

**KILLER T-CELLS**  White blood cells that ingest and remove possible pathogens

**LAV**              The particles thought possible to cause AIDS virus according to the Institut Pasteur – LAV stands for Lymphadenopathy (Swollen Lymph Gland) Associated Virus

**LENTIVIRUS**       A virus said not to cause harm to infected cells until many hundreds of healthy cellular generations have taken place since the infection.

**LEUKAEMIA**      Cancer of blood cells

**LIPOATROPHY**     A localised loss or malformation of fat cells that is a common side effect of certain antiretroviral drugs.

**LYMPHADENOPATHY**        Swollen Lymph Glands – often associated with activation of lymph system in fighting disease.

**LYMPHOCYTE**               White blood cell associated with immune system, includes T-Cells and B-Cells

**LYSOSOME**        Organelles produced within the cell by the Golgi apparatus that contain digestive chemicals used to dispose of waste, including that from dying or dead cells.

**MESSENGER RNA**         A strand of RNA carrying instructions

**METHEMOGLOBINAEMIA** A disorder in which the blood's capability to carry oxygen is reduced, producing cellular malnourishment and starvation.

**MICROGRAPH**         Image produced with electron microscope

**MICROPARTICLES**     Non-organic particles between 0.1 and 100 μm in size

**MicroRNAs**          A very short strand of RNA.

**MICROTUBULES**   A tubular component of the cell's cytoskeleton with a diameter of 25 nm and length varying from 200 nanometres to 25 micrometers. They provide a network for transport of materials with the cell and are thus involved in many cellular processes.

**MITOGENIC**         Chemical or other agent that encourages cell division.

**MITROCHONDRION** A cell component encased in a membrane with its own DNA that originated with independent bacterial cells that came to live by symbiosis within other cells. Today it provides most of the cell's supply of energy by generating adenosine triphosphate (ATP).

**MOV** A name used by Gallo and Popovic for the French virus LAV

**mRNA** See Messenger RNA

**MYCOBACTERIA** A very common and varied bacteria family that has a particularly protective cell wall membrane enabling them to survive long exposure to acids and antibiotics. A member of this family is m. tuberculosis but billions of people host these bacteria without having tuberculosis.

**MYCOBACTERAEMIA** A person with a high number of mycobacterium. This condition can be a symptom of severe illness. As mycobacteria can produce false positive results with the HIV test, this condition may frequently be mistaken for an HIV infection.

**MYCOPLASMA** A genus of small bacteria that can change shape and pass through filters designed to prevent passage by bacteria. They cannot make cholesterol but need it, so live harmlessly as parasites within organisms.

**NANOTUBES** Actin fibres used for transporting vesicles within cells and between cells.

**NUCLEOSIDES** An organic molecule out of which DNA and RNA are constructed. There are 5 – adenine, guanine, cytosine and thymine in DNA, with uracil replacing thymine in RNA.

**ORGANELLES** The 'small' organs of cells e.g. mitochondria

**ONCOGENE** A gene said to cause cancer.

**ONCOVIRUS** A virus said to carry an oncogene

**OXYHAEMOGLOBIN** An oxygen-transporting protein found in red blood cells.

**P24** A protein with the molecular mass of 24 kiloDaltons

**PCR** Polymerase Chain Reaction – a laboratory technique used to make short strands of genetic code clone themselves many millions of times so they can better be studied.

**PERMANENT CELL LINE** *see Continuous Cell Line*

**PHA** Phytohaemagglutinin – a protein substance found in plants, especially red kidney beans. In animals it induces cell division (mitosis) and the beans can be toxic if incorrectly cooked. It is used in laboratories to induce cells in cultures to produce RT activity - which some see as indicating HIV production.

**PHAGE** An inter cellular particle, or virus, produced by bacteria

**PLASMA** In biology, the yellow fluid left after removing cells from blood. In physics, an ionised gas in which electrons of the atom are separated from the nucleus.

**POLYMERASE CHAIN REACTION** *see PCR*

**POLYPEPTIDE** A chain of amino acids. Proteins are polypeptide molecule chains containing more than 50 amino acids.

**PRIMER** In molecular biology, a short strand (perhaps 30 nucleotides) of genetic code for which matches are sought using PCR.

**PROTEASE** Any enzyme that digests proteins.

**PROTEIN** A large intricately folded molecule made up of amino acids that is a basic building block of cells and intercellular vesicles/viruses

**PROVIRAL DNA** The genetic code (RNA) of a retrovirus after being turned into DNA within the recipient cell

**READING FRAME** Genetic code with instructions for building a protein.

**REDOX** 'Reduction Oxidation' – the change of a molecule's oxidative state by the addition or subtraction of electrons.

**RETROELEMENTS** A generic term for intracellular particles that carry RNA

**RETROTRANSPOSON** A transposon that utilises RNA rather than DNA. It translates a segment of the cell's DNA into RNA, manipulates this, changes this back into DNA and reinserted into the cell's genome in a new position.

**RETROVIRUS** A virus that moves genetic codes between cells, with these being incorporated into the nucleic DNA of the recipient cell. It also carries RT.

**REVERSE TRANSCRIPTASE** An enzyme molecule utilised within cells to change RNA into DNA. Abbreviated as RT

**RNA** Ribonucleic Acid. A form of genetic code that is easier to change than DNA.

**RNA Polymerase** Translates in the cell's nucleus a segment of DNA into messenger RNA.

**RIBOSOMES** Messenger RNA travels from the nucleus to the surrounding cytoplasm where it instructs some of the many thousands of tiny ribosome organelles to assemble ('translate') specific protein molecules out of amino acids. Ribosomes are not bound by an envelope and are made of RNA (60%) and protein (40%).

**ROUS SARCOMA VIRUS**      A virus said to cause cancer in chickens.
**RT**                  *See Reverse Transcriptase*
**SELENIUM**              A mineral used by cells as an anti-oxidant.
**SERUM** Blood from which red blood cells and other clotting elements have been removed.
**T-4 CELL**              *See Helper T-Cells*
**T-8 CELL**              *See Killer T-Cells*
**T-CELL LINE**          A culture of T-cells. 'T' refers to the Thymus Gland where these immune cells
are processed and stored after being created in the bone marrow.
**TRANSPOSON**          A class of cellular mobile genetic elements that manipulate and transport
sequences of DNA to new places within a cell's genome.
**TRYPSIN**    A protease enzyme in the digestive system. Used in laboratories to break down proteins
  – and to encourage viral production.
**VACCINE**              A medicine given to stimulate the production of specific antibodies.
**VESICLE**              Hollow particles produced by a cell that are used in the transport of cellular
material both within a cell and to other cells.
**VIRAL LOAD**          An estimate of the number of specific genetic code sequences in a unit of
blood.
**VIRION**              A single virus
**VIRUS**                Vesicles produced by a cell capable of carrying genetic codes and cellular
material to other cells. The absorption of this material into a recipient cell is commonly called
infection although it is not necessarily harmful.
**WESTERN BLOT**    A test of blood serum that separately records the attachment of antibodies to
specific antigens.


# Approximate widths in the nano-world.


IN NANOMETRES, 1 nm = thousand millionth of a meter; $1 \times 10^{-9}$ m)
0.1 nm diameter of a hydrogen atom
0.8 nm Amino Acid
2 nm DNA Alpha helix width
4 nm Globular Protein
6 nm microfilaments within cells
10 nm thickness of cell membranes
11 nm Ribosome within cells
25 nm Microtubule width within cells
50-200 nm Nanotube bridge width between cells
100-120 nm average large virus or exosome


IN MICROMETRES, 1 μm = 1 millionth of a metre; $1 \times 10^{-6}$ m)
0.2 – 0.5 μm lysosome organelles within cells
0.5 to 5 μm bacterial cells
3 μm Mitochondrion (within cells)
10 - 30 μm Most Eukaryotic animal cells
10 - 100 μm Most Eukaryotic plant cells
90 μm smallest Amoeba
100 μm Human Egg

# Index

Lightning Source UK Ltd.
Milton Keynes UK
22 November 2010

163249UK00005B/15/P